KU-538-858

Psychology for Nursing

Edited by Alison Torn and Pete Greasley

polity

Copyright this collection © Polity 2016

The right of Alison Torn and Pete Greasley to be identified as Authors of this Work has been asserted in accordance with the UK Copyright, Designs and Patents Act 1988.

First published in 2016 by Polity Press

Polity Press
65 Bridge Street
Cambridge CB2 1UR, UK

Polity Press
350 Main Street
Malden, MA 02148, USA

All rights reserved. Except for the quotation of short passages for the purpose of criticism and review, no part of this publication may be reproduced, stored in a retrieval system, or transmitted, in any form or by any means, electronic, mechanical, photocopying, recording or otherwise, without the prior permission of the publisher.

ISBN-13: 978-0-7456-7148-2
ISBN-13: 978-0-7456-7149-9 (pb)

A catalogue record for this book is available from the British Library.

Library of Congress Cataloging-in-Publication Data

Torn, Alison.
 Psychology for nursing / Alison Torn, Pete Greasley.
   pages cm
 Includes bibliographical references and index.
 ISBN 978-0-7456-7148-2 (hardback : alk. paper) – ISBN 978-0-7456-7149-9 (pbk.: alk. paper)
1. Nursing–Psychological aspects. I. Greasley, Peter. II. Title.
 RT86.T67 2016
  610.73–dc23
2015019882

Typeset in 10.5 on 13pt Minion Pro by
Servis Filmsetting Ltd, Stockport, Cheshire
Printed and bound in the UK by CPI Group (UK) Ltd, Croydon, CR0 4YY

The publisher has used its best endeavours to ensure that the URLs for external websites referred to in this book are correct and active at the time of going to press. However, the publisher has no responsibility for the websites and can make no guarantee that a site will remain live or that the content is or will remain appropriate.

Every effort has been made to trace all copyright holders, but if any have been inadvertently overlooked the publisher will be pleased to include any necessary credits in any subsequent reprint or edition.

For further information on Polity, visit our website:
politybooks.com

Contents

Tables, Figures and Boxes

Boxes

Contributors

Paul Buckley is a family and systemic psychotherapist accredited to the UK Council of Psychotherapy. He currently works within the NHS as part of a Community Mental Health Team. With a first degree in psychology, he is trained in person-centred, psychodynamic and systemic counselling and therapeutic approaches.

Dr Sue Elmer is an associate principal lecturer in the Institute of Childhood and Education, Leeds Trinity University, where she is programme leader of the MA family support and the BA child and family welfare studies degrees and supervises PhD students. She is a social worker registered by the Health and Care Professional Council, a Relate-trained counsellor and a full member of the British Association of Play Therapists (BAPT). Sue is experienced in teaching and training students registered on professional awards as part of their continuing professional development (CPD), including professionals in the teaching, health and social care sectors. Her research interests cover social work, domestic abuse, integrated practice, practitioner research and play therapy.

Dr Pete Greasley is a research tutor on the doctorate in clinical psychology at Lancaster University. He has conducted research and published academic articles on a range of topics, among them psychology, nursing, education and sceptical inquiry. He has also published two books: *Quantitative Data Analysis Using SPSS: An Introduction for Health and Social Science* (Maidenhead, Open University Press, 2008) and *Doing Essays and Assignments: Essential Tips for Students* (London: Sage, 2011).

Patricia Green is an assistant professor in clinical skills in the Faculty of Medicine at Bond University in Queensland, Australia. She is a UK-trained midwife and nurse and has worked across a range of hospital, education and training contexts since emigrating in 1989. Her research interests are in medical education, where she is currently investigating medical student identity, and also in the area of women's health, in which she is involved in a collaborative study that aims to examine, using self-reported data, the association between mode of birth and perinatal and psychosocial risk factors in the maternal and infant physical and emotional health outcomes.

Dr James Jackson is a chartered psychologist and an associate fellow of the British Psychology Society, as well as an associate principal lecturer at Leeds Trinity University. An active member of the British Tinnitus

Association, he speaks regularly at tinnitus information days and to self-help groups across the north of England. His research interests include how people cope with tinnitus distress, how tinnitus affects individual sufferers, and how individual differences affect appraisal of the tinnitus sensation. He is also interested in the concept of 'mental toughness' and how personality and environment can affect pain tolerance.

Dr Patricia Johnson has held senior positions in both the clinical and the academic arena. Currently she is employed as an associate professor and simulation manager in the clinical skills area of the medical programme at Bond University, Queensland. Before this, she managed the international programmes and postgraduate critical care nursing programmes at Griffith University, Queensland. Patricia maintains her currency of practice as a visiting clinical academic in the intensive care unit of a local private hospital.

Dr Gabrielle Tracy McClelland is a registered mental and physical health nurse with a professional background and special interest in substance misuse and youth sexual exploitation. She took a master's degree in research methods for the social sciences while working as a lecturer at the University of Bradford. Before this Gabrielle managed a substance misuse service in Bradford and studied to become a health professional educator. Currently she is a senior lecturer/postdoctoral researcher at the University of Bradford in the Division of Nursing.

Dr Joe MacDonagh is a chartered psychologist and an associate fellow of the British Psychological Society. He is also a chartered scientist and a former president of the Psychological Society of Ireland. In addition to lecturing at the Institute of Technology, Tallaght, Dublin, he works as a consultant to various hospitals around Ireland. His research interests include the dialogical construction of nursing identity and the nature and genesis of depression.

Beverley Norris is a lecturer within the School of Nursing at the University of Bradford. She has a clinical background in palliative care and has expertise in quality assurance, having facilitated peer review audits within specialist palliative care settings. She leads on communication skills education for nurses and other health professionals at the university and teaches on end of life care issues within the pre-registration and continuing professional development programmes. Among her research interests is the care of families of those receiving palliative care.

Raghu Raghavan is professor of mental health at De Montfort University, Leicester, where he is head of research at the Nursing and Midwifery Research Centre in the Faculty of Health and Life Sciences. He has a background in health psychology and learning disability nursing. His research addresses several important issues in disability, mental health and wellbeing – improving access to services/ interventions, user involvement, practice and service development, cultural diversity and inclusion – and a major theme is the mental health needs of people with intellectual disabilities. He has published widely, including books, book chapters, peer reviewed journals and research reports.

Dr Sally Sargeant is a senior lecturer in behavioural sciences at Bond University in Queensland. She also holds an adjunct post in the research cluster for health improvement within the University of the Sunshine Coast, also in Queensland. Her research is in the fields of communication in healthcare, psycho-oncology and medical education. Sally is also interested in the health of Aboriginals and Torres Strait Islanders and contributes to initiatives in medical curricula that incorporate indigenous health and wellbeing.

Dr Peter Spencer is a registered practitioner health psychologist. He gained a BSc at Aston University, during which time he spent a year working with patients who were suffering from brain damage following trauma. Following a PhD in psychology at the University of Wales (Bangor), he worked in rehabilitation. Currently he is associate principal lecturer in psychology at Leeds Trinity University. He has served as external examiner for the BSc psychology with counselling course at Hull University and MSc in disability at Huddersfield University and works with patients with chronic pain and fatigue.

Claire Surr is professor in dementia studies at Leeds Beckett University. She has worked in the field of dementia education and research for over fifteen years and has undertaken a wide range of research studies concerned with improving care for people living with dementia, both in the community and in formal care settings. She is an expert on the use of dementia care mapping in research, with a particular focus on care homes and acute hospital care. Claire was named a prestigious national teaching fellow by the Higher Education Academy in 2014 for her contribution to dementia studies education for the health and social care workforce.

Dr Vanessa Taylor is senior lecturer/academic lead for quality enhancement within the School of Nursing, Midwifery and Social Work at the University of Manchester. With a clinical background in cancer and palliative care, she has research interests in the evaluation of cancer, palliative and end of life education, workforce development and service evaluation, including the challenges of delivering cancer and palliative care within non-specialist settings. Vanessa has led projects identifying the cancer-specific learning needs of the primary, community and palliative care workforce with the Macmillan Cancer Improvement Project and has developed end of life care outcomes for Health Education Yorkshire and the Humber.

Dr Gillian Tober is consultant psychologist and head of training and clinical service manager at the Leeds Addiction Unit, part of the Leeds and York Partnerships NHS Foundation Trust, and associate senior lecturer at the University of Leeds. Her research, training and clinical practice are concentrated on the development, delivery and rating of protocol-led and manual-based cognitive behavioural and network treatments of substance misuse and dependence. She has also undertaken research on the nature and measurement of dependence and its treatment outcomes.

Dr Jane Toner is a consultant clinical psychologist and is head of therapy for Meadows Care, a company specializing in complex therapeutic care for children. She is also an honorary lecturer at Lancaster University on the clinical psychology programme and has a master's degree in CBT. Jane worked for ten years as a mental health nurse using CBT in primary care and with early psychosis.

Dr Alison Torn is senior lecturer at Leeds Trinity University, where she teaches social psychology and critical mental health on the undergraduate psychology degree programme. Before this she spent nine years working as a psychiatric nurse, followed by eight years at the universities of Leeds and Bradford as a qualitative researcher on a diverse number of health-related projects. Her PhD used a narrative analytic approach to explore first-person accounts of madness and examine the relationship between identity, social positioning and recovery. She has published articles relating to nursing, mental health and narrative psychology. Current projects include narratives of resistances to psychiatry and narratives of early educational experiences.

Steve Williams is a lecturer-practitioner and field lead for mental health nursing at the University of Bradford. He teaches pre-registration mental health nursing with a focus on recovery-oriented practice and post-registration courses in applying cognitive behavioural therapy in practice. A registered nurse since 2002, he has worked predominantly in adult community mental health teams as a community nurse specialist and clinical nurse specialist. He is currently employed as a group therapist for his local trust. His interests are in applying psychological therapies within nursing and working with people with experiences of psychosis and long-term personality difficulties.

Preface

Nurses are increasingly under both public and political scrutiny. With failures of care leading to high mortality rates in Mid Staffordshire Hospital, some nurses and care staff were accused of showing a 'disturbing lack of compassion towards patients' (Francis, 2013). One of the key recommendations following the inquiry was that 'there should be an increased focus on a culture of compassion and caring in nurse recruitment, training and education' (ibid.). Reflecting this core concern for a more compassionate approach to care and a need for a deeper understanding of patients, the Nursing and Midwifery Council (NMC) heads up their essential skills cluster for graduate nurses with skills centred around 'care, compassion and communication' (NMC, 2010). High-profile cases such as Mid Staffordshire highlight how the ability to listen, respond and engage therapeutically with patients is pivotal to delivering person-centred and collaborative care. It should be emphasized that such problems are not limited to the high-profile case of Mid Staffordshire, which was subject to two major inquiries, but may occur at any institution where there is poor management and lack of resources. As the UK Health Secretary Jeremy Hunt commented, concerning a later investigation into another NHS hospital, 'To those who have maintained Mid Staffs was a one-off "local failure", today's report will give serious cause for reflection' (Hunt, 2015).

In relation to engaging in compassionate care, the question of how nurses can understand the subjective experience of being a patient is a central theme of this book. Together with the importance of subjectivity, a second important theme concerns the binary concept of health and illness – that is, to view people as either healthy or ill, diseased or disease-free, is a fundamentally flawed perception. We all exist on a continuum of health (or ill health, if you like) that constantly changes. Our subjective experience of our health and wellbeing is influenced both by internal factors (e.g., our personalities, perceptions, beliefs) and by external factors (our environment, relationships, finances) and the interaction between these two. As our circumstances change, so does our subjective experience of our health status. In order to understand the shifting nature of patients' health experiences, this book draws not only on psychology as a generic discipline but also on health psychology as a means of understanding how nurses can work in partnership with patients in order to deliver high-quality patient-centred care.

With nurses increasingly being held to public and professional account, the importance of understanding a clinical encounter, in particular its psychological aspects, together with developing a skillset to respond to patients, has never been greater. This book covers a range of clinical situations nurses may encounter in their professional career, offering and providing insights into the psychological processes underlying what can be challenging patient – and colleague – encounters. It aims to broaden the reader's understanding and application of psychology in relation to health, illness, wellbeing and healthcare within modern nursing practice. While aimed at pre-registration nurses in all four branches, the book is also relevant to post-registration nurses, in particular those who are interested in the field of psychology and how it applies to everyday nursing practice. That said, the book makes no assumptions that readers come from a psychological background or possess psychological training and practice, and therefore it is written from the perspective of the naïve reader.

Features of the book

The book is divided into four parts. Part I considers why psychology is relevant to nursing. It starts by introducing some key psychological theories and studies that have specific relevance to nursing practice and the delivery of care. It continues by introducing some of the core models that underpin much of what follows in the book: the biopsychosocial model and health models related to personality, decision-making and behaviour change, all of which are key to influencing the field of health psychology.

Part II takes a developmental approach following patients at different stages of the life cycle, from the child and young person through to the older person and those at the end of their life. This second part aims to discuss some of the more challenging situations nurses may encounter, such as caring for an individual with learning difficulties or managing extreme pain. At the heart of each chapter is developing an understanding of the patient's experience, with personhood, identity and self-esteem providing a common theme throughout. Application of psychological theories to practice is also addressed by considering key psychological approaches that can equip nurses with the skills to respond to challenging patients and situations.

Part III moves onto mental health, an area that many nurses encounter on a regular basis in their practice but may know little about. Many mental health states that are discussed may be recognized in ourselves or others – for example, depression and anxiety, which are common conditions encountered in healthcare settings. This section also pays attention to a phenomenon that is increasingly seen in general healthcare settings, that of an individual with an altered mental state – for example, those experiencing delusions or hallucinations. There are many reasons that may underpin altered mental states, with a complex interaction between the physical and the psychological. Drawing on the biopsychosocial model, this section looks at theories of causation and responses to mental health issues.

Part IV introduces more specific communication and interpersonal strategies that nurses can use in their everyday practice. The emphasis in this section is about understanding the psychological principles behind different therapeutic approaches and providing the reader with simple but useful strategies that can facilitate the nurse–patient relationship. Recognizing the increasing focus within the nursing profession of care, compassion and communication, the chapters here focus on therapeutic engagement and how to listen and respond to patients on the basis of warmth, sensitivity, compassion and trust.

The book draws to a close with a chapter on reflective practice, which explores the challenges of making the transition from student to qualified nurse; there is a particular focus on the dynamics of intra- and interprofessional communication and relationships. This conclusion also addresses the challenges and need for continuing professional development.

The book features a single case study throughout. Beth is a student nurse whom we follow through different placements during her training. As she encounters a diverse range of patients in different healthcare settings, we reflect on her experiences in relation to the psychological issues covered. Each chapter is structured to enable you, the reader, to reflect on the psychological issues discussed and apply them to nursing practice.

- Each chapter begins with a list of key issues that will be covered, allowing you to identify the salient points quickly.
- The key issues are linked to a list of learning outcomes – what you can expect to have learnt having read the chapter and engaged in the activities.
- The case study of Beth is integrated into each chapter, illustrating how the psychological issues covered can be applied to everyday nursing practice.
- Activity boxes and discussion points form an important part of the chapters, enabling you to reflect not only on what you have learnt from the reading but also on your own practice.
- Each chapter ends with a short listed summary of the key areas covered.
- To expand your knowledge further on the issues raised, questions for discussion and further recommended reading are given at the end of each chapter.

Different readers may use this book in different ways. Some may read the introductory chapters and then the chapters that are pertinent to their clinical placement, while others may read the book in its entirety. Lecturers may use it to provide their students with an introduction to psychology that has a strong application to practice as well as a source for classroom exercises. Whichever way you use it, our hope is that it adds value to your everyday nursing practice, deepening your knowledge and understanding of the reasons why people may behave in particular ways. Having read this book, you should feel more confident in managing some of the challenging situations you may encounter and be able to develop more meaningful relationships with both patients and colleagues.

Acknowledgements

We would firstly like to thank the contributing authors for their hard work and dedication to this book as well as Emma Hutchinson, Pascal Porcheron and Clare Ansell from Polity for their support in bringing it to publication. Our copy-editor, Caroline Richmond, had a meticulous eye for picking up on details overlooked by us, and our thanks also go to her. We are grateful to the three reviewers who gave helpful and constructive feedback on previous versions. Particular thanks go to Sue Elmer, for stepping in at extremely short notice with chapter 3, and Anne Goodman, for her support and attention to detail in the final checking of the manuscript. Alison would like to thank Richard, Tom and Joe for giving her a much needed work–life balance; Pete would like to thank Wendy.

Steve Williams and Gabrielle Tracy McClelland, the authors of chapter 11, 'Altered Mental States', would like to thank Dr Sally Barlow of City University, London, for her work on an earlier version of this chapter.

Part I

Nursing and the Psychology of Health and Healthcare

CONTENTS

The ability to understand human behaviour underpins the discipline of psychology, and if we can increase our understanding of why people behave in the way that they do, we can develop a flexible range of responses for dealing with different behaviours. Many behaviours faced by nurses in their professional career can be challenging and incomprehensible. This book aims to shed light on the diversity of behaviours you may encounter as a nurse, and this first part introduces you to the core theories of both psychology as a broad discipline and health psychology as a more specific area aligned to nursing, thus providing the theoretical foundations for the rest of the book.

Chapter 1 aims to give an overview of psychology, how it developed as a discipline, how the main approaches were formed and why psychology is relevant to nursing. It goes on to cover how psychology emerged as one of the most dominant disciplines in healthcare research, with particular reference to the rise of the biopsychosocial model. In so doing, the chapter includes key landmark studies in psychology and how they relate to twenty-first-century nursing. It concludes by providing an outline of the four main psychological approaches that have driven the development of psychology: Freud's psychodynamic approach, behaviourism, humanistic psychology and the cognitive approach.

The introduction of specific health models and the relationship between personality and health form the core of chapter 2. The first part looks at the role of psychological models in our everyday behaviours relating to health, appraising models such as the health belief model, the health locus of control and the theory of planned behaviour. The chapter then goes on to focus on how theories of personality have contributed to the psychological understanding of illnesses such as coronary heart disease and cancer. Throughout, the relevance of health models to nursing practice is discussed, together with how practising nurses may become informed about the choices and risks people take with their own health.

What is Psychology and Why is it Relevant to Nursing?

Pete Greasley

KEY ISSUES IN THIS CHAPTER:

▶ The potential relevance of key studies from social psychology to nursing

▶ 'Expressive' elements of care and the biopsychosocial approach to health and wellbeing

▶ Four key perspectives in the development of psychology: psychodynamic, behavourist, humanist, and cognitive

BY THE END OF THIS CHAPTER YOU SHOULD BE ABLE TO:

▶ understand how psychology is relevant for nursing

▶ appreciate the difference between the biomedical model and the biopsychosocial perspective to health

▶ be aware of key historical perspectives in psychology and their approach to health, wellbeing and behaviour.

1 Bad things happen when good people do nothing

When the Healthcare Commission in the UK was alerted to unusually high mortality rates at Mid Staffordshire Hospital in 2007, an inquiry was launched which uncovered some 'harrowing personal stories' from patients and their families about the 'appalling care' received at the hospital. In many cases the accounts related to basic elements of care and the quality of the patient experience (Francis, 2013: 18):

- patients were left in excrement in soiled bed clothes for lengthy periods
- assistance was not provided with feeding for patients who could not eat without help
- water was left out of reach
- in spite of persistent requests for help, patients were not assisted in their toileting
- wards and toilet facilities were left in a filthy condition
- privacy and dignity, even in death, were denied
- triage in A&E was undertaken by untrained staff
- staff treated patients and those close to them with what appeared to be callous indifference.

The inquiry highlighted a variety of reasons for these incidences of poor care, including prioritizing financial targets over patient experience, understaffing, and a culture of denial: many people working at the hospital knew what was going on, but they did nothing. And, yes, there was a lack of compassion in some care staff but as the Royal College of Nursing points out in their response to the Francis inquiry report:

> When a culture is not right in an organisation, it has an impact on the professional attitudes and behaviours of the staff who work for it. Put simply, a toxic culture can pollute good people. The RCN acknowledges that a very small but distinct minority of staff in the NHS exhibits attitudes and behaviours that are detrimental to patients ... [but] ... [t]he RCN believes that the NHS often sets up good people to do bad things; through constant change, chronic under-staffing and unrelenting pressure, staff have kindness and compassion eroded from them ... more must be done to tackle the burnout associated with the constant emotional labour of caring and to support staff who chose to give their working lives to our NHS. (RCN, 2013)

What do you think would have happened if you had been working as a nurse in an environment like the one described above? Might you have been one of the care staff accused in the inquiry of showing a 'disturbing lack of compassion towards patients?' Hopefully not, but there are

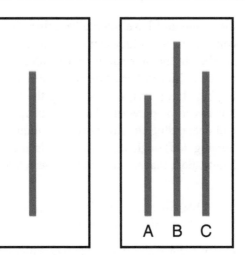

Figure 1.1 Cards used in the Asch experiment; the card on the left shows the 'reference' or 'standard' line, the card on the right the comparison lines.

some classic experiments in social psychology which show that we may all struggle to resist the influence of others and, perhaps, conform to a toxic culture.

1.1 Conformity: would you agree with others even if you knew they were wrong?

Take a look at the two diagrams in figure 1.1 and decide which one of the lines on the card on the right matches the one on the left. It should be obvious that line A is shorter and B is longer, so the match is clearly C. And when the psychologist Solomon Asch (1951) asked thirty-six people to judge twenty similar versions of this task, they agreed: out of a total of 720 judgments (36 people × 20 tasks/cards = 720), 717 were correct. So the task is clearly very easy, with one obvious correct answer.

But now imagine that you've been asked to do this task with a group of seven other people, *all of whom agree that the answer is not C but A or B*. What would you think? What would you *say*? Well, when Asch conducted his famous experiment in which the group had been instructed to give the wrong answer, it was found that thirty-seven of the fifty participants (74%) *yielded to group pressure* at least once: they conformed.

When participants in the experiment were asked *why* they conformed, the most common reason they gave was the 'painfulness of standing alone against the majority' (Asch, 1956: 70). And, while some said they doubted their own eyesight and others wondered if they'd misunderstood the instructions, it became clear that, 'as the opposition persisted ... subjects expressed fear of conspicuousness ... and of group disapproval; they felt the loneliness of their situation' (ibid.).

When people behave in ways to gain acceptance in a group, they are submitting to what psychologists call a 'normative social influence' (Deutsch and Gerard, 1955). This doesn't mean they actually agree with the group and have internalized these beliefs; rather, they are merely conforming to avoid rejection and gain acceptance. Might you have succumbed to the 'normative social influence' reflected in poor standards of care at Mid Staffordshire Hospital? I suspect the answer is a resounding 'no'; but perhaps, after seeing the results of the Asch experiment, it is easier to appreciate that some people who are working in stressful and demanding circumstances (the inquiry noted a chronic shortage of nursing staff) might come to accept 'standards of care, probably through habituation, that should not have been tolerated' (Francis, 2013: 86).

1.2 Obedience: would you do as you're told even if it might kill someone?

In 1963 the psychologist Stanley Milgram placed an advert in local newspapers asking for volunteers to take part in a study at Yale University about the effects of punishment on learning. Forty men from a variety of backgrounds (teachers, salesmen, etc.) responded. When they arrived at the university they were met by the experimenter and introduced to another person who they were told had also volunteered for the study. The experimenter asked them to draw lots from a hat to decide who would be the teacher and who would be the pupil. Once this was decided, the pupil was taken to another room and strapped into a chair with his arms attached to electrodes; these would deliver an electric shock from the 'shock generator' in another room. The 'teacher' was given a 45-volt shock just to experience what it was like.

The task for the pupil was to remember the second word in a series of pairs that had been read out by the teacher (e.g., blue-girl, nice-day, fat-neck). The teacher would say the first word of each pair, followed by five words of which only one was the correct answer. If the pupil got the answer wrong, the teacher would deliver an electric shock. Each time the pupil got the question wrong the electric shock was increased by 15 volts. The generator had switches labelled with voltages and a description of the shock, rising through:

15–60	'Slight shock'
75–120	Moderate shock
135–180	Strong shock
195–240	Very strong shock
255–300	Intense shock
315–360	Intense to extreme shock
375–420	Danger: severe shock
435–450	XXX

Note that, in the UK, household voltage is 240 volts.

Now it transpired the pupils weren't very good at this task, but, despite protests of 'I can't stand the pain', 'Get me out of here', banging on walls, screaming and, eventually, deathly silence, all the teachers administered shocks up to 300 volts, *and 65 per cent (26 out of 40) continued to the maximum 450 volts.* Thankfully, but unknown to the 'teachers', the pupils were not actually receiving electric shocks; they were acting as part of the experiment. Writing later about the results of this study, Milgram (1974: 6) said:

> This is, perhaps, the most fundamental lesson of our study: ordinary people, simply doing their jobs, and without any particular hostility on their part, can become agents in a terrible destructive process. Moreover, even when the destructive effects of their work become patently clear, and they are asked to carry out actions incompatible with fundamental standards of morality, relatively few people have the resources needed to resist authority.

When the 'teachers' were interviewed after the study, they said that they obeyed instructions to turn up the voltage because the experiment was conducted at a prestigious university and they were following the orders of a scientist. And, indeed, variations in the experiment did show that, when the experiment was conducted in a run-down office building in a downtown shopping area, obedience levels dropped to 48 per cent; and when orders were given by a person in plain clothes who was not a scientist, only 20 per cent of people went all the way up to the maximum 450 volts. So the extent of obedience may depend on where the experiment is conducted and by whom. Would this level of blind obedience have occurred outside the laboratory setting in a more naturalistic setting – a hospital, for example?

1.3 Obedience in nursing

Hofling et al. (1966) were curious to know if nurses would administer an excessive dose of an unauthorized drug to a patient if a doctor told them to do so over the phone. They therefore conducted an experiment in which a fictitious drug called Astroten was planted in a cabinet on the ward. The drugs, which were actually pink placebo tablets filled with glucose, were placed in labelled boxes.

> **ASTROTEN**
>
> 5 mg. capsules
> Usual dose: 5 mg.
> Maximum daily dose: 10 mg.

The experiment was conducted on medical, surgical, paediatric and psychiatric wards between 7 and 9 p.m.; this time was chosen to ensure minimal support from other staff so that 'the nurse would have to make her own immediate decision regarding the telephone calls' (ibid.: 172). A doctor-observer on the ward signalled an appropriate time for the phone call to be made and would stop the administration of the drug should the nurse comply with the order – e.g., 'when the nurse had poured the medication and started for the patient's bed' (ibid.). Twenty-two nurses were telephoned, and *all but one complied with the instruction.* Hofling and his colleagues provide a transcript of a typical telephone call from the doctor to the nurse (with names changed):

Nurse:	Ward 18; Miss Rolfe.
Caller:	Is this the nurse in charge?
Nurse:	Yes it is.
Caller:	This is Dr Hanford from Psychiatry calling. I was asked to see Mr Carson today, and I'm going to have to see him again this evening.
Nurse:	Yes.
Caller:	I haven't much time and I'd like him to have received some medication by the time I get to the ward. Will you please check the medicine cabinet and see if you have some Astroten.
Nurse:	Some what?
Caller:	Astroten. That's ASTROTEN.
Nurse:	I'm pretty sure we don't.
Caller:	Would you take a look, please?
Nurse:	Yes, I'll take a look, but I'm pretty sure we don't.
[45 seconds pause]	
Nurse:	Hello.
Caller:	Well?
Nurse:	Yes.
Caller:	You have Astroten?
Nurse:	Yes.
Caller:	OK. Now will you give Mr Carson a stat dose of 20 milligrams – that's four capsules – of Astroten. I'll be up in about ten minutes, and I'll sign the order then, but I'd like the medicine to have started taking effect.
Nurse:	Twenty cap … Oh, I mean, 20 milligrams.
Caller:	Yes, that's right.
Nurse:	Four capsules. OK.
Caller:	Thank you.
Nurse:	Surely.

Activity 1.1 Comply or question?

What do you think you would have done if you were a nurse in the experiment set up by Hofling and his colleagues? Would *you* have complied? Your answer is probably 'no' on account of the discrepancy in the dosage. When Hofling et al. asked twenty-one student nurses what they would do in a similar situation, all twenty-one *said* they would not have given the medication – mainly because of the discrepancy in the dosage. But, in the actual experiment, twenty-one out of twenty-two nurses did comply.

Reflecting on their experiment, Hofling et al. comment that compliance reflects the need for trust and efficiency in healthcare, which may be 'of inestimable value to physicians and to the patients. It is easy to recall crisis situations in which the nurse's loyalty to the physician, her appreciation of the value of his judgment, and her willingness and ability to act promptly and efficiently without wasting precious time in discussion have made the difference between life and death for the patients' (Hofling et al., 1966: 178). However, they also point out that this need for efficiency and professional courtesy should not have 'precluded the nurses' making some sort of appraisal of the situation and then arriving at a conscious decision instead of an automatic response' (ibid.: 179).

But does Hofling's experiment reflect what happens in practice? Does it have what psychologists call 'ecological' or 'external' validity – that is, would the same thing happen in real life, in the real world? In this respect, Rank and Jacobson (1977) were concerned that the results from the Hofling experiment were misleading because they tested nurses' compliance under unusual circumstances: firstly, the nurses had no medical knowledge of the drug, so they were completely dependent on the physician as a source of information; secondly, it would be unusual not to have anyone to contact of equal or superior rank. So Rank and Jacobson set up a similar experiment where the nurses were familiar with the drug to be administered and were allowed to interact naturally with other nurses. Under these more normal circumstances, they believed, nurses would not administer an overdose merely because a physician ordered them to do so.

In this experiment the doctor phoned the medication order to the nurse on the ward, saying: 'This is Dr __, I've been asked to see __ this evening/morning. I'm afraid I don't have much time so I'd like the patient to have had some medication by the time I get to the ward. Will you please give (him/her) a stat [immediate] dose of 30 milligrams of Valium I.M.? I'll be up in a little while to sign the order.' The dose of 30 mg was selected because it would definitely be a recognizable, though non-lethal, overdose (2 to 10 mg being the recommended dosage in the prescription guide). In these circumstances sixteen out of eighteen nurses tested in two hospitals refused to administer the valium: two nurses broke open the drug and prepared to give it, but the other sixteen attempted to check the dosage/order in some way (twelve attempted to recontact the doctor; three attempted to contact their supervisor and one attempted to contact the pharmacy). Rank and Jacobson did note, however, that seven of the nurses said they would have gone ahead if the doctor had insisted when they phoned back to check, suggesting that the power of authority may override personal doubt.

These studies were conducted over thirty years ago (for more recent commentaries, see Krackow, 1995; Martin, 2013), and we have since witnessed the increasing professionalization of nursing. But the hierarchy of power remains, as does our inherent desire to avoid confrontation with others, especially those more powerful than ourselves.

1.4 Summary

We have focused on some classic experiments from social psychology which provide an insight into our capacity for conforming and complying with others. While the problems at Mid Staffordshire Hospital were clearly symptomatic of systemic issues, these experiments might also provide us with an insight into how some staff at the hospital might conform to, and comply with, the appalling levels of care that were outlined in the inquiry. In such circumstances, patients may be treated as 'objects' known by their physical ailments that require treatment; this is why it is important to maintain a holistic approach to care.

2 A biopsychosocial approach to care

It is better to know the patient who has the disease than it is to know the disease which the patient has.   Hippocrates, quoted in Straub (2007: 8)

Hippocrates (460–377 BC), regarded as the 'father of medicine', placed a great deal of emphasis upon the psychological and social aspects of health and illness:

> For example, to learn what personal habits contributed to gout, a disease caused by disturbances in the body's metabolism of uric acid, he conducted one of the earliest public health surveys of gout sufferers' habits, as well as their temperatures, heart rates, respiration, and other physical symptoms. Hippocrates was also interested in patients' emotions and thoughts regarding their health and treatment, and thus he called attention to the psychological aspects of health and illness. (Straub, 2007: 8)

In this respect, Hippocrates may be said to have taken a holistic approach to medicine rather than simply focusing on the illness as a biomedical reaction.

Activity 1.2 Traditional Chinese medicine: a proactive approach to healthcare?

The holistic approach continues to be a feature of traditional Chinese medicine (TCM), with an emphasis on maintaining harmony and balance in life and promoting wellbeing more generally. Indeed, historically, while most TCM practitioners were paid at the point of care, some of the more affluent patients paid a retainer to their doctor to keep them healthy; if they became ill, the doctor would have to return part of the fee (Daemmrich, 2013).

What do you think of this approach?

In Western civilizations the holistic approach to healthcare declined during the age of Enlightenment, when the belief in tradition and faith was superseded by the promotion of scientific discovery and a more objective approach towards the body. The influential French philosopher René Descartes (1596–1650) came to see the body as a machine, separate from the mind, and he proceeded to construct mechanical models to demonstrate bodily reflexes. For Descartes, disease occurred when the machine broke down – the physician's task was to *repair the machine*. Thus, in what is termed Cartesian dualism, the mind and the body are two separate entities.

This perspective on treating the body as separate from the mind was reinforced by discoveries in the nineteenth century (e.g., by Louis Pasteur, 1822–1895), when diseases were found to be caused by viruses, bacteria and other germs or cell abnormalities. By the end of the nineteenth century, scientists had discovered microorganisms responsible for major diseases such as malaria, pneumonia, diphtheria, leprosy, syphilis, bubonic plague and typhoid, and this biomedical approach to health became the standard model for Western medicine.

Ogden (2007: 2) provides a basic outline of the biomedical model in terms of its approach to health and illness.

- Disease is the result of a pathogen (bacteria, virus) that invades the body, causing internal physical changes.
- Individuals are not responsible for their illnesses, which arise from biological changes beyond their control; people who are ill are victims.
- Treatment should be vaccination, surgery, etc., which aims to repair the physical state of the body.
- Responsibility for treatment rests with the medical profession.
- Health and illness are two different things – you are either healthy or ill – there's no continuum. Thus, health is viewed as nothing more than the absence of disease, placing the focus on causes of physical illness rather than factors that promote physical, psychological and social health (under which 'healthcare' might be more appropriately labeled 'disease care' – a reactive rather than a proactive approach).
- Mind and body function independently of each other; the abstract mind relates to feelings and thoughts and is incapable of influencing matter.
- Illnesses may have psychological and social *consequences* but not psychological or social *causes*.

Psychology and sociology, however, promote what is referred to as the biopsychosocial model of health and illness, recognizing that illness is often due to a combination of, and interaction between:

- biological factors (e.g., genetics, viruses, bacteria)
- psychological factors (behaviours, beliefs, attitudes, expectations, emotions)
- social factors (e.g., environment, culture, ethnicity).

The problem with the biomedical model is that it concentrates on biological causes of illness, disregarding the fact that most illnesses are the result of an interaction of social, psychological *and* biological factors. The biomedical model promotes the idea that physicians need not be concerned with psychosocial issues because they lie outside their responsibility and authority.

Activity 1.3 Applying the biopsychosocial model

Think about how you could apply the biopsychosocial model to a person with alcohol problems in terms of possible biological, psychological and social factors that might contribute to the development of the 'disease' and its maintenance.

Can you think of any examples where you feel that the biomedical model might be too dominant in the *diagnosis* and *treatment* of particular health issues?

In the biopsychosocial approach it is therefore important that nurses recognize, and address, the psychological (and social) needs of a patient: caring is not only about practical, clinical tasks that address the physical needs of patients but also about the emotional, spiritual and psychological aspects of being a patient (Greasley et al., 2001; Priest, 2012). In this respect it is important to highlight a distinction between two components of caring that have been drawn in the nursing literature:

- 'instrumental' elements of care, which are the practical aspects of care, such as dressing a wound or administering medication
- 'expressive' elements of care, which are patients' needs for comfort, information, reassurance, empathy, dignity and self-esteem, and general attentiveness.

Activity 1.4 Barriers to 'expressive' care?

In a survey of nearly 3,000 nurses across thirty-one NHS Trusts in England (Ball et al., 2012), 66 per cent reported that they did not have enough time to talk to and comfort patients. 'Expressive' activities such as these were most likely to be forgone due to time pressures related to staffing levels.

What is your own experience of visiting a friend/relative in hospital or of being a patient? Were there any aspects of nursing that were particularly valued or criticized? Could you relate these to 'instrumental' and 'expressive' elements of care?

---

3 Four key perspectives in the historical development of psychology

As an academic discipline, psychology evolved through conflicting perspectives and theories about motivation and behaviour. In this final section of the chapter, we will look at four key perspectives or 'schools of thought' that have driven the development of psychology:

* psychodynamic
* behavioural
* humanistic
* cognitive.

3.1 The psychodynamic perspective of Sigmund Freud

In the early twentieth century, Sigmund Freud (1922 [2011]) developed a psychodynamic theory of personality which proposed that our motivation and behaviour is determined by three conflicting aspects of our personality:

* the id – the instinctual, primitive component of personality motivated by instinctual drives to meet our basic needs for food and sex (the pleasure principle)
* the superego – the part of our personality that comes from our parents throughout childhood, and society generally, which serves to moderate and repress the instinctual drives of the id
* the ego – which mediates between the demands of the id and the restrictions imposed upon it by the superego, balancing our basic urges with the demands of society.

Freud believed that we are all living with the constant conflict between the expression of our animal instincts (the id) and the artificially imposed constraints, customs and morals of society (represented by the superego): the virtuous person was one who repressed his impulses, while a sinful person enjoyed them! For most people, however, our behaviour is a compromise between what the id wants and what the superego will allow, and this may lead to anxiety and neuroses through the repression of issues that are pushed back into the unconscious.

In order to uncover these issues, Freud believed that it was necessary to unlock the unconscious by means of hypnotism, the interpretation of dreams, and 'free association' – encouraging patients to say whatever came into their heads. Hence Freud's psychoanalysis was known as the talking cure, aiming to bring unconscious issues to the surface where they might then be acknowledged and addressed. Activity 1.5 provides a list of psychodynamic mechanisms that we may use to avoid, repress and deal with traumatic issues.

Activity 1.5 Strategies to deal with traumatic issues

Freud identified a variety of strategies that people use to deal with traumatic issues. Can you think how these might apply to patients – or nurses?

Activity 1.5 (continued)

- *Denial*: the refusal to acknowledge 'reality' or the feelings associated with it – e.g., 'I'm not an alcoholic, I just drink two bottles of gin a day because it helps me to concentrate.'
- *Repression*: where traumatic incidents or unacceptable feelings, thoughts and emotions are moved into the unconscious so they don't have to be dealt with.
- *Regression*: where a person is said to regress to an earlier childhood state during times of stress and anxiety as a source of comfort – e.g., sucking their thumb, comfort eating, having a temper tantrum.
- *Projection*: where a person 'projects' their own thoughts, feelings or insecurities onto another – e.g., when a person who is insecure about their abilities accuses others of thinking that they are not capable of the task; or, if a patient dislikes a nurse, they may accuse the nurse of not liking him/her (and vice versa).
- *Reaction formation*: where a person may conceal their true feelings by behaving in the opposite way.
- *Displacement* – also referred to as 'kick the cat syndrome' – where anger or frustration is displaced onto a non-threatening object or person.
- *Rationalization*: where a person justifies their own behaviour or provides excuses for their shortcomings which serve to avoid criticism.

3.2 Behaviourism

Psychoanalysis came to prominence during a time when psychology was striving to become an experimental science (Hornstein, 1992). For the behaviourist psychologist John Watson (1878–1958), Freud's psychodynamic theory was too speculative and subjective to constitute a scientific approach to psychology: the explanation for people's motivation and behaviour relied on the interpretation of the analyst, based on unseen theoretical entities such as the 'id' and the 'superego'. Watson wanted psychology to become an objective experimental branch of natural science which would be able to predict and control behaviour. He believed, like Freud, that we are merely another form of animal, but, while our behaviour may be more complex and refined, it could still be reduced to basic stimulus and response mechanisms:

- stimulus: any event, object or action of another which causes a response
- response: any activity or behaviour which occurs as a result of that stimulus.

This led behaviourists to focus on two ways in which behaviour is conditioned by environmental stimulus. The first of these is classical conditioning, where an *association* with a stimulus produces a response. Watson was influenced by the work of the Russian psychologist Ivan Pavlov (1848–1936), who showed that dogs may be 'conditioned' to salivate in response to the ringing of a bell because they associated it with the provision of food (see activity 1.6).

Activity 1.6 Classical conditioning and the power of association

Can you think of any other examples where the power of association might apply? For example, research has shown that patients undergoing chemotherapy often experience anticipatory nausea and vomiting *before treatment* because it has become associated with going to the hospital (Morrow et al., 1998).

The second is operant conditioning, where an *action* produces a response. The behavioural psychologist B. F. Skinner (1904–1990) used operant or 'instrumental' conditioning to shape behaviour. For example, when a rat presses a lever in a cage and receives some food, it will press the lever again to get the reward. This is known as positive reinforcement and is similar to when, for example, a parent or teacher rewards a child for good behaviour. However, unwanted behaviours may also be inadvertently rewarded – e.g., the disruptive child who gains attention by misbehaving (see activity 1.7).

Activity 1.7 The power of reinforcement

In operant conditioning, desired behaviour is positively reinforced with a reward, and undesired behaviour is negatively reinforced with removal of the 'reward'. Can you think of some other situations in which reinforcement is used to shape or modify behaviour? This might involve humans or animals (dogs in particular) and the reinforcement might take many forms – e.g., treats, money, praise.

But, clearly, learning is not *just* a matter of reinforcement and conditioning; we also learn through observing and imitating others. This is the focus of social learning theory, which originated from the work of Albert Bandura (1965), who set up an experiment in which children watched a film of adults hitting an inflated doll. When the children were later left in a playroom with a similar doll, they imitated the adults' aggressive behaviour towards the doll, whereas those in a control group who had not watched the film were not aggressive towards the doll. So social learning theory emphasizes the importance of observation and imitation of others, particularly role models (see activity 1.8).

Activity 1.8 Role models at Mid Staffordshire Hospital?

Could social learning theory help to explain the poor levels of care at Mid Staffordshire Hospital?

3.3 Humanistic psychology

For Abraham Maslow (1908–1970), the problem with Freud and the behaviourists was that they placed too much emphasis on our continuity with the animal world, leading them to ignore the very characteristics that make the human species uniquely different from all other animals:

> the use of animals guarantees in advance the neglect of just those capacities which are uniquely human, for example, martyrdom, self-sacrifice, shame, love, humour, art, beauty, conscience, guilt, patriotism, ideals, the production of poetry or philosophy or music or science. Animal psychology is necessary for learning about those human characteristics that humans share with all primates. It is useless in the study of those characteristics that humans do *not* share with other animals or in which he is vastly superior. (Maslow, 1954: 178)

Maslow took a more humanistic approach to psychology, focusing on the positive attributes of humans rather than the negative. In this respect he was also critical of Freud's theories of human behaviour because they were based on the study of neurotic and psychotic clients: 'Freud supplied to us the sick half of psychology', said Maslow, 'and we must now fill it out with the healthy half.' And so Maslow decided to study the most successful, high achievers he could find and, as a result, provided us with his famous hierarchy of needs (see figure 1.2). Maslow argued that more basic needs must be satisfied before we move onto higher needs. For example, food, water and security are more fundamental than 'higher' needs for creativity, respect, self-esteem and self-actualization (see activity 1.9).

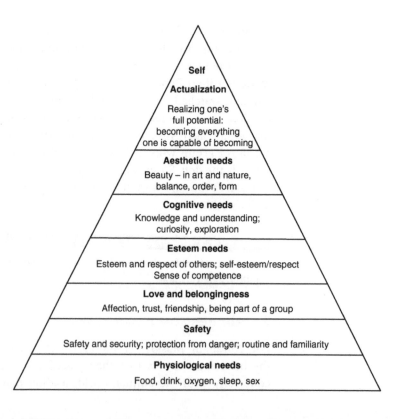

Figure 1.2 Maslow's hierarchy of needs

Activity 1.9 Applying Maslow's hierarchy of needs to patients

Can you relate Maslow's hierarchy of needs to people who are acutely ill or chronically ill? To what extent do you think the standards of care at Mid Staffordshire Hospital addressed Maslow's hierarchy of needs?

1

Carl Rogers (1965) also believed that we have an 'actualizing tendency', as we aim to make our 'actual self' as close as possible to our ideal self, but this may be thwarted for a variety of reasons, including illness. Rogers developed an approach to counselling, particularly relevant to nurses in their role as carers, which emphasized three key elements:

- *genuineness*: being truly genuine, open and transparent; being yourself and not hiding behind a detached professionalism – dealing with the patient 'person to person'
- *empathy*: trying to see things from the patient's point of view by putting yourself in their situation
- *respect*: viewing the patient with 'unconditional positive regard' – dignity, acceptance and respect; not judging the person for their behaviour, attitudes or opinions; the counsellor 'feels this client to be a person of self-worth; of value no matter what his condition, his behaviour or his feelings. He respects him for what he is, and accepts him as he is, with his potentialities' (Rogers, 1965: 22).

In Rogers's client-centred therapy, the emphasis is on seeing things from the client's perspective, allowing them to express themselves without feeling that they are being judged for the things they say. This approach may be particularly useful for nurses in encouraging patients to talk about their feelings and anxieties and to facilitate rather than block communication (cf. Wilkinson, 1991). This counselling approach is discussed in chapter 13.

3.4 The cognitive approach

The problem with the classical behaviourist approach is that it ignores anything that goes on in between the stimulus and the response – i.e., what the person is thinking and feeling about the stimulus. This can, of course, lead to very different types of response – for example, what is stressful to some is not to others. The importance of what is happening inside a person's head, their appraisal of events, is the concern of the cognitive approach. This is illustrated by the ABC model proposed by Albert Ellis (1962), which points out that it is not events themselves which cause particular reactions but our personal appraisal of events (see figure 1.3):

- Activating event: an event or the action of another person that has triggered the response

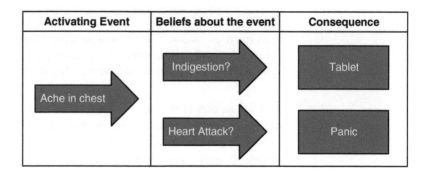

Figure 1.3 The ABC approach

- Beliefs about the event: how the person appraises this
- Consequence: emotional or behavioural reaction.

So the key point here is that A does not directly cause C; rather, B causes C – emotions are a consequence of the individual's beliefs and reaction to events. The focus in cognitive therapy is therefore on addressing the dysfunctional beliefs that people may hold which lead to distress. For example, some people may be accused of interpreting events in a particularly negative way (a negative cognitive bias), leading to 'catastrophic thinking' ('catastrophizing'): an unpleasant event that might be perceived by some as a minor inconvenience (e.g., losing some keys, missing a train) is blown out of all proportion into a tragedy from which the individual may never fully recover. Focusing on how a person is appraising a situation in this way allows the therapist, or the nurse, to reflect on how a patient's beliefs and attitudes, rather than the events themselves, may be responsible for their emotional state (chapter 12 on cognitive behavioural therapy provides a more detailed account of this approach).

3.4.1 Think positive?

This approach influenced the 'positive psychology' movement (Seligman 2002), which rekindles the humanistic critique of a psychology that focuses on the negative aspects of humanity. Rather than focusing upon disease and remedial treatment, they argue, psychology should centre on positive human attributes such as hope, optimism and perseverance. This is relevant because maintaining a positive outlook can act as a psychological buffer to ward off catastrophic thinking and maintain health and wellbeing. Studies have suggested, for example, that people who maintain a positive attitude to life are healthier and happier, and have higher survival rates from illness (e.g., recovering from coronary artery bypass surgery (Scheier et al., 1989)) and a better quality of life, compared to people who are more pessimistic (Diener and Chan, 2011). According to Carver, Scheier and Segerstrom, 'there is evidence that optimism is associated with taking proactive steps to protect one's health, whereas pessimism is associated with health-damaging behaviors' (2010: 879).

But, before we get carried away with the power of positive thinking, it is important to exercise some caution (Ehrenreich, 2009). Firstly, regarding the research evidence, we need to distinguish between correlation and cause: are people healthy because they are happy or happy because they are healthy? Secondly, the 'all in the mind' approach puts the emphasis firmly on the individual for the state of their health and recovery from illness, which borders on the magical thinking promoted by some quack alternative practitioners (Greasley, 2010). Thirdly, and more generally, this approach promotes subjective adjustment to what may be an unhealthy environment rather than addressing the situation that is causing the problem – e.g., workplace stress due to inadequate staffing at Mid Staffordshire Hospital.

Summary

- ▶ Classic experiments from social psychology illustrate our capacity for conforming and complying with others. These provide some insight into the failings of care that were uncovered by the inquiry at Mid Staffordshire Hospital in 2007.
- ▶ Studies examining the propensity for obedience in nursing highlight the potential consequences of the power hierarchy in hospitals.
- ▶ Nurses should adopt a holistic approach to care, recognizing the importance of biological, psychological and social factors. It is also important not to neglect the 'expressive' elements of care that patients value.
- ▶ Caring is not only about practical, clinical tasks that address the physical needs of patients ('instrumental' elements of care) but also about the emotional and psychological aspects of being a patient ('expressive' elements of care). It is often these 'expressive' elements that are compromised by organizational pressures (e.g., staffing).
- ▶ Psychology has evolved through conflicting perspectives (psychodynamic, behavioural humanistic, cognitive) which provide different interpretations and approaches to health and wellbeing.

Questions for discussion

1 Psychological experiments can provide us with interesting insights into the behaviour of people in unusual circumstances, but it is important to keep in mind that observations are drawn from particular samples, often in very artificial experimental situations, and, as such, the results should be treated with some caution.

For example, the studies on conformity and obedience have been replicated many times and revealed some interesting variations in the results (e.g., Bond and Smith, 1996). Do you think, for example, that the same results would be found with people from different social and cultural backgrounds?

2 How might a patient's attitude impact on their recovery? To what extent do you think that the mind can affect the body in terms of susceptibility to illness and recovery from illness?

3 If there is a link between 'positive thinking', optimism, and health and wellbeing, how do you think this might relate to more general social circumstances such as education and income?

4 Can you make a case for adopting a more pessimistic outlook rather than maintaining an optimistic outlook?

5 The humanist psychologists have been criticized for ignoring the wider social and environmental context in which behaviour takes place. To what extent do you think the failures of care at Mid Staffordshire Hospital, in respect of empathy, respect, etc., relate to particular individuals who were accused of showing a 'disturbing lack of compassion towards patients' rather than to wider social and structural issues at the hospital, such as problems with staffing levels?

Further reading

Ballatt, J., and Campling, P. (2011) *Intelligent Kindness: Reforming the Culture of Healthcare*. London: RCPsych Publications.
This is essential reading for nurses. It examines the organizational reforms in the NHS, highlighting the increasing alienation of health service staff and the demise of compassionate care. It includes discussion of the Mid Staffordshire inquiry with reference to psychological perspectives that provide some insight into 'how good staff become bad'.

Diener, E., and Chan, M. Y. (2011) Happy people live longer: subjective well-being contributes to health and longevity, *Applied Psychology: Health and Well-Being* 3(1): 1–43, http://internal.psychology.illinois.edu/~ediener/Documents/Diener-Chan_2011.pdf.
This article provides a good summary of research on 'positive psychology'.

Ehrenreich, B. (2009) *Smile or Die: How Positive Thinking Fooled America and the World*. London: Granta.
This very interesting and accessible book provides a critical look at the 'positive psychology' movement.

Psychology and Models of Health

Sally Sargeant

KEY ISSUES IN THIS CHAPTER:

▶ Psychological theories and models relating to health, including decision-making and behaviour change
▶ Internal and external influences of control
▶ The relationship of personality to health

BY THE END OF THIS CHAPTER YOU SHOULD BE ABLE TO:

▶ outline the key theories relating to perceptions of health, including biopsychosocial and biomedical models
▶ understand health behaviours according to social cognition models
▶ understand factors that contribute to decision-making processes about health
▶ appreciate the relationship between personality characteristics and health.

1 Introduction

The aim of this chapter is to introduce key theories and models of health psychology that are of relevance to the health professions, together with their significance to nursing practice. It discusses general models of health and illness and specific theories that address individual decision-making processes, including the health belief model and the theory of planned behaviour. The chapter closes by examining how personality relates to health and the extent to which our physical wellbeing influences our personality.

1.1 Psychological models and health behaviours

Before delving into the intricacies of theory, let us take a moment to consider what health psychology specifically comprises. Many of the theories associated with health behaviours are drawn from the wider area of social psychology and have subsequently been refined to address properties of health and illness. A simplified definition of health psychology is the study of cognitive, behavioural and emotional factors that can influence how we maintain our health, how illness occurs, and the courses that illnesses can take, alongside our responses to them. There are various theories and models that can assist us to investigate these areas of inquiry at a detailed academic level. However, it is also useful to have a basic awareness of them as a practitioner in any health discipline. When trying to understand how individuals make decisions about their health, and act on them, there are a number of ways we can break down people's thoughts and reasons that may contribute to these actions. What may at first seem to a health professional like an irrational or ill-judged decision may have a totally different meaning or explanation for a patient. A patient may have rationalized their behaviour based upon their emotional needs or familial or social influences. A clinical agenda does not always correspond with how a person manages their health outside of a clinical setting. It is therefore helpful to look at attitudes, beliefs and

Case Study 2.1:

Student nurse Beth is on placement in a busy accident and emergency department. David, a 20-year-old male university student, is admitted after his friend, Tom, found him in bed and in a somewhat confused state earlier in the day. Tom admitted that they had been out drinking the night before but he became concerned, as David hadn't got out of bed by mid-afternoon. Beth and her colleagues establish that David is diabetic and that he has taken quite a risk by drinking excess alcohol. He also has not been taking his insulin and his blood sugars are dangerously low.

Why might David have behaved in this way knowing that he has a chronic illness?

norms surrounding our complex relationship with health and wellbeing. To do this there are several theoretical frameworks that we can use. Such frameworks not only broaden our understanding of health behaviour at individual and collective levels but also form the bases of interventions that motivate health behaviour change or adherence to recommendations made by health professionals. The models that are discussed here converge on the nature of illness and health, theories of health limiting/enhancing behaviour, and the role of personality in determining health.

2 The biopsychosocial model of health

To begin to understand how individuals think and make decisions about their health, it is helpful to understand wider societal concepts attributed to health and illness. To consider what it is to be healthy and ill in an historical context can help establish how people's perceptions relate to how they behave with respect to their own health. It also helps cement the shift from the notion of individuals as being passive 'victims' of illness to that of being responsible for their own health to a greater or lesser degree. This shift, alongside many other components, is intrinsic to the biopsychosocial model of health, which was first proposed by Engel (1977) and is very much the basis of health professionals' education in many occupational and academic contexts.

As the name suggests, this model asserts that health and illness are determined by biological, psychological and social factors. While this may seem logical today, this was not always historically the case. Many years before Engel advocated a new model of health, medicine and nursing were influenced primarily by a biomedical model of health. Again, as the name suggests, such a model asserted that only biological and physiological factors accounted for presentations of health and illness, while psychological and social influences were not considered. Table 2.1 demonstrates some of the key ideological differences between the biomedical and biopsychosocial models.

Although the biopsychosocial model is seen as a more fitting account for how illness presents or is talked about, it is surprising how many assumptions are made about treatment and/or management that

Table 2.1 Differences between the biomedical and biopsychosocial model of health	
Biomedical model	**Biopsychosocial model**
Mind and body are separate	Mind and body influence each other
Psychosocial factors are irrelevant	Psychosocial factors are integral
Medical professionals are responsible for health	Everyone is individually and collectively responsible for health
Treatment is biologically focused	Treatment considers psychological and social factors as in addition to biological ones

defer to the biomedical model. Indeed, it is documented in medical education that students training to be doctors often seek biological explanations and understandings of illness rather than considering additional factors that might easily contribute (de Visser, 2009). However, it is preferable and more beneficial for health professionals to look towards understanding how individual and collective presentations of illness occur within a biopsychosocial framework.

While generally seen as an improvement upon the biomedical model of health and illness, the biopsychosocial model is not without problems. Some arguments assert that health professionals may be too quick to assume that individuals have more control over their health/ illness trajectory than is actually the case, thereby erroneously overestimating patients' responsibilities for their health (Street and Haidet, 2010). Yet, despite such shortcomings, the model is useful to draw parallels with the other models that this chapter considers, in particular the social and cognitive influences that affect health presentations and behaviour. These will now be discussed in turn.

3 Behaviours and beliefs

At this point it is appropriate to move from generalist perceptions of health and towards social cognition models and consider how such models can account for more specific behaviours – for example, patterns of healthcare utilization, illness presentation/representation, and health risk-taking.

3.1 The health belief model

The first is the health belief model (HBM) proposed by Rosenstock (1974). The model is based on the principle that people consider the benefits and disadvantages associated with health behaviours, before acting accordingly. More importantly, it was based upon a principle within social psychology which argued that people are likely to behave in a certain way if they believe their behaviour will lead to a particular valued outcome. Overall the HBM attempted to predict and explain the likelihood of individuals engaging in (or ignoring) certain health behaviours. The model is represented graphically in many different ways, but, for the purpose of beginning to understand the basics, is shown in its simplest form in figure 2.1.

The terms in the model are applied to any health behaviour, be this positive or negative. Let us take an example of a positive behaviour and refer to the case study with David's medication for Type 1 diabetes. The first point, perceived susceptibility, involves an assessment of the chances of getting a disease or an associated symptom, in which case, David might appraise his situation as '*I will become hypoglycaemic if I do not take my insulin.*' In the same way, his perceived severity position

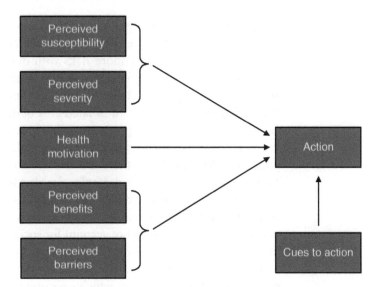

Figure 2.1 The health belief model

might be '*Diabetes is a serious illness*' – a cognition that will also act as a motivator to adhere to a medication regime. The 'cost–benefit analysis' part of the model involves exactly that – in this case, David might believe the cost of adhering to his medicine might be having to disclose his illness to others at inopportune times, while a perceived benefit might be the belief that he will save himself the difficulties of additional physical complications and possible hospitalization.

As well as these assessments of belief, the HBM contains cues to action which contribute to the likelihood of behaviour. These may be external cues, such as information leaflets or advertisements, or internally embodied symptoms that prompt action. The combination of all of these elements in the HBM attends to the beliefs and perceptions that individuals hold about their health and wellbeing and result in behaviour.

Activity 2.1

Using the HBM, consider how David might appraise the benefits and barriers of taking his medication. Consider how other health behaviours might be aligned to this model, such as smoking or not attending hospital appointments. Also consider how the model applies to positive health behaviours, such as eating a healthy diet or maintaining regular exercise.

The HBM has been used extensively in research and continues to enjoy considerable interest. It has been used particularly to assess patterns of health screening behaviours for various cancers (e.g., Yoo et al., 2013) and especially to determine the extent to which women practise breast self-examination (Umeh and Jones, 2010). However, the model also attracts criticisms.

One of the main limitations is that there is an assumption that the deliberation of barriers and benefits does not change over time.

We cannot expect to hold the same beliefs across the many different contexts of our lives as we mature or as our circumstances change. For example, we may take more risks with our health when we are younger, as we do not perceive the dangers or disadvantages as much as a more mature person. The specific health context is also important. It is highly possible that, in an isolated area of decision-making (such as attending a screening procedure), individuals might cognitively process a clearly defined set of pros and cons that fit within the components of the HBM. Yet there are also unconscious actions related to maintaining health – for example, cleaning teeth to maintain oral hygiene: such everyday actions, or omissions, are not necessarily accompanied by a conscious decision-making process. Another weakness is that the model does not account for social influences on behaviour and how the views of others may shape a person's own attitudes and beliefs. Above all, the model assumes a level of rationality in all individuals to make decisions which we cannot guarantee. To address these difficulties, other theories have included additional elements that consider societal influence and our individual thresholds of self-control. These will be discussed in turn.

3.2 The theory of planned behaviour (TPB)

The HBM is a cognitive model of health behaviour, but it largely excludes the societal and emotional influences that can and do play significant roles. A theory that accounts for these influences and advances the work of the HBM is the theory of planned behaviour (Ajzen, 1985). This is a widely used theory within behavioural medicine, and it is a useful basis in assisting all health professionals to understand health behaviours.

The principles that inform the components of the theory are in some ways similar to the HBM. However, where the HBM focuses on points that are quite far advanced along the decision-making trajectory, the TPB extends our understanding of behaviour by taking a person's *intentions* into account. In other words, the development of the TPB strongly indicated that health behaviours are not simply a matter of consciously evaluating one's susceptibility to and severity of illness. By including intentions, the TPB adds another contributory factor to the decision-making processes and, in addition to the evaluation of perceived benefits and barriers that are intrinsic to the HBM, asserts that *attitudes* determine intentions (see figure 2.2).

Another component of the TBP is that, in conjunction with attitudes, the perceived beliefs of other people also carry considerable influence. This determining factor is the subjective norm, an especially pertinent consideration when planning health interventions that are based upon the TPB: for example, young people are more likely to respond positively to interventions targeted at their peer group rather than those which are targeted towards older people. The subjective

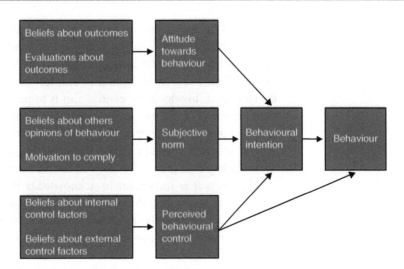

Figure 2.2 The theory of planned behaviour

norm further allows us to consider the social demands that influence behaviour: peer pressure to engage in health-limiting behaviours such as smoking or recreational drug use is an obvious example.

The consideration of peer pressure and other circumstances that comprise the subjective norm influences how much control we have over our own actions, and perceived behavioural control is the third factor in the TPB that is deemed to influence our intentions. The word 'perceived' is very important here, as this relates to an individual's belief that they have a certain level of control over their behaviour. It does not refer to actual control, which may mean that there are practical, concrete factors that determine whether or not a person engages in certain behaviours. Such factors might, for example, involve prohibitive costs of medication.

While the TPB advances our ability to access reasons why people adopt certain health behaviours, it is not without limitations. A major obstacle is the conceptual leap between intentions and behaviour: we all have good intentions in various contexts, but, for a myriad of reasons, this does not mean we necessarily carry them out. This limitation alone poses difficulties for the TPB as a predictor of behaviour. It serves to enhance our understanding of behaviour but not necessarily to explain it to a more precise level.

More recently, there have been strong calls to 'retire' the TPB, despite its wide application in empirical studies. Sniehotta, Presseau and Araújo-Soares (2014) argued that research utilizing the TPB as the theoretical framework was largely dependent on correlational studies (lacking predictive power) in which many of the subjects were university students, and that such studies were not suited to longitudinal designs (though see Conner (2014) for a critical commentary on this paper). Furthermore, a similar criticism of the HBM is levelled at the TBP in that it is based on conscious rather than unconscious reasoning.

Recent developments in health behaviour change theory now seek to integrate different theories to try and account for the variability in observed behaviour that is not always captured by more established models. The Theoretical Domains Framework is an example of this development, in which the central aim is to provide a more evidence-based framework for measuring behaviour change from a wider theoretical context (Michie et al., 2011): by amalgamating constructs from several different theories rather that selecting one, the possibility of omitting key factors or influences on health behaviour is minimized.

However, it is important to acknowledge the dominant presence of the TPB in the last thirty years within health behaviour research and useful to think about certain aspects such as perceived behavioural control. When contemplating how much control a person has on their health behaviour, it is useful to consider how we can define control more specifically. Control is determined by many psychological dynamics, such as conformity, obedience and social roles. Chapters 1 and 4 address these areas in more detail, but, for the purpose of introducing control as a key element in health behaviour, it is more helpful at this stage to simplify it to a locus of control and, more specifically, consider internal and external loci.

3.2 The health locus of control

The extent to which people hold beliefs about their levels of self-control varies. However, this variability can be broadly divided into different areas. Individuals who believe that they actively manage and determine their own outcomes by the decisions they make are seen as having an internal locus of control. Conversely, those who have an external locus of control position themselves as being a passive recipient of circumstance and do not assume full responsibility for their circumstances. These perspectives have been explored and measured by the development of the health locus of control (HLOC) scale (Wallston et al., 1978). Explorations of how HLOC beliefs may influence health have been extensively researched within many clinical specialties and conditions. One example lies in HIV/AIDS research, in which healthy survivors in an HIV-positive group were found to have significant differences in strengths of HLOC beliefs to those of a matched control group (Ruffin et al., 2012).

This leads appropriately to a third dimension in the HLOC – *powerful others*. The inclusion of this element recognizes that the actions and communications of health professionals can also determine the level of internal or external locus of control within individuals. When thinking of the control that we as individuals exert over our health in relation to our behaviour, the issue of taking medicines as directed, or maintaining behaviour according to health professionals' guidance demands considerable attention. In case study 2.1 we saw that David does not take his insulin as directed, which could have serious consequences. However, such behaviour is not uncommon and leads to poor clinical outcomes; it can reduce quality of life and increase the likelihood of disease. This begs the question why people choose not to take medicines or adhere to recommendations. Social cognition models such as the HBM and the TPB can help to explain this in terms of appraising benefits and barriers to health, intentions and motivations. But there are other psychological factors at work, which suggest there are more specific reasons influencing why we may or may not adhere to medication.

4 Adherence and compliance

Another influential model in health psychology that helps us to address these issues is Ley's (1988) model of adherence, which suggests that adherence is largely dependent on three factors: understanding, memory and satisfaction. Before explaining the model in more detail, it is interesting to note that, when it was first developed, it was initially called a model of *compliance*. This word is still used in some academic spheres relating to patients sticking to their prescribed medicines or recommended actions. However, 'adherence' is used more frequently because 'compliance' refers mainly to doctors' desire for patients to comply with their instructions about treatment – i.e., 'patients should do as they are told'. 'Adherence', on the other hand, is a more neutral term and is more representative of the extent to which a patient's behaviour coincides with the advice that they are given. 'Compliance' also carries with it the implication that non-compliance is a deliberate act of defiance or resistance, and the dynamic between health professionals and patients is of course not as simple as that. Ley's model demonstrates the complexities involved in most instances where patients don't take their medicine.

Let us return to the factors of understanding, memory and satisfaction. If a health professional suggests that a patient follows a particular treatment regime and the patient does not *understand* the causes of their illness or the processes involved in treatment, this is likely to have a negative effect on adherence. Similarly, from research into memory, we know that recall of verbal information is poor and that patients are unlikely to remember all of the information that they are given. Information that is conveyed earlier on in a consultation is generally remembered best – known as the 'primacy effect'; the 'recency effect' also applies to information that is conveyed towards the end of a consultation. In addition to the order in which information is presented, recall can be affected by the way a patient feels at the time, particularly if increased levels of anxiety are involved. In a focus group study examining factors that affected adherence to osteoporosis medication, the three components of Ley's model were clearly supported, as participants cited lack of understanding, failure to remember instructions, and dissatisfaction with doctors' visits as key contributors to their non-adherence (Iversen et al. 2011).

While the other models and theories cited so far can allow for a greater understanding into how and why patients engage in health-enhancing or -limiting behaviours, Ley's model is especially useful in that it lends itself to practical changes that nurses and health professionals can undertake to maximize patient adherence and subsequent wellbeing. It is possible to increase understanding of conditions and their treatment by encouraging patients to be actively involved in the consultation. It is also possible to facilitate increased recall capacity by providing information in structured form, avoiding medical jargon, or providing written information where appropriate. In addition, there are many ways of increasing satisfaction, but clarity of communication and building rapport are key components that contribute to adherence.

5 Stages of change model

A successful relationship between nurses (and other health professionals) and their patients depends on many things, and efforts to understand why individuals enact certain health behaviours will naturally contribute to continued positive clinical outcomes and mutual trust. All of the theories and models addressed so far have assumed a continuing position taken towards health behaviour. However, there are also circumstances in which health professionals, including nurses, are involved in encouraging behaviour change. Among these might be programmes to stop smoking, to initiate exercise, to change diet, and to practise safe sex, to name a few. In these contexts, it is more useful to consider individual cognitions as staged processes rather than being on a continuum.

The stages of change model (SoC), also known as the trans-theoretical model of behaviour change, was developed by Prochaska and DiClemente (1984) and focused principally upon smoking cessation. The model assumes that people go through various stages as they make behavioural changes:

- *Pre-contemplation*: no intention of changing behaviour
- *Contemplation*: beginning to consider change at some non-defined point in the future
- *Preparation*: getting ready to change in the near future
- *Action*: engaged in change now
- *Maintenance*: steady state of change has been reached.

If we return to our case study of David and his reluctance to take insulin and adopt health-enhancing behaviours in managing his diabetes, it is safe to say that he would be at the pre-contemplation stage. Following his hospital admission he might start to contemplate changing his behaviour by wanting to prevent such incidents occurring in the future. To prepare, he might set individual goals, such as identifying times when he can discreetly inject his insulin or working out sensible strategies for drinking alcohol when out with friends, which would be followed by carrying out those actions and displaying overt behaviour change. Unfortunately, the fifth stage of maintenance is often broken by relapses into health-limiting behaviour. Indeed, the process is not always linear as, depending on their motivations and individual circumstances, someone may begin to prepare but may still return to the contemplation stage.

Like the HBM and the TPB, the SoC has also been used as a basis for interventions that help people change their behaviour, and the advantage of the model's staged structure is that interventions can be targeted to reach people at different stages. Health promotion material such as leaflets or television programmes may be used effectively to target people in the pre-contemplation stage. The stages of contemplation, preparation and action can all be addressed in health professionals' direct communication with patients, in discussing strategies of how to prepare for and maintain change. Of course, motivation and self-efficacy on the patient's part is crucial to achieve positive change, but there are communicative strategies that are directly aligned to the principles of the SoC model that can be used to great effect. Motivational interviewing is a key example and will be discussed in more detail in chapter 14.

As with all the theories and models mentioned here, the SoC does not escape criticism. Empirical studies have identified the difficulties in allocating participants to discrete stages of the model, which suggest that continuing models of readiness or preparedness may present more useful frameworks with which to consider an individual's disposition towards behaviour change. There is also evidence to suggest that past behaviour can predict the likelihood of change. A lengthy history of a health-limiting behaviour which is firmly established renders the first two stages of pre-contemplation and contemplation somewhat redundant if there is no motivation. However, the SoC is still widely acknowledged to be a significant contribution towards interventions that facilitate change that are deployed by nurses and other health professionals. How motivated people are and the levels of self-efficacy they possess are of course dependent on individual differences, internal and external. It is fair to assert that our personalities play a considerable role in our ability to effect change and control our health status, and at this juncture it is appropriate to expand on the role and influence of personality in health.

6 Personality types and health

The models in this chapter can partially account for beliefs and behaviours about health. They are not without criticism, but they can offer explanations as to why individual perceptions vary when it comes to health and illness. However, they do not explicitly account for personality or emotion. Chapter 3 will examine the role of emotion in nursing care in more detail, but this section will introduce the wider areas of personality psychology and how this contributes to our concepts of mental and physical health.

The relationship between personality and health is a complex one. Do our personalities determine how healthy we will be? Or does our health influence what type of person we are? Can we assume that our personality is the same over time and in different contexts with different people? These are questions that are very relevant to how healthy we are; they are also important for health professionals to consider when engaging with patients at a level other than a clinical encounter.

To begin, it is helpful to draw attention to some key theories of personality in psychology that have been influential in health-related research. Many people have investigated dimensions of personality, but there are two major theories that continue to be widely used in health and social psychology research.

The first proposes that there are essentially three individual personality traits. Eysenck (1970) proposed a three-factor model consisting of psychoticism, extraversion and neuroticism. At first glance this might appear to be an alarming set of traits, but it is worth remembering that these personality traits relate to their opposite dimensions too. Therefore neuroticism (a nervous or anxious disposition) sits opposite traits of emotional consistency, such as contentment. Similarly, psychoticism, indicative of antisocial or aggressive personality, sits opposite pro-social and considerate behaviour. Eysenck's three-factor model has been used extensively to research specific populations. One example is the role of personality within criminal cognitions and social identity (Boduszek et al., 2012), in which extraversion was found to be a strong mediator of criminal thinking styles among prisoners with learning difficulties.

Another model that has been widely used is the five-factor model of personality, often referred to as the 'Big Five' (McRae and Costa, 1987). The five factors here are openness, conscientiousness, extraversion, agreeableness and neuroticism. The model has been validated in many cultures, and the five personality factors, which are deemed to be stable and permanent, have been deployed to many areas of health research. For example, examinations of dietary behaviour and food preference using the five-factor inventory identified that conscientiousness and agreeableness were highly associated with healthy eating behaviours, while preferences for sweet foods were aligned with low levels of openness (Mõttus et al., 2013). It is, however, reasonable to question whether everyone incorporates a certain number of traits and to argue that individual differences can significantly alter the ways in which such traits manifest and impact upon our individual and collective health.

In addition to the broader factor analyses of traits, it has been suggested that there are three 'personality types' that have a bearing on particular health conditions: Type A, Type B and Type C. Historically,

Type B personalities were designated as relaxed and with low levels of aggression (Rosenman et al., 1976), while Type C personalities were deemed to suppress emotions and be prone to certain diseases such as cancer (Grossarth-Maticek et al., 1985). However, the Type A behaviour pattern, with its link to coronary heart disease (CHD), is perhaps the best known. Type A behaviour is typically associated with individuals who are of a highly strung nature, competitive, impatient and easily annoyed/irritated. Before this pattern was explicitly named, there were earlier indications at the start of the twentieth century that such personality characteristics were linked to ill health. As early as 1910, Sir William Osler coined the term hurry sickness. It was not until the 1950s, when research into such personality characteristics became more focused, that this led to the discovery of a group of behaviours collectively known as 'Type A' (Friedman and Rosenman, 1959).

The further classification of a Type D personality historically identified patients as being overly distressed and prone to worry and was also closely linked with CHD (Denollet et al., 1995). Associations between this personality type and prognosis in cardiovascular disease have continued to generate research interest, albeit questioning the strength of the relationship as time has passed (Grande et al., 2012). While some of the evidence concerning personality types in relation to specific diseases is contradictory, there is little doubt that such typologies have an established place in health psychology and that they can assist practitioners' understanding of patients' behaviour. Such models and theories do not dictate that we as individuals have only a certain number of personality factors or that our personalities remain static over time. However, they may act as useful frameworks within which to contextualize some of the determinants of our health. (There is further discussion of these personality types and their particular relation to stress in chapter 9, 'Stress and Illness'.)

7 Conclusion

This chapter has journeyed through several theories and models that can account for healthy and unhealthy behaviours. But how can they assist with nursing practice at policy and individual levels? Given the wide reach of the aforementioned models and theories across a variety of illness, contexts and behaviours, it is evident that the relevance here is not confined solely to nursing practice that lies specifically within the domain of mental healthcare. At the beginning of the chapter, the issue of conflicting agendas between health professional and patient was raised. Staged and continuum models of health behaviour, alongside research into personality and health, can greatly assist us to understand why patients may make what seem to be questionable choices about their health or why they may be anxious about it. This is of particular relevance to nursing; nurses are more likely to engage in patient interactions that provide opportunities for discussing psychosocial elements of health and illness. Nurses may be witnesses to disclosures that are not aired to other health professionals, and knowledge of the psychological theories that can underpin health choices and behaviour is advantageous in establishing trust and rapport. The final chapter in this book ('Psychology and Working as a Nurse') will deal specifically with occupational challenges and how other psychological theories can assist and explain them. Such knowledge is also beneficial for interprofessional understanding and can greatly assist in daily communications, such as handover or documenting information for patient safety. Overall, being able systematically to appreciate and apply elements of the psychological models included in this chapter will equip nurses with enhanced ability to communicate, evaluate and monitor interventions for patients.

Summary

▶ Perceived benefits and barriers, susceptibility and severity are important influences on individuals' health behaviours.
▶ Society and attitudes greatly influence our intentions relating to our health.
▶ There is evidence to suggest that our personalities contribute to our physical and mental wellbeing.

Questions for discussion

1 How might the theory of planned behaviour be applied to smoking cessation?
2 How might nurses use their skills to encourage someone to adhere to medicines?
3 Give examples of what might be the internal and external HLOC contributors to the case study 2.1 (David not taking medication).

Further reading and resources

Ogden, J. (2012) *Health Psychology: A Textbook.* 5th edn, Maidenhead: Open University Press.
Now in its fifth edition, this book will provide more detail about the theories and models described in this chapter that will also broaden an understanding of health psychology.

Marks, D. F., Murray, M. P., Evans, B., and Estacio, E. V. (2011) *Health Psychology: Theory, Research and Practice.* 3rd edn, London: Sage.
As well as addressing models of health psychology, this book takes a critical approach and pays particular attention to community psychology and health promotion.

Part II
Being a Patient

CONTENTS

Part II takes a developmental approach, as it follows our case study of Beth on her placements with children and young people, adults, those with learning disabilities, older people, people in pain and those at the end of life. The chapters in this section look at the psychological issues pertinent to particular patient groups, but there are also common themes that feed through them relating to personhood, identity, self-esteem and the role of stories in the continual evolvement of the self.

Chapter 3 explores the relevance of psychology in nursing children and young people. It begins by focusing on the infant as an active participant in the formation of the self, which is based on interaction with others. The chapter raises key issues in child development, such as dependency, trust, autonomy, attachment and control – themes that are important from the beginning of life and are experienced, worked through and repeated in each developmental phase. The implications of nursing children and young people are considered in the light of this perspective, with brief vignettes to illustrate the abilities and capacities that define developmental phases. The chapter also addresses how the emotional needs of both the child and the family can be met alongside their physical health needs, which can help increase satisfaction with care.

Being an adult patient may not initially seem problematic, and yet there is a paradox within the term whereby an autonomous, independent individual may suddenly be in a position of dependency and need. The difficulties of being faced with a serious or chronic illness or disability as an adult are explored in chapter 4. Using a health psychology model as a framework, the chapter discusses the psychological factors regarding how an individual comes to terms with illness, from the initial point of recognizing symptoms and seeking advice through to receiving a diagnosis and treatment. It also introduces the role of narrative psychology in relation to how people make sense of their experiences through the stories they tell. Chapter 4 ends by looking at the shifting roles and power dynamics that come into play between patients and healthcare professionals and the impact this has on the patient experience in the twenty-first century.

Chapter 5 moves on to the psychological aspects of nursing those with learning disabilities. This is relevant not only to those studying within this branch of nursing but for all nurses. Individuals with learning disabilities today have an increased life expectancy, so that more children and young people reach adulthood with complex and multiple needs. Added to this, there is an increase in the numbers of school-age children who are identified with autistic spectrum disorders. This chapter focuses on how psychology can be applied in order to respond sensitively but effectively to individuals with learning disabilities. The behavioural, cognitive and psychodynamic approaches introduced in Part I are discussed in relation to the management of anxiety, depression and challenging behaviours – behaviours which are likely to be exacerbated when individuals with learning disabilities are placed in unfamiliar healthcare settings.

Moving forwards through the life trajectory, chapter 6 explores cognitive decline. The focus here is nursing patients with dementia, the treatment of which has traditionally been dominated by a medically driven perspective. Over the last twenty years psychology has contributed significantly to providing an alternative person-centred, biopsychosocial model that can help to support the diagnosis, treatment and care of people living with the condition, with person-centred care as recognized best practice. This chapter explores how the psychosocial aspects of a person and their life are essential in interpreting behaviours, in successful communication and in providing appropriate nursing support for people with dementia in a range of health and social-care contexts.

Chapter 7 looks at pain, a phenomenon encountered by us all. Drawing from the psychology of pain, it discusses the motivational importance of pain and how the perception of pain is vital in keeping us safe. It considers failure of the body system – for example, fatal illnesses that produce limited sensation of pain – as well as the many less threatening conditions that result in intense pain and real distress. Drawing on the biopsychosocial model, the chapter illustrates how mindset and personality affect pain perception, with the emphasis that pain is perceived in the brain and not the body. By understanding such factors, nurses can more readily reassure many of the patients in their care and so allow them to assist in pain reduction, whether that pain is chronic or acute.

Part II closes with a chapter that looks at the psychological needs of those who require palliative and end of life care and their families, as well as health professionals. The significance of social support in relation to increased control, healthy coping abilities, reduced depression, recognition of self-worth and psychological wellbeing are explored within the philosophy and principles of palliative care. As with other chapters in this section, the role of the nurse in delivering person-centred and holistic care is central. The chapter considers how individuals can be helped to adapt to the palliative end of life phase of their illness, as well as considering the support needs of the family and loved ones. Importantly, it also addresses the psychological needs of professionals, examining the stressors involved in end of life care and identifying the knowledge and skills required to support patients, families and colleagues effectively.

Nursing the Child and Young Person

Paul Buckley and Sue Elmer

KEY ISSUES IN THIS CHAPTER:

▶ The ability of nurses to communicate effectively with children and young people depends upon understanding their changing capacity and ability over time.
▶ Infants need to be seen as active participants in interaction with adults and their environment as they construct their own perspectives in the world.
▶ Developing children are situated in multiple contexts (individual, family and the wider culture and society) which need to be considered in order to understand their needs.

BY THE END OF THIS CHAPTER YOU SHOULD BE ABLE TO:

▶ explain some of the major changes in the psychological development of children and young people
▶ critically describe aspects of key debates in developmental psychology and some of the major theorists' contributions
▶ consider the adaptation of nursing practice when working with children and young people
▶ identify some ways in which psychological interventions can be used by the nurse with children to enhance compliance and reduce the anxiety and stress associated with health problems.

1 Introduction

Implicitly or explicitly, theories of development influence nursing practice. The aim of this chapter is to capture the key features of the rapidly expanding field of developmental psychology, knowledge of which has been shown significantly to improve interventions. Some 20 per cent of the 12 million children and young people (0 to 19 years of age) in England present for healthcare in a typical year, between 10 and 30 per cent of whom are affected in some way by chronic illness (Underdown, 2007; Craig and Mindell, 2014). These conditions may have consequences for the emotional, educational and social development of the young person as well as impacting their families and schools. While many children and families cope well with the demands of much illness, the emotional and psychological needs of people with acute and long-term conditions can be described on a continuum from healthy coping, through disease-related distress, to psychological and psychiatric conditions. Through preventive and restorative means (such as immunization and health promotion), social care (education, local authority) and healthcare (surgery, accident and emergency departments, maternity/neonatal services, specialist services such as paediatric oncology, cardiology and child and adolescent mental health services), nurses are at the forefront.

The broad aim of emotional and psychological care is to support the individual with the condition, their carers and their family to prevent and reduce any distress that has a negative impact on the individual's general wellbeing and ability to self-manage their illness, and the impact of that illness, effectively (NHS Confederation, 2012). There is an ever increasing and good evidence base to support the clinical effectiveness of psychological interventions for a number of medical conditions and illnesses (Edwards and Titman, 2010; Eccleston et al. 2015). Psychologically informed interventions may result in better medical outcome (quicker recovery and increased levels of adherence); better psychological functioning (reduced anxiety, improved mood, and less distress and anger); better family functioning; reduced levels of disability, pain and distress; and better communication between the medical team and the family (see www.cochrane.org). Nurses have a vital role in the care of children and young people, and their application of such knowledge has been researched in forming positive relationships with youngsters, preparing parents and children for hospital admission, and facilitating appropriate emotional expression (Siegel and Conte, 2001). All of these have been found to reduce anxiety, improve children's coping behaviour, and lead to quicker recovery after minor surgery (Keiling et al., 2011).

The present chapter is divided into four parts. It begins with a general discussion of current developmental psychology before turning to a case example. The systems theory perspective will be described, and the following three sections focus on children of different ages in order to explore particular features of cognitive and emotional development. The major states of mind – feelings in infancy, narratives in early childhood, and identity formation in adolescence – are discussed. Each of these parts ends with key summary points. The chapter concludes with some suggested reading and useful weblinks.

3

2 An overview of contemporary developmental psychology

Developmental psychology aims to describe and explain the changes found in human beings from the beginning of life to its end. It is a scientific endeavour, seeking answers to questions and testing ideas or theories. While the term 'growth' refers to quantitative changes, the term 'development' includes such changes in size or quantity but also refers to qualitative changes, shifts in type or kind. 'Maturation' refers to the biological unfolding of the individual and the ways in which experiences result in more or less permanent changes in thought, feeling and behaviour. Hence, developmental psychologists are interested in questions about the domains of development (physical, cognitive, emotional-social); the relative influence of genes and learning (nature and nurture); whether development occurs through small steps or stage-like shifts; and typical and atypical development. Although such variables are often researched separately, most psychologists adopt a holistic perspective and understand the several areas as being interdependent. This chapter is focused on the earlier stages of life, but the discipline itself has expanded to encompass the changes that occur over the whole of the lifespan.

A multitude of theoretical perspectives influence current developmental psychology. It has been the rapid acquisition of complex physical, emotional and cognitive skills that largely occupied the pioneers. Besides his theory of evolution, Charles Darwin (1809–1882) wrote a baby biography of his infant son, keeping a typically detailed record of observed behaviours, and evolutionary psychology is now an established discipline. Sigmund Freud (1856–1933) attempted a complete psychology and drew attention to children's inner lives with his psychosexual stages, the powerful emotions undergone, and the ways in which such experiences are interpreted or given meaning. Freud's emphasis on the individual was modified by Erik Erikson (1902–1994). Famous for the term 'identity crisis', Erikson came to understand our sense of self or self-identity as the result of the important choices we make and our relationships with others. Lev Vygotsky (1896–1934) was interested in the ways in which information and cognitive skills are transmitted from one generation to the next. He and his colleagues developed the idea of learning taking place first between people and only then internalized by the individual. The founder of behaviourism in America, John B. Watson (1878–1958), emphasized nurture over nature by asserting that children's ideas, skills and preferences were a product of experience – even going so far as to state that, given healthy infants and a controlled environment, he could guarantee the outcome on the basis of learning: doctor, lawyer, beggar or thief. Arnold Gesell (1880–1961) upheld that both nurture and nature are important. Besides contributing to public hygiene, education and child-rearing, Gesell also studied biological maturation in human development, charting a series of milestones (physical, motor, etc.).

Perhaps still best known is the work of Jean Piaget (1896–1980). His cognitive-developmental stages were developed from his research (initially on his own children) and detailed the progression from infancy to adulthood. The child is viewed as a 'little scientist', actively constructing categories of experience (though 'schema' is Piaget's (1950) term) to enable adaptation. The stages of development through which every child was thought to progress are discrete and move from immediate, sensory activity, through an egocentric stage, to logical reasoning, which is acquired in adolescence. Talking with children at length and using thought experiments and tasks, Piaget made careful observations of infants and children as exemplars of the stages shown in table 3.1.

Whether it was physical maturation, as for Gesell, the strong emotions and interpretation of experience of Freud, or Piaget's cognitive mechanisms, the pioneers of developmental psychology sought what was universal, offering the idea of development progressing through a series of stages. Subsequent research has raised many criticisms – for example, the idea of stages comes with the assumption of linear, unvarying steps that are universal (Morss, 1995; Jarvis et al., 2014). Having been a dominant figure in the mid-part of the twentieth century, Piaget has been criticized for underestimating younger children's abilities and

Table 3.1 Piaget's stages of cognitive development and age	
Age	Skills and abilities
Sensorimotor stage: 0–2 years	Sounds, smells and sights are used along with touch and taste. Gradually objects become familiar, and the infant learns that they continue to exist when out of sight.
Pre-operational stage: 2–7 years	Language is acquired, making self-awareness possible as well as symbolic thought. Children are strongly influenced by the appearance of things, rather than by logical thinking. At this stage children are egocentric, unable to take another's perspective into account.
Concrete operational stage: 7–11 years	Both logical reasoning and understanding others' perspectives is possible. Causality is comprehended, but difficulty with abstract concepts is experienced.
Formal operational stage: 11 years onwards	Children are capable of using abstract thought. They can form ideas and pursue hypothetical arguments.

for his neglect of emotion and culture (Burman, 2008). Further, it is implied that there is only one developmental path to maturity which (if we are to be considered normal) everyone must follow – a view which seriously neglects the importance of culture and history. As Rutter and Rutter (1993) state, this way of thinking about development is insensitive to the dynamics of change and individual variations. Contributions from other approaches, such as the information-processing, contextual and affective-neuroscience viewpoints, shed important light on facets of development, some aspects of which are included in this chapter.

What are the signs of emotional and psychological wellbeing in children and young people? Although deficit models may make such a question hard to think about, we can all probably readily imagine children who have a zest for life, enjoy secure relationships, and have a healthy curiosity and a strong imaginative capacity (Waddell, 1998). Confident, adaptable and assertive children have 'space' in their minds for new experiences and ideas – they are open to maturation and learning (Underdown, 2007; Howe, 2011). Protective factors such as being healthy and safe and having enjoyment, economic wellbeing and security of attachment relationships are crucial. But poverty, neglect, trauma, abuse and witnessing domestic violence are frightening and painful realities for many (Elmer, 2013). Even in such circumstances some children are resilient and find ways to cope, whereas others suffer various forms of physical and mental health problems. Simple and static constructions of childhood have – through empirical and theory research – given way to complex, dynamic-interactionist models. Integrative models are most useful in approaching this complexity, and the ecological systems paradigm will be adopted for the purposes of this chapter.

Many introductory texts now include the ecological model (e.g., Levine and Munsch, 2011) developed by Urie Bronfenbrenner (1917–2005). Ecology is perhaps usually associated with plants and animals, but we can just as easily think about human ecology. Systems theory holds that an individual's genetic wealth, inherited temperament, and thoughts, feelings and behaviours have to be considered within the multiple contexts of our lives – family, school, community and wider society – if they are to be understood. The implications of nursing children and adolescents are considered in the light of this intersubjective perspective, with a composite case study to illustrate the abilities and capacities that define both developmental lines and phases.

Activity 3.1

Ask yourself what children of differing ages are capable of: infancy (0–18 months), early (2–6 years) and middle (6–10) childhood, and adolescence (10–17+). How confident would you feel about nursing any of these children? What influences in the treatment setting could influence the child's emotional wellbeing and recovery?

To counter the tendency to describe isolated individuals, the systems perspective enables us to map the family within the wider contexts of community, society and historical time period. Nurses seek to work in partnership with families, and, to support this aim, ecological systems thinking was introduced into British nursing in the 1990s (Hemphill and Dearmun, 2006). This paradigm holds that families can be viewed as a system of humans in continual interaction with one another and with their community and society. While within-individual processes are important, so are the interactions that take place between self and other, which include groups and organizations, as changes in one part impact other parts. One debate in psychology has been whether the child is an active agent or reflexively programmed to adapt and passively respond to environmental stimuli. Theorists such as Piaget and Erikson took the active view: children are small scientists seeking to understand their world and are agents who make decisions about what they want. On the other hand, Freud, Watson and Skinner viewed children as largely passive, subject to inner drives, parents, culture or reinforcers – rewards and punishments. Instead of having to choose between such opposing emphases, the systems paradigm allows us to see children both as active agents and as influenced by others. For researchers such as Vygotsky and Bronfenbrenner, effects are bi-directional: from the child to others and from the environment to the child.

To appreciate the various contexts which are useful to consider as actively influencing states of mind and behaviour, Bronfenbrenner (1979) uses five technical terms, but (following Herbert, 2003: 7) only three are used here.

- The *microsystem* refers to the child's characteristics and immediate environment of family, peers and school (shown in figure 3.1 by dark and mid-green ovals).
- The *exosystem* comprises factors such as father's work, government and school systems, which are not experienced by the children directly but which affect development.
- The *macrosystem* is the larger cultural context, such as systems of belief, customs, values, laws, lifestyles and opportunities.

The model is dynamic, and each part of the system, being nested within others as with a set of Russian dolls, is open to influence with what happens at other levels. Take the example of child-rearing behaviour. This depends on attitudes derived from culture and values, but is also affected by family stresses (poverty or illness), age, social contacts, and so forth. The importance of respecting culture and diversity is a requirement for all healthcare professionals and is embodied in the UK Nursing and Midwifery Council Code (NMC, 2015; for further guidance, see www.nmc-uk.org/Documents/EandD/EandD%20annual%20 report%202012-2013.pdf). Considering this model, case study 3.1

explores some of the key features of each stage of development and their implications for nursing care.

> **Case Study 3.1:**
>
> Ram and Lesley began living together five years ago when they were expecting Sanjit. Lesley is a 33-year-old mother of three children. Having returned part-time to her job as a library assistant, she is worried about her two older children. Her eldest is Anne, born from a brief relationship with John when Lesley was seventeen. They have had no contact with John for many years. Anne was diagnosed with cystic fibrosis in infancy but, remarkably, has been largely symptom-free until several recent hospital admissions. She has stayed out late, not done her homework, seems increasingly chaotic in her behaviour, and is withdrawn. A decision is pending with the Cystic Fibrosis (CF) Team as to whether or not antibiotic injections are the best way to help manage future chest infections. Lesley and Ram have two children together; a third (a twin daughter) died in utero. Sanjit is four and a half years old and had settled into his reception year at school but has said in an upset and angry way that he doesn't want to go anymore. The youngest, Jamie, who is ten months old, has begun standing and walking with aid, can say a few words and seems contented. In the preceding year Ram was made redundant and was out of work for five months, during which time the family experienced food poverty despite the help of family and friends. He now has a new job which is better paid but it entails longer hours.

The people described in case study 3.1 and their relationships can be represented visually in a modification of the map of the family, the genogram, the ecogram or 'ecomap' (Hemphill and Dearmun, 2006) (see figure 3.1). This valuable picture of individuals (females are represented by circles, males by squares), their connections to others (solid or broken lines for relationships that are current or broken) and the impact of other socio-historical factors attends to the complexity of life and aids effective case formulations.

This case example has relevance for nursing practice in a number of ways. The nursing of children and young people presents specific challenges. Family-centred care is important, as it recognizes that family life is both fundamental in a child's life and a system that is open to a wide variety of influences. The various issues and ages of the children modify how problems are presented, the required nursing intervention and the type of psychological care. Competence in communicating with children and young people, understanding their needs, involving them and their parents/carers in decision-making, and assisting children to care for themselves (RCN, 2004) can be greatly enhanced by an understanding of the psychology of development.

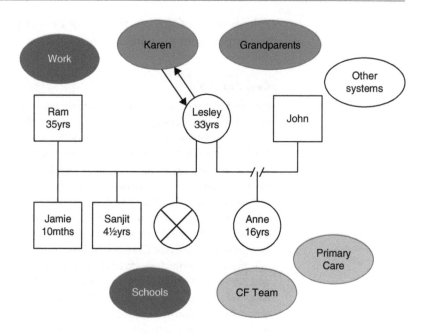

Figure 3.1 Ecomap of case study

3 Infancy – the world of feelings

We can further our exploration of key developmental ideas by considering the youngest child, Jamie. Already, by the time he is ten months of age, richly complex changes have taken place. From conception there is a rapid growth of neurons, which continues over the first year of the infant's life. More neurons are produced than are actually needed, and they are 'pruned' in response to experience with the environment. Even though the newborn's brain is only one-third of the size of an adult's brain, it already contains many of the subcortical structures that are important in early communication (Trevarthen, 2003). These structures are functioning from the embryo stage (the first two months of life) – long before the formation of the cerebral cortex – and infants around six weeks after birth routinely act to engage adults in 'chat'. This type of verbal behaviour was termed 'proto-conversation' by Mary Catherine Bateson and is more usually referred to in psychology as the babbling stage. Through careful analysis of video recordings, Trevarthen shows how intricate and sophisticated this form of interaction is. Coordination of rising and falling pitch in cycles lasting around thirty seconds were found, and mothers' responses were contingent – that is, appropriate and attuned to the intensity, type and timing of their children's behaviour. Historically, fathers were neglected in developmental accounts – so much so that the kind of talk carers employ with infants has been termed 'motherese' – but fathers, family members, childhood friends, teachers, and so on, are included in modern psychological accounts. Trevarthen goes on to comment that similar cycles of excitement occur in music and baby songs, and Bateson suggests that proto-conversation is the precursor not only of speech and language but also of ritual healing practices.

Piaget would locate Jamie in the early state of mind, the sensory-motor stage. As he lacks language, reflexive responding is dominant, and the world is explored through smell, touch (particularly via the mouth) and vision. But Daniel Stern (1985) holds that the infant is active in organizing the sensations, mobility and feelings in the first two months after birth. This aspect is retained throughout life as emergent forms of self, which entail interest and excitement as well as, at turns, calm and quiet states. John Bowlby's (1907–1990) attachment theory has provided a useful way of viewing parent/carer–child relationships. While 'bonding' refers to the way a parent may bind to a child, 'attachment' refers to the emotional tie of the child to the caregivers. Research has underscored the importance of the parent–child relationship for children's sense of security, curiosity about their world, interactions with others, balancing their own emotions, and resilience to stress (Siegel, 1999). Regulation of the infant's state (contented, hungry, bored, sad) through contingent communication is the priority in this early, pre-attachment phase (i.e., before around seven months of age). Arguably, such responsive communication is important to us throughout life.

In typical development, the sense of a core self is established between two and six months of age and a subjective self from seven months, accompanied by memory development and the increasing grasp of language. The set of emotions evident at birth include interest, distress, disgust and contentment (Gerhardt, 2004). If intense and unregulated, emotions can result in behavioural problems and interfere with reasoning but, for the majority, where the care provided is good enough, affects and emotion support reasoning and social competence (Damasio, 1999). Infants become increasingly coordinated and purposeful: six-month-olds will roll or pat a ball depending on what mother was observed to do; they follow the eyes of another person (joint attention), not head direction (though not if the eyes are closed); the joint attention facilitates language development (infants who follow a gaze more accurately learn language faster); a new toy will be avoided if mother exhibits disgust but will be played with otherwise (Levine and Munsch, 2011). The infant is an active participant in construing its own world, highlighting that the formation of the self is always based on interaction with others. In his work on the development of playfulness, Trevarthen (2003) came to similar conclusions to Winnicott (1971), arguing that play develops in the space between mother and baby. Trevarthen (2003) concluded that, when the mother fails to develop 'motherese' and is unresponsive to her baby in terms of vocalizations and gestures, the baby will eventually stop reaching out to her. In these circumstances, the baby's attempts to be playful will be inhibited.

Unfortunately, many children who are subjected to abuse and neglect may have an unreliable attachment relationship with their mother or other important carers (Bowlby, 1980; Crittenden and Ainsworth, 1989). The consequences for the child can be poor or faulty attachment relationships, which create anxiety and result in an inability to play to the child's satisfaction (Elmer, 2010).

The senses of self continue to feature and function throughout life; themes such as dependency, trust, autonomy and control are important from the beginning and are experienced, worked through and repeated in each developmental phase (Johnsen et al., 2004). Through tone of voice, facial expression, gestures, and so on, we communicate non-verbally. Schore (2003) presents evidence that the right hemisphere of the brain is dominant during the first three years of life. Furthermore, he argues that this is the site of the system unconscious which Freud ([1922] 2011) equated to infantile mental life. According to Schore (2003: 12), the right hemisphere is experience-dependent and open to adapting to the particular environment into which the baby is born. With its strong links to the autonomic nervous system, the right hemisphere is closely involved in survival, coping with stress and emotional regulation. While the infant is reliant upon caregivers for restoring emotional and physical equilibrium, as we mature, we become able to act to regulate our own inner states.

Case Study 3.2: Jamie

While the health visitor talks to Lesley, student nurse Beth is left alone with Jamie. Having crawled towards her, he supports himself using Beth's leg, reaches up and firmly grasps one of her fingers. Jamie looks intently into Beth's eyes before turning away. Seeing a soft toy beside her, Beth gently says, 'Shall we play?' She waits, and when Jamie returns his attention to her again she uses the toy slowly to play 'peek-a-boo'. Beth talks in a sing-song voice and smiles broadly, and the two gaze into each other's eyes when the toy is moved to one side. Both Jamie and Beth are smiling and giggling when Lesley and the health visitor return. Jamie turns, smiles at his mother and waves.

In this vignette, Beth is able to make use of an age-appropriate game to engage Jamie's attention. She is aware of the importance of play for children and unconsciously moderates her vocalizations and expressions, as well as the timing of her actions, to match Jamie's interest. Her communication is contingent. Their game brings in Piaget's notion of object permanence – Jamie has hit just the right age to be aware that the object does not disappear if it is out of sight – and he is comfortable with his mother's absence. In approaching and interacting with Beth, Jamie appears trustful and autonomous. There are signs of the attachment phase. Without being aware of it, they have all participated in a strange situation test – Ainsworth's (1978) classic design to gauge security of attachment. In this test, a child is placed in the presence of a stranger with the caregiver but is then briefly left alone with the stranger before being returned to the caregiver. There were marked differences between the behaviour of securely attached children and that of insecure children when reunited with the caregiver. The latter show a range of behaviours – distress at separation, avoidance of the caregiver on their return, or some combination of the two. Like the securely attached child, Jamie greets his mother warmly when she comes back and is not anxious to return to her immediately.

3

Summary points of infancy:

- Nurses need to be sensitive to the greater importance of non-verbal communication in pre-school children and adjust to their developmental level, attending to gestures, facial expressions and actions.
- Verbal language must be simplified and accompanied by expressions and gestures.
- Under fives tend to be more immediate in their focus of attention and may be concrete and literal in their understanding.
- Play and musicality are important aspects of behaviour and are usually incorporated into child-focused work.

4 Middle childhood – the world of stories

Around three years of age, while still remaining themselves, the average child experiences yet another leap in development. Here we consider the capacity for autobiographical narratives. As with the other major shifts, the developmental changes affect nearly all areas of experience, but now human actions are additionally understood as psychological story plots. Children now go beyond having words for things and tell stories, simple at first, both to others and to themselves in play, either individually or with other children. Where there is a disability such as hearing impairment or sight problems, sign language and touch are essentially symbolic and allow children to begin to make sense of their experiences, observations and feelings. Although the speed of language acquisition varies from child to child, between the ages of two and four there are marked improvements in grammar. Past and present tenses, singular and plural, and link words such as 'because' or 'if' are used appropriately as cause and effect becomes better understood. Piaget was fascinated by the errors children made in language and logic at this age. We may be amused at a child saying 'You bring-ed my toy', but he or she is applying a rule about the use of the past tense.

Cognitive development refers to thought and understanding. For Piaget (1952), the pre-operational child is still impressed by how things appear. One experiment has an equal amount of liquid presented to children aged three to five, but either in a short and wide container or in a tall, thin one. Typically, the response was that the taller container held more fluid. In the well-known 'three mountains' experiment (Piaget and Inhelder, 1956), Piaget finds evidence for the term 'egocentric' for this period of childhood – not a pejorative term but a descriptive one. Seated in front of a table on which rested a model of three mountains, a doll was placed at various points as if it was looking at the mountains. Children of varying ages were then asked to choose from a selection the photograph of the view that the doll is likely to see. While young children were unable to understand the task, children around the age of seven tended to choose the photograph of what *they* could see, rather than what it was the doll would see; at this stage they were egocentric – i.e., unable to take the other's perspective. However, Margaret Donaldson (1978) later showed that some of the effects were to do with the language used by Piaget as well as the situation presented to the child. When appropriate language and a scenario where a policeman was looking for a child or the child's soft toy was used, younger children could accurately identify others' perspectives.

Case Study 3.3: Sanjit

While she was shadowing a school nurse, Beth recalled a lecture on the family life cycle and forms the hypothesis that Sanjit's distress over attending school is most likely to be related to recent events. She noted that previously he had been settled and happy at school, had made friends and seemed to be a cheerful, outgoing child. Beth's two main ideas were that Sanjit had been affected by Anne's recent illnesses and/or Ram's new job keeping him away from home more. Mindful of communication with pre-operational children, she approached her ideas indirectly. Beth invited Sanjit to help her complete a drawing of the family. Sanjit reported on his own actions as he took pencils from her to draw an outline of a house with Lesley, Anne and Jamie inside. There was occasional conversation between the two, and Beth risked asking about Daddy, who was not included in the drawing. Sanjit said simply, 'Daddy is gone', and carried on drawing intently. Beth suppressed her urge to disagree and asked Sanjit to make a second drawing explaining where Sanjit was now, reassuring the child that Daddy comes home from work and will be back later. Beth is aware that children express feelings through symbolic play and won't necessarily draw people but objects to represent family members. Sanjit eventually drew Daddy on the other side of the picture but had difficulty imagining what work is. Beth studied both pictures, complimented the detail and said to Sanjit, 'Yeah, Big Man, we all miss Daddy… but not as much as he misses you.'

Focused on the recent changes in Sanjit's behaviour, this vignette illustrates the sensitive use of psychological developmental knowledge. Using the systemic approach, Beth can appreciate that redundancy led to Ram being more present, but now the long hours of his new job mean he is out of the home for over twelve hours a day. During his working week, Sanjit will not get to spend time with his father; he is 'gone' until the weekend. It is literally so. Aware of Piaget's concrete operational stage, Beth resists trying to reason with Sanjit. Guessing that he is only just beginning to understand probability, cause and effect, she stops herself from imposing her adult logic on to the situation and remains empathic, trying to attune herself to the child's experience.

Beth has the presence of mind not to attempt anything 'wild' and keeps to her strengths. Had she been able to recall the details, she would have found that the social learning perspective of Vygotsky offered another possibility to help (see Levine and Munsch, 2011: 248–9). Vygotsky added an important corrective to Piaget's thinking about development – social relationships. He was interested in social interactions, arguing that children look to others for help and learn from them. Vygotsky realized that the type of help offered, say, by an adult had to be within a certain range that is not too far above the level of ability of the child. When it is pitched at the right level, children readily behave confidently and competently. The small gap was termed the 'zone of proximal development' and is therapeutically a very useful idea. Understanding the developmental level of a child enables the nurse to plan interventions in this area. The term 'scaffolding' was added to describe the activities of the helper, referring to actions that support the child in achieving a goal. In the case of Sanjit, this may have been the use of drawing to think ahead to when Daddy would be back or to think back to when he was last there. Without a good working relationship, however, it would be unwise to attempt such an intervention because there are too many uncertainties, and a child may become more distressed. Beth showed good judgement in this regard.

Summary points of middle childhood:

- Children between the ages of five and ten have greater vocabulary and cognitive abilities but may find it difficult to respond to adult questions about internal states such as feelings and intentions.
- There is a preference for play and imaginative and symbolic activities. An understanding of these peculiarities enables the nurse to adapt their skills accordingly to deliver safe, child-focused interventions.
- Children at this stage may attend more to appearances and may be literal and concrete in their thinking.

5 Adolescence – the world of identity

The term 'adolescence' is derived from the Latin *adolescere*, meaning to grow to maturity, and is usually constructed as a transitional period between childhood and adulthood. It is difficult to make generalizations about this important period of development because the form it takes depends on many factors – social class, gender, sexuality, ethnicity and culture, to name only a few. Individuals mature at different rates and in different ways. The ecological model allows these multiple factors to be held in mind. Initiation rites are clear markers of the end of childhood in some cultures, whereas Western culture, for example, has biological and legal markers (e.g., the right to marry, vote, drink alcohol, drive). Previously held ideas that adolescence is inevitably a period of 'storm and stress' are not supported by research. Beginning with puberty, the striking physical changes of adolescence led earlier researchers to the view that physiological and emotional changes coincide. Further findings, however, revealed that bodily changes at puberty occur before emotional ones. For instance, girls may menstruate as well as develop secondary sexual characteristics from the age of nine or ten, long before the important themes of adult identity are encountered (Rutter and Rutter, 1993).

Alongside growth and hormonal changes, adolescence is characterized by brain development (Music, 2011). Rapid changes take place, with the complex reorganization of neural networks. More aggression, impulsivity and risk-taking may be features – behaviours which can impact others negatively but which also open up possibilities for development. But, besides possibility, this is a period of vulnerability for some, with stress, increased mental health worries, and the impact of substances such as alcohol and drugs. According to a 2007 UNICEF report (see www.unicef.org.uk/Latest/Publications/Child-well-being/), Britain and the USA were rated the worst places for children to live of all the economically developed countries, with children being described as unhappier and feeling less loved than in economically similar countries (Layard and Dunn, 2009).

The period of adolescence is most usually divided into phases such as early (ages 11–14), middle (14–17) and late (17 onwards), each phase being associated with different tasks and with the overall hoped-for outcome of maturity. Adolescents are expected to gain the cognitive, economic and social skills of adults in their community. As in the first period of life, themes of trust, dependency, autonomy and control are important in early and late adolescence but in more complex forms. Beyond the achievement of the ability for abstract thought (as in table 3.1, Piaget's formal operations wherein ideas can be manipulated in hypothetical arguments in accordance with logic), phase-specific tasks are to form identities and roles and to develop one's own values and relationships with peers. Social experimentation and new forms of social identity are common. But attachments remain important, and containing relationships both support development and protect against adolescent turbulence. Young people who enjoy safety, security of attachment, the meeting of basic needs for food, and opportunities for friendships, play and learning form new identities which are unique.

Beth's patient, empathic and 'mind-minded' stance helps Anne clarify issues around self-efficacy and identity. Anne's recent illnesses and episodes under hospital care had deprived her of her usual sense of self-direction, and she felt low, seeing herself as 'defective'.

Case Study 3.4: Anne

While attending the cystic fibrosis service for an outpatient appointment, Anne abruptly asked if she could speak to 'somebody'. Unless she was prepared to wait, the only available person was student nurse Beth. Surprised when Anne agreed to talk with her, Beth felt privileged but also unsure of her role and worried about 'getting it wrong'. Despite her nerves, Beth was able to reflect in action (Schon, 1990). She could see a parallel between adolescence and her own thoughts and feelings, chuckling inwardly that she 'felt like a teenager' again, not sure who she was or what to do. Remembering how she hated to be told what she was thinking and feeling by her parents, Beth began conversationally, saying 'Hi. What's going on?' Hesitantly at first, but then more confidently, Anne tells her how she 'loathed' feeling helpless and having to stay in hospital. She thinks exam stress made her ill and she again 'hated' her cystic fibrosis and wanted to be normal. Anne was worried about not being able to study and had reluctantly agreed to try 'weed', as she was told by some friends it would help her 'chillax'.

3

Consequently she had been less motivated to study, which led to her feeling worse – a vicious cycle which also resulted in withdrawal – and she had tried cannabis under pressure from peers. Yet in some ways Anne felt liberated, and she enjoyed a sense of acceptance from a group whom she sees as high in status. By speaking directly with Anne, eliciting information, modifying technical language, using good listening skills and demonstrating empathy, Beth creates a satisfactory experience. Kelsey and Abelson-Mitchell (2007) found that poor experiences included inadequate non-verbal communication, power imbalances, being excluded from conversation and judgemental attitudes.

As above, nurses have a very important, multi-faceted role to play when working with young people. Primary is foregrounding the best interests of adolescents, encouraging autonomy and self-reliance, and ensuring that the young person's voice is heard. A good knowledge of physical and psychological development at this age, along with competence to communicate effectively, is required for engagement and intervention.

Summary points of adolescence:

- Adolescence is a period of rapid and significant changes, both physically and psychosocially. A minority of individuals experience this as problematic, even turbulent, and possible difficulties can be complicated by chronic illness.
- The needs of adolescents are distinct and differ from persons in other age categories. Nurses will be aware of the stereotyped and stigmatizing images of young people and maintain a holistic and person-centred focus.
- Nurses should base their conversations with adolescents on empathy, genuineness and acceptance of the young person. Where

possible, they should use problem-free talk and appropriate humour and maintain their own self-awareness.

• Nurses aim to work as far as possible in partnership with children and young people. They work to build on family members' understandings and to develop their particular strengths and resources to help each other.

Summary

Nurses are ideally suited to provide psychologically informed care to children and young people. A systems approach commends itself to embracing the complexity of factors involved in individual development. Piaget's model of cognitive development can still be useful in orienting the nurse to age-appropriate understanding and intervention but needs critical appraisal to avoid confusing the map with the territory. Other contributions can enhance both understanding and intervention with children of differing ages and needs.

Questions for discussion

1 While you will most likely have come across the genogram tool, the ecological systems view may not be so familiar. Take a moment to map your own system and your current ideas of identity, family and culture. How might this have looked when you were a baby, a toddler or a teenager?

2 Non-verbal communication is a crucial dimension of interpersonal relating. Watch a short sequence from a film or television programme where people are talking, but without any sound. Can you identify the participants' feelings?

3 Commencing around four years of age, the narrative self is richly important to our identities. Think of one of your own narratives – of you as skilled (perhaps with an ability to drive a car), of showing courage, or of being a nurse. Can you recognize dominant parts of your stories? What of past, present and future parts? What of private, smaller stories or sub-plots?

Further reading

Levine, L., and Munsch, J. (2011) *Child Development: An Active Learning Approach.* Thousand Oaks, CA: Sage.

There are a number of excellent introductory texts on developmental psychology. This is one which covers all the main theorists and approaches as well as including the stage of adolescence. The authors adopt an active learning approach and include numerous interactive exercises for the reader to apply the topics and test their knowledge.

Kitzinger, S., and Kitzinger, C. (2000) *Talking with Children about Things that Matter*. London: Pandora Press.
Very readable accounts of literary accounts and conversations with children on subjects such as being 'good', sex, friends, death, politics and religion.

Lovegrove, M., and Bedwell, L. (2012) *Teenagers Explained: A Manual for Parents by Teenagers*. Richmond, Surrey: Crimson House.
This is a highly readable account of young people's views of being a teenager.

3

Seidenfaden, K., Draiby P., Christensen, S. S., and Hejgaard, V. (2011) *The Vibrant Family: A Handbook for Parents and Professionals*. London: Karnac Books.
Beautifully illustrated, this book makes use of the ecological systems approach to families.

Stern, D. N. (1990) *Diary of a Baby*. New York: Basic Books.
This clear and fascinating account of typical children's development is an excellent introduction to the main themes of Stern's research.

Weblinks

The website Academic Earth has complete lecture series on psychology available. Recommended are Dr Paul Bloom's series, especially the lectures on Piaget and Freud: see www.academicearth.

For a systematic review of thirty-five studies concerned with the psychological support of parents whose children have long standing or life threatening conditions, see Eccleston, C., Palermo, T. M., Fisher, E., and Law, E. (2015) *Psychological Therapy for Parents of Children with a Longstanding or Life-Threatening Physical Illness*, www.cochrane.org/CD009660/SYMPT_psychological-therapy-for-parents-of-children-with-a-longstanding-or-life-threatening-physical-illness.

Very helpful regarding cultural differences with some activities to help develop our understanding is *Transcultural Health Care Practice with Children and their Families* (2004), www.rcn.org.uk/resources/transcultural/childhealth/sectionone.php.

UCL provides a yearly *Health Survey for England*; see www.ucl.ac.uk/hssrg/studies/hse.

Nursing the Adult

Alison Torn

KEY ISSUES IN THIS CHAPTER:

- ▶ The common sense model of illness
- ▶ Attribution and causality
- ▶ Self-belief and self-esteem
- ▶ Narratives of illness
- ▶ Roles and power

BY THE END OF THIS CHAPTER YOU SHOULD BE ABLE TO:

- ▶ explore psychological theories regarding how people recognize and come to terms with serious illness
- ▶ develop an awareness of how attributing causes of an illness can affect health outcomes
- ▶ understand the importance of self-belief and self-esteem in relation to health outcomes
- ▶ understand the importance of stories as a means of coming to terms with illness
- ▶ understand the importance of roles and the ways in which power operates in healthcare settings.

1 Introduction

This chapter focuses on the experiences of being an adult patient. It is important at the start to define what adulthood means for the purposes of this chapter. Traditionally, it has been perceived as being between the ages of eighteen and sixty-five. However, the UK has an ageing population, and it is estimated that there will be a doubling of people aged sixty-five and over, from one in six currently to one in four by 2050 (Cracknell, 2010). Not only are people living longer, our perception of what is meant by older adulthood is shifting, with later retirement ages and more active 'third-age' lives after retirement (Carr and Comp, 2011). Many people over the age of sixty-five lead full, active and healthy lives, rejecting the identity of the 'older person'. With this in mind, when this chapter refers to nursing the adult, we refer to adulthood as not being constrained within age parameters.

When as adults we become patients, we may be encountering new experiences to which we may react in very different ways. We may feel vulnerable, frightened, insecure, disempowered, alone, anxious, angry, depressed. Depending on why we're in hospital, we may feel uncertain about what our future holds. Studies demonstrate that hospitalized patients experience high levels of psychological distress compared with the normal population (Johnston, 1997). Volicer and Bohannon (1975) developed the Hospital Stress Rating Scale, which identifies forty-nine potentially stressful events that result from being a patient in hospital. These include undergoing investigations and treatments, being away from family and the home environment, being in an unfamiliar environment, dependency on others, and the anticipation of communication difficulties with hospital staff. Critically, this research concluded that the behaviour of hospital staff was an influential factor in relation to high stress events. All healthcare professionals need to understand and respond to the different ways in which patients may present, but, as the people who have the most contact time with them, nurses need to understand the reasons why patients behave in certain ways in order that they can respond to them appropriately.

Case Study 4.1:

Student nurse Beth is one year into her studies and is currently on placement on a cardiac ward. Simon, a 47-year-old married father of three young children, is admitted for investigations after suffering severe chest pain and a possible myocardial infarction. This is his first admission to hospital. He works full time as a solicitor and describes himself as very sporty and regularly competes in triathlons.

Using the potential stressful events listed above as an example, outline the potential stressors Simon faces following his admission.

2 Understanding illness

When people are admitted to hospital, they may not only have to negotiate a new identity or sense of self; they may also develop their own understanding of the way that they feel (i.e., symptoms) and what those feelings may indicate. One of the key models that informs psychologists about how people understand their illness experience comes from Leventhal and his colleagues (1980, 1997; Leventhal and Cameron, 1987). Based upon the analysis of open-ended interviews with patients with different diagnoses, Leventhal et al. (1980) proposed a cognitive model of illness beliefs, which was developed further by Lau and Hartman (1983). Referred to as the common sense model of illness (CSM), this model offers a cognitive framework for understanding illness. The model suggests that individuals have a set of beliefs which are used to interpret symptoms and form a lay understanding of chronic conditions such as hypertension and asthma and acute conditions such as myocardial infarction. These beliefs guide health-related behaviours and are strongly associated with the development of effective coping mechanisms. The model encompasses five dimensions, which will be discussed in turn in this section of the chapter.

1 *Identity*: signs, symptoms and the illness label – 'What is the name of the illness I have?'
2 *Consequence*: the possible physical/psychological/social effects of the illness – 'What will happen to me?'
3 *Time line*: rate of onset (sudden or gradual); fluctuations and perceived time frame about how long the illness will last – 'What is the duration of the illness?'
4 *Causes*: perceived causes of the illness, which may be biological, psychosocial or environmental – 'Why has this happened to me?'
5 *Cure/Control*: whether the illness can be cured or controlled by self or others – 'What can be done about it?'

2.1 Identity

Within Leventhal's model, identity refers not to the person but to the identifying and naming of an illness – in other words, the process of making a diagnosis. Before this, however, the individual needs to identify perceived symptoms as deviating from personal norms in a meaningful as opposed to a minor way (Leventhal et al., 2011) – for example, severe chest pain accompanied by pain radiating into the shoulder and arm, as opposed to chest pain that feels like indigestion. Receiving a diagnosis is often the primary objective underpinning the question 'What is wrong with me?' Shontz (1975) suggested that, if it has potentially serious or long-term consequences, there are a series of stages that patients go through after receiving their diagnosis:

- *shock*: feelings of bewilderment and detachment from the situation; behaving as if on autopilot
- *encounter reaction*: disorganized thinking, feelings of loss, grief, helplessness and despair
- *retreat*: denial of the illness and its consequences; retreat into the self as a means of coping with the diagnosis.

Shontz's model is short-term, addressing the initial reactions as a means of coping with a diagnosis. Its stages reflect a mourning process, but for most people the stages are relatively temporary as denial is difficult to maintain. The final retreat stage enables the individual to come to terms with and face up to the reality of their illness.

2.2 Consequence

Following a diagnosis, a common question is 'What will happen to me?' For most patients this refers not only to the development of the illness and their physical wellbeing but also to the impact of the illness on their work, family, social activities and finance. Crisis theory has been used as a framework for examining the impact of physical illness on an individual's personal and social identity (Moos and Schaefer, 1984). More generally, crisis theory emerged from examining major life transitions such as bereavement, parenthood and divorce. Its underlying premise is that a crisis occurs when a problem outweighs the resources needed to deal with it, necessitating the development of coping strategies outside of the usual repertoire (Caplan, 1964). The theory suggests that, when in crisis, individuals are motivated to maintain some form of psychological equilibrium or stable state, and, in this respect, crises are self-limiting events. Serious physical illness or trauma is often perceived as a significant event and as such can be considered a crisis. Moos and Schaefer (1984) identified five changes that occur following serious physical illness:

1 *changes in identity* – e.g., from provider to dependent, from parent to child
2 *changes in location* – e.g., a new environment such as hospital
3 *changes in role* – this is related to changes in identity; a shift from being an active, independent adult to a passive dependent will inevitably result in changed roles
4 *changes in social support* – e.g., separation from friends/family
5 *changes in the future* – the future may become uncertain; such uncertainty may be short term or long term, depending on the nature and duration of the illness.

In relation to the concept of the self discussed at the beginning of this chapter, crises that threaten core roles or identities (e.g., parent, provider) are argued to be more psychologically disruptive than crises that threaten peripheral roles (e.g., friend, son) (Thoits, 1991).

> **Activity 4.1**
>
> Reflect on how the five changes outlined by Moos and Schaefer (1984) impact on Simon. How could you help Simon to manage his crisis?

When the crisis is acute and coping mechanisms are compromised, quality of life is impaired. Resolution of the crisis, which may include physical and psychosocial adaption to a severe or chronic illness, has been demonstrated to lead to a similar level of quality of life relative to healthy individuals (Sprangers et al., 2002). The psychological literature acknowledges that, when successfully resolved, crises can be beneficial – for example, promoting personal growth and effectiveness (Caplan, 1964). Schaefer and Moos (1992) report that over 50 per cent of people describe positive consequences as a result of experiencing a crisis. Examples are closer relationships with friends and family, new coping skills, and a shift in perspective on what is important in life.

2.3 Time line

Data from CSM studies shows that the model evolves over time as patients move from an acute or time-limited frame of reference to a chronic one (Meyer et al., 1985). From a series of studies on MI and congestive heart failure (CHF) patients, Leventhal et al. (2011) identify two time lines: rate of onset and duration. These authors suggest that rapid onset of symptoms stereotypical of MIs (severe chest pain, radiation to shoulder and arm) and rapid increase in severity of symptoms is associated with seeking healthcare more promptly. Conversely, a slower onset of symptoms (suggestive of CHF) which tend to be chronic in nature and more ambiguous in their relation to cardiac problems (e.g., swollen legs, breathing difficulties) is associated with a slower call for professional help.

The acuteness and chronicity of a condition has also been associated with compliance (Meyer et al., 1985). For example, individuals with acute asthma have been identified as being less compliant with medication than those with chronic asthma (Horne and Weinman 2002). Moreover, patients new to treatment are more likely to drop out if they believe their illness to be acute as opposed to chronic (Meyer et al., 1985). That said, belief in the chronicity of the illness has been associated with increased anxiety and depression, leading to lower physical functioning (Rozema et al., 2009). The evidence related to time line is therefore mixed. If a patient believes their illness to be acute, compliance with treatment is lower, but they may have better psychological wellbeing than those patients who believe their illness to be chronic.

2.4 Causes

Identifying a reason behind an illness is an important initial process in adjusting to it and is often reflected in a seemingly existential search for meaning – 'Why did this happen to me?' Even when illnesses are fundamentally biological in their nature (e.g., multiple sclerosis), the individual will carry out a search for meaning, not only to understand the causality of their illness but also to understand and come to terms with its implications (Taylor, 1983; Taylor et al., 1984). The search for causality is underpinned by attribution theory (Heider, 1958), which suggests that people are motivated to make sense of, predict and control their environment. We don't like to think of events such as sudden illness occurring to us randomly, and so we try and find reasons as to why they happened. Explaining events helps us not only to understand what has happened but also to predict what might happen in the future, and therefore we can take action to avoid similar occurrences.

Psychological research has examined the relationship between how people attribute the causes of their illness and health outcomes. For example, evidence suggests that patients who attribute the causes of their illness to biomedical and lifestyle factors (e.g., genetics, poor diet) are more likely to follow biomedical and lifestyle treatment plans, whereas patients who attribute illness to stress-related factors are more likely to engage with stress-reduction behaviours (e.g., meditation). Examining a cohort of hypertension patients, Hekler and his colleagues (2008) found some support that belief in biomedical and lifestyle causation was related to lower systolic blood pressure, unlike stress-related causation, where no association was found. This suggests that changes in lifestyle, such as an improved diet, can have a greater impact on health improvements compared with stress-reduction behaviours (the impact of stress on health is addressed in depth in chapter 9).

Interventions aimed at exploring patients' attributions, in particular their misconceptions of an illness, and aligning understanding with medical knowledge have been shown to improve outcomes. Petrie et al.'s (2002) research demonstrated that MI patients who received interventions based on the CSM – for example, being taught about the condition and equipped with illness management strategies – felt better prepared when returning home, returned to work sooner, and had significantly fewer MI-related symptoms one month post-hospital discharge than control patients. Taylor (1983) argues that, however people attribute, the process of searching for a cause ('Why did this happen?') becomes less of an existential question and more of a critical factor in coming to terms with or cognitively adapting to an illness. He goes on to state that understanding illness causation and its implications gives the illness meaning. This is a critical feature of CSM and a theme returned to later in this chapter when we look at the work on illness narratives.

2.5 Cure/control

Taylor identifies two further processes that relate to Leventhal et al.'s (1997) common sense model of illness – a search for mastery and the process of self-enhancement – both of which are related to cure/control. The search for mastery may be related to preventing the reoccurrence of an illness or controlling a longer-term condition. From his research on women with breast cancer, Taylor (1983) identified that control could be either internally located ('I can do something about my cancer') or externally located ('They can do something about my cancer'). This attribution of control is reflected through psychological practices (e.g., positive attitude, meditation) and behavioural practices (e.g., searching for information, changing diet, changing medications, changing therapies). Belief in the controllability of a condition such as breast cancer has been associated with improved physical and mental wellbeing (Rozema et al., 2009), although such evidence has been open to criticism (see chapter 1 and chapter 9, which questions the true outcomes of positive thinking). Belief in control is also related to compliance, with results from cardiac rehabilitation programmes suggesting that attendance is significantly associated with a strong belief that the condition can be controlled or cured (Petrie et al., 1996). Furthermore, Lau-Walker (2006) argues that increased levels of personal control can favourably influence the course of some illnesses.

Taylor's final process in adjusting to illness relates to self-enhancement, a concept central to self-esteem. Self-enhancement is the process by which we develop and promote a favourable image of ourselves through self-affirmation (e.g., boasting or fishing for compliments) (Sedikides 1993). It is a particularly strong motive when self-esteem is damaged or low, as, generally, having high self-esteem is psychologically adaptive and has been strongly related to the acceptance of physical trauma such as disability (Li and Moore, 1998). When it comes to self-esteem, we like to think well of ourselves and, as such, we tend to overestimate our good points and our control over events, as well as being unrealistically optimistic (Taylor and Brown, 1988). This is known as the positivity bias. For patients who have encountered a severe illness, having a strong positivity bias is fundamental to bolstering self-esteem and regaining a sense of control over an uncertain future. Specifically, Taylor (1983) suggests that it is the process of self-enhancement that is key to the rebuilding of self-esteem. One way in which individuals self-enhance and raise their self-esteem is by comparing themselves with other people – what is known in social psychology as social comparison theory (Festinger, 1954). Comparing ourselves with others not only validates our perceptions, attitudes, feelings and behaviours, it also boosts our self-esteem, as the tendency is to make downward social comparisons. Put simply, comparing ourselves with people whom we judge to be slightly worse off or less skilled than us makes us feel better about ourselves.

Case Study 4.2:

Both Simon and student nurse Beth may make downward social comparisons in order to feel better about their own situation, boosting their self-worth. Simon may compare himself with a patient in close proximity who has a more severe condition or perhaps less social support; Beth may compare herself with a peer from her cohort who is performing less competently than herself.

However, we not only compare ourselves with others, we also compare within the self – how we actually are and how we would like to be. Higgins (1987), in his self-discrepancy theory, suggests we have three types of self in relation to self-awareness:

4

- actual self – how we are
- ideal self – how we would like to be
- ought self – how we think we should be.

He argues that we are motivated to reduce the discrepancy between how we are (actual self) and how we would like to be or how we think we should be (ideal or ought selves).

Activity 4.2

What might be Simon's perception of his actual self following his MI and admission to hospital?

Using Higgins's three types of self, identify some of the discrepancies Simon may have between his actual and ideal self and between his actual and ought self. How might you as his nurse help to reduce these discrepancies?

Research demonstrates that failure to resolve either discrepancy can result in different emotions: if we fail to bridge the gap between our actual and ideal selves, this leads to disappointment, dissatisfaction and sadness; if we fail to resolve the discrepancy between our actual and ought selves, this leads to anxiety, agitation, threat and fear (Higgins et al., 1986). The discrepancies between actual, ideal and ought selves have been studied in relation to health. Good examples are discrepancies in relation to recovery. For life-changing illnesses, a discrepancy between an actual and an ideal self which is focused on an insistence on recovery has been identified as a maladaptive state, a form of denial which is thought to reduce motivation for physically and psychologically adapting to a changed state – in other words, accepting the actual self (Fink, 1967). Unrealistic hope towards an ideal self – for example, being able to walk again after spinal cord injury – may prevent adaption to new physical circumstances (Lohne and Severinsson, 2005; Smith and Sparkes, 2005). However, there is some evidence that suggests a low to moderate degree of insistence on recovery can lead to functional improvements and lower levels of depression and apathy in some conditions, such as following a stroke (Hama et al., 2008). Even having unrealistic hope has been identified as an important psychological function in coming to terms with changed circumstances (Smith and Sparkes, 2005). So, while the practitioner may view beliefs of full recovery oriented towards an ideal self as unfounded and even irrational, evidence suggests that having hope can be related to increased physical and psychosocial adjustment to serious or life-threatening illness and a better prognosis. Hope is therefore an important coping mechanism in relation to both recovering from illness and adapting to a new physical and psychological being.

2.6 Evaluation of the common sense model

Evidence suggests broad support for the CSM in relation to positive patient outcomes. Developing interventions that help increase patients' knowledge of what the diagnosis is, what the diagnosis means in relation to how long the illness will last, how it will be treated, and its impact on daily life has been associated with increased compliance with treatment plans and swifter resolution of the medical problem (Leventhal et al., 2011). Lau-Walker (2006) suggests that patients' beliefs about their illness and treatment have greater impact on their recovery than the severity of the illness. Addressing misconceptions about the illness representations is central to improving communication between patient and healthcare provider and improving outcomes. It is argued that exploring the patient's illness experience and the behaviours associated with it facilitates both interpersonal communication and trust, bridging the gap between patient and practitioner (Leventhal et al., 2011; Phillips et al., 2011). According to Leventhal et al., 'Acceptance of the reality of patient experience will be critical …These experiences are real, central to patient models that drive behaviour, and need to be understood' (2011: 131–2). It is this focus on the patient experience and the joint search for understanding that underpins the next section on narratives of illness.

3 Narratives of illness

Experiences of suffering are a profound part of what it means to be human. Research into the role of patients' stories in relation to their illness experiences has become increasingly popular over recent years. Examples include exploring patients' experiences of motor neurone disease (Brown and Addington-Hall, 2008), chronic pain (Williams, 2004), HIV (Ezzy, 2000), breast cancer (Murray, 2009), rheumatoid arthritis (Bury, 1982) and madness (Torn, 2011). The aim of such research is to allow the voice of the patient to be heard unimpeded by professional or academic accounts, thus helping all parties reach a deeper understanding of the lived experience of the patient.

Much of the work on illness narratives is premised on the argument that physical illness or psychological trauma often leads to a critical juncture in someone's life story – what is referred to as a 'biographical disruption' – whereby our understanding of everyday life and all it entails is disrupted (Bury, 1982). Charmaz (1991) argues that such significant events become turning points and constitute a shift not only in life biography but also in self-understanding and the sequence of events, delineating a 'before' and an 'after', a 'past' and a 'future' (Charmaz, 1991, 1999). Simon from our case study, for example, will separate his life story into 'before the heart attack' and 'after the heart attack', 'how life used to be' and 'how life will be in the future'. It is argued that, by exploring, examining and putting the crisis of illness into words – that is, in constructing a story around the illness experience – it ceases to be a meaningless, incomprehensible, random event (DeSalvo, 1999). Such stories can be verbal, captured by researchers in semi-structured interviews, or they can be written narratives. Pennebaker (1997) details how writing about significant experiences, especially those that have a strong emotional component, can reduce stressors related to mental health. In a similar vein, Smyth et al. (1999) demonstrated how writing about life stressors reduced symptoms and uptake of hospital services in both asthma patients and rheumatoid arthritis patients. Possible explanations underlying such positive impact include writing as both a cathartic and cognitive process and the narrative restructuring of experience.

Frank's (1995) theory on illness narratives is among the leading work in this area. He suggests that there are three types of illness narrative:

- *the restitution narrative* – illness is considered to be a temporary interruption. It is a story of health restored and a return to a former healthy self, encapsulated by the phrase 'good as new'.
- *the chaos narrative* – illness is considered to be a crisis, catastrophe or trauma that is almost beyond words. It is characterized by a fragmented, confusing account of an event, as the individual struggles to deal with an unexpected and difficult illness experience.
- *the quest narrative* – illness is considered to be a challenge that can be overcome. It is characterized by a search for deeper meaning, personal growth and change.

A patient such as Simon may move in and out of these typologies numerous times in the process of coming to terms with their illness, so, in this sense, such narrative typologies should not be considered progressive stages.

Activity 4.3

Reflect on a recent day in practice. Is it hard to listen to patients' stories?
Why is it hard to listen at times? If it isn't hard to listen, why might that be?

Listening and paying attention to patients' stories of their illness can be a powerful therapeutic tool, playing a significant part in facilitating a coming to terms with an illness and ultimately enabling physical and/or psychological recovery. Smith and Sparkes (2005), in their study of males who sustained spinal cord injuries, explored how concepts of hope were constructed through narratives, mapping these onto Frank's narrative typologies. Concrete hope was shaped by the restitution narrative ('Everyday I tell myself that I'll walk again'; 2005: 1097). Here patients drew on a range of narratives, both medical ('Technological advancements will enable me to walk') and cultural (biographical examples of cure). The second narrative of hope, transcendent hope, was based around Frank's quest narrative ('I don't view disability as a crisis. I'm on a different path, and I think a better, more fulfilling one'; ibid.: 1099). Such counter-narratives of disability and illness are pivotal to reconstructing identities and restoring the self and the life narrative. Smith and Sparkes's final narrative of hope is despair or loss of hope, which is shaped primarily by the chaos narrative. This reflects the despair over the trauma and difficulty envisioning a future ('My life, it's, it's, not here. It's over. I have nothing left to live. I have no hope of a life. I have nothing'; ibid.: 1101). Traumatic experiences are often difficult to put into words, and the chaos narratives that emerge from trauma are difficult to hear.

4 Roles and power

So far in this chapter, the focus has been on understanding the experience of illness. However, there is another important aspect of being ill, and that is the experience of being a patient. When we become a patient we take on a role constructed and given to us by our culture or society. Simon starts to 'act' the role or behave in the way he expects a patient to behave. His knowledge of how to act will be embedded in a variety of sources – for example, observation of friends and family who have been patients, his previous contact with medical professionals and institutions, TV drama and documentaries. Other ways in which 'the patient' is represented through language and images (what psychologists refer to as discourses) may also influence Simon's perception of being a patient – for instance, the way in which the NHS and patients are talked about by politicians and the media (Leventhal et al., 2011). This process of role-taking and 'acting the part' has received substantial academic attention, most notably by Erving Goffman. Goffman (1959) argued that the multiple roles we take on in everyday life are comparable to enacting a drama – what is known as dramaturgical theory. For example, the setting of the hospital becomes the background scene in which the roles of patient, nurse, relative, doctor, and so on, are performed. Supporting these roles are the props that individuals use (thermometer, stethoscope, bed, drip), the costume (uniform, scrubs, nightwear) and the behaviours (which may differentiate a good patient from a bad patient). When an individual is admitted to hospital, their everyday props and costumes are removed (in Simon's case, this might be his briefcase and business suit). Consequently, the individual is rapidly shifted from one role (solicitor, breadwinner) to another (patient, dependant). Perhaps for the first time since childhood, an adult is dependent on others, not only for their knowledge and expertise but also for their basic requirements, such as self-care and financial support.

Loss of role and identity through, for example, the removal of personal effects can contribute to a process of depersonalization, or what Goffman (1961) referred to as 'non-person treatment'. The individual is perceived as a 'patient with a disease' or even 'a case'. Rather than being treated as a person, the patient becomes a problem to be fixed or an educational tool (e.g., in ward rounds). Being treated as an object of medicine leads patients to feel vulnerable and insecure, contributing to the 'sick role' they adopt.

4.1 The sick role

A seminal theory around the experience of being a patient was put forward by the sociologist Talcott Parsons in 1951 and has been central to the development of thinking in both health psychology and social psychology. Parsons argues that, when they become ill, people adopt a 'sick role'. His theory suggests that, when ill, an individual is unable to perform their usual social roles, so relief is given until they are restored to health and able to return to their everyday roles. Within this theory, the role of practitioners is to aid recovery, thereby acting as a form of resocialization, thus maintaining social order. From this perspective, medicine and all it encompasses are viewed as an integral part of the functioning of society. The sick role has four key features. Sick people:

- are exempt from their social duties (e.g., as employee, parent)
- are not responsible for their illness
- must want to get well, as illness is undesirable
- must seek professional help and co-operate with treatment to enable their recovery (Parsons, 1951: 436–7).

According to the theory, sickness is perceived by society as an undesirable state involving deviant behaviour. If sickness goes on too long, the privileges and benefits of the sick role (what are known as secondary gains), together with societal costs (e.g., prolonged extra workload for colleagues), are judged to be too high. Therefore exemption from social duties is conditional upon the individual making concerted efforts to get better.

Implicit in Parsons's theory is that the sick person gives up their usual roles and rights, accepting constraints on their activities and behaviours (e.g., staying in bed, complying with requests from medical staff). This dependence leads to feelings of powerlessness and helplessness, as the individual takes on not only the role of the patient but also the behaviours society ascribes to being a patient.

4.2 Power and resistance

Medical roles are based upon expertise, and within this expertise lies authority. Nursing works within the realms of medicine, and this same authority underpins the power relationships between practitioner and patient. At this point, it is important to distinguish between authority and power. While medicine may have authority in terms of knowledge and expertise, power resides in the relationship between practitioner and patient. For example, a nurse may exercise her power in encouraging adherence to prescribed physical exercises, but equally the patient may exercise their power through resistance. In relation to adherence to medical and nursing regimes, patients may comply not because they are forced or even persuaded to do so, but because there is a valid reason to comply, a reason accepted on the practitioners' authority (Latham, 2002).

As Parsons (1951) suggests, when patients are admitted to hospital, certain rights and freedoms are relinquished, compromising the individual's agency and autonomy. Reactance theory (Brehm, 1966; Wortman and Brehm, 1975) suggests that withdrawal of freedom will result in one of two behaviours: either there is an attempt to regain control and prevent further loss of freedom (resistance) or there is an acceptance of loss of freedom resulting in helplessness (compliance). This is reflected in two polarized constructions of patient behaviour: good patient behaviour (adherence to the medical regime and prescribed treatment, facilitating practitioners' work) and bad patient behaviour (resistance, demanding, complaining, obstructing practitioners' work) (Lorber, 1975; Taylor, 1979). The polarization of good patient/bad patient is mediated by the severity of the illness. The more serious the illness, the more tolerant staff are to demands and complaints (Lorber, 1975). That said, seriously ill patients who are co-operative, undemanding and uncomplaining are judged by practitioners to be the 'ideal' patient (ibid.). In her classic paper, Taylor (1979) suggests that the polarization of good patients and bad patients poses health risks to individuals, with the former having an underlying anxiety or depressed helplessness and the latter displaying anger towards their lack of freedom. She suggests that informed and participatory roles can ameliorate these implicit health risks, improving physical and psychological wellbeing (see chapter 2 for further discussion on compliance and adherence).

The authority previously automatically afforded to healthcare professionals is not as it once was. The ways in which medicine and nursing are portrayed in the media (fictional and factual), together with the ever expanding availability of medical knowledge on the internet, means that patients are not only more circumspect about medical knowledge, but they also have increased levels of knowledge about their illness and potential treatments. This expansion of the presence of medicine in media and technology has contributed to the construct of the patient as the consumer, an individual with rights who can legitimately challenge the perceived authority of others. High-profile individual cases involving murder or abuse (e.g., Beverley Allitt, the paediatric nurse convicted of murdering infants through insulin overdose), together with institutional cases such as the neglect endemic in the Mid Staffordshire NHS Trust and the case of Alder Hey Hospital, where human tissues and organs from children were retained after post-mortems without parental permission, have further eroded public confidence in the healthcare profession, prompting the questioning of the power, rights and responsibilities of both practitioner and patient. However, the evidence is mixed in relation to patients taking on a more proactive, consumerist role vis-à-vis their health. Studies suggest that age and education predict non-adherence, with younger, more educated people questioning medical authority more than older, less educated people (Lorber, 1975; Lupton, 1997). However, even those who fully adhere to medical authority still want an active role in their treatment. Over the past twenty years, patient-focused services and the notion of the expert patient, particularly in relation to chronic illness, have gone some way in shifting the power from practitioner to patient (Bury, 2004). This represents a welcome shift for all parties from consumerism to partnership.

Summary

▶ The common sense model of illness is one framework which psychologists use to understand the patient's experience of coming to terms with an illness.
▶ The ways in which patients attribute the causality of their illness can impact on health outcomes.
▶ Having a strong sense of self-belief and high self-esteem can improve health outcomes.
▶ Narratives and storytelling are used both to help patients come to terms with their illness and for the practitioner to gain a deeper understanding of the meaning of the illness for the patient.
▶ The roles people occupy and the power that operates in healthcare settings critically impact on the patient experience, with the emphasis in more recent times on practitioner–patient partnerships.

Questions for discussion

1 Considering each of the five elements of the common sense model of illness, identify ways in which nurses can help patients come to terms with a serious and/or chronic illness.
2 What can nurses do to help patients' stories be realistically integrated into their care?
3 In what ways has the shift from 'patient as recipient of healthcare' to 'patient as consumer of healthcare' impacted on the nurse–patient relationship?

Further reading

Marks, D. F., Murray, M. P., Evans, B., and Estacio, E. V. (2011) *Health Psychology: Theory, Research and Practice*. 3rd edn, London: Sage.
This book introduces models of health psychology and is useful in the critical stance it takes.

Ogden, J. (2012) *Health Psychology: A Textbook*. 5th edn, Maidenhead: Open University Press.
Ogden's classic text provides a broad understanding of health psychology, applying theories to different health-related behaviours.

Radley, A. (1998) *Making Sense of Illness: The Social Psychology of Health and Disease*. London: Sage.
This text gives an overview of the social psychology of health and illness, looking at how people make sense of illness in everyday life.

Nursing Those with Learning Disabilities

Raghu Raghavan

KEY ISSUES IN THIS CHAPTER:

▶ Nursing people with learning disabilities
▶ Learning disability nursing and psychological interventions
▶ The evidence base for clinical practice

BY THE END OF THIS CHAPTER YOU SHOULD HAVE AN UNDERSTANDING OF:

▶ learning disability and comorbidity issues
▶ behavioural interventions
▶ cognitive interventions
▶ the application of psychotherapeutic approaches.

1 Introduction

The past three decades have seen a major shift in the model of learning disabilities (LD) from a medical model to that of social model, concerned with ordinary citizens with rights of equal access to and use of ordinary community services. The closure of long-stay hospitals in the UK has led to the expansion of wide-ranging patterns of services in the voluntary and independent sectors. Services for people with LD in the NHS tend to be specialized, to do with health facilitation, assessment and intervention for behaviour, and mental health. This chapter will explore applied psychology covering behavioural, cognitive and psychodynamic approaches to address anxiety, depression and management of behaviour disorders in people with LD.

1.1 What is learning disability?

In the United Kingdom the definition of learning disability includes the presence of:

- a significantly reduced ability to understand new or complex information or to learn new skills (impaired intelligence), along with
- a reduced ability to cope independently (impaired functioning) and/or
- cognitive impairment before adulthood, with a lasting effect on development (DoH, 2001b).

The term 'learning disability' should not be confused with the term 'learning difficulties', as the latter is concerned more with problems of learning in educational settings. However, many people with LD would classify themselves as having learning difficulties and wish to be described in this way. Recently, the term 'intellectual disability' has become widely used internationally. The American Association on Intellectual and Developmental Disabilities suggests that intellectual disability is characterized by significant limitations in both intellectual functioning and adaptive behaviour, which covers many everyday social and practical skills. This disability originates before the age of eighteen.

The International Classification of Diseases and Disorders (ICD-10) published by the World Health Organization is the system of classification commonly used in the UK, although some countries use the *Diagnostic and Statistical Manual*, DSM-5 (American Psychiatric Association, 2013) being the most recent version. The ICD-10 defines 'mental retardation' (or learning disability) as 'a condition of arrested or incomplete development of the mind ... characterised by impairment of skills manifested during the developmental period, which contribute to the overall level of intelligence, i.e. cognitive, language, motor and social abilities' (WHO, 1992).

1.2 Prevalence

According to recent estimates, in the UK the prevalence of learning disability is about 2 per cent of the general population (DoH, 2001b; Emerson et al., 2010). A report from MENCAP suggests that around 200 babies are born with LD every week. Recent reports also suggest a much higher prevalence rate projection for adults with LD in England, to around 14 per cent by 2021 (Emerson et al., 2010), as a result of:

- increased life expectancy, especially among people with Down's syndrome
- a growing number of children and young people with complex and multiple disabilities who now survive to adulthood
- a sharp increase in the reported numbers of school-age children with autistic spectrum disorders, some of whom have LD
- a higher prevalence among the minority ethnic population of South Asian origin.

People with LD have a number of comorbid conditions, such as autism, challenging behaviour and mental illness. There is a highly significant association between LD and autism, with epidemiological studies reporting prevalence of between 14 and 40 per cent (Gobrial and Raghavan, 2012). Such persons also have severe or challenging behaviours which pose serious problems for health and social care services. Challenging behaviour is defined as culturally abnormal behaviour of such intensity, frequency and duration that the physical safety of the individual or others is likely to be placed in serious jeopardy, or behaviour that is likely seriously to limit or deny access to and use of ordinary community facilities (Emerson, 1998). People with LD, like any other people, experience mental health disorders. The nature of manifestation of mental health disorders in this population is complex and confusing and poses severe challenges for professionals in terms of detection, diagnosis and appropriate interventions.

1.3 What is learning disability nursing?

Learning disability nursing has a long history going back to the history of LD itself and the institutional models of care that prevailed during the last two centuries. Nursing roles span community support specialists, liaison between services and agencies, and positions in secure or forensic health settings, all of which offer support across the age continuum (Manthorpe et al., 2004). Thus learning disability nurses work in partnership with users, carers and services for health assessment, health improvement and health promotion.

Teaching people to improve their lifestyle is an essential part of therapeutic nursing. This is an area that is not congruent with the traditional forms of nursing, which lay heavy emphasis on the model of caring for the sick person. However, in learning disability nursing the development of personal competence through teaching and empowerment is seen as an integral part of practice. Helping people to acquire skills of self-care, personal control, and management of feelings and emotions such as anger and anxiety are pillars of therapeutic nursing activities with people with LD.

The facilitation of therapeutic care depends on having knowledgeable and skilled practitioners. The therapeutic care for people with LD is delivered in a range of settings, such as in the person's own home, in mainstream mental health services, in group homes, and in specialist units designed to facilitate and monitor assessment and treatment. The following sections explore a number of psychological approaches for nursing people with LD.

Case Study 5.1:

Pat is thirty-four and lives in a group home, which she shares with two other clients. She has moderate learning disabilities, Prader Willi syndrome, and challenging behaviour consisting of both verbal and physical aggression, to the extent that her placement is at risk. She has been progressively deteriorating in this regard over the past six months, and her carers have found it increasingly difficult to cope with her difficult behaviour. Student nurse Beth has noticed that Pat has become much more irritable, with frequent temper outbursts consisting mainly of verbal abuse. She seems to be excessively tired all day and when angry is very difficult to reason with or support. She has had recent medical problems with a fistula between her large bowel and bladder, which has resulted in pain and repeated infections.

Activity 5.1

What are the complexities of learning disability and associated syndromes?

What are the possible psychological intervention approaches that Beth could consider to help Pat?

---

2 Behavioural approaches

Behaviour therapy is based on the behavioural school of thought in psychology through the works of Pavlov, Watson, Skinner and others (see chapter 1). It has dominated the treatment realm for people with LD because of its objective principles and methods and through its commanding role in teaching and maintaining adaptive behavioural skills. The key principle is the assumption that behaviour is affected primarily by conditions existing in the person's environment rather than by the psychic/mind dynamics. It is believed that behaviour is a spontaneous response in relation to environmental stimuli, and a person learns to use these responses through reinforcement, which increases the probability of the response to occur repeatedly.

The intervention strategies using behaviour therapy principles consist of key stages:

- objective/operational definition of the target behaviour (to be increased or decreased)
- assessment of the target behaviour using the Antecedent, Behaviour, Consequence framework (A–B–C) in identifying its pattern, frequency and duration
- functional analysis, which helps to formulate hypotheses of the causative factors of the target behaviour and to approach this systematically through the use of a range of skills teaching and/or techniques of reinforcement schedules
- intervention plans and strategies, which are constantly evaluated against baseline measures of the target behaviour.

Over the years behaviour therapy has undergone modifications, and current principles tend to address the issues of intervention from a biopsychosocial perspective, emphasizing the rationale for the objective of behaviour as well as identifying the causative or trigger factors for inappropriate behaviours or emotional problems. Behaviour therapy focuses on teaching adaptive skills and social behaviours, thus promoting physical, psychological and social wellbeing.

2.1 Systematic desensitization

Developed by Joseph Wolpe (1958), systematic desensitization (SD) is a useful therapy for treating fear and anxiety in people with learning disabilities. This is a behavioural treatment procedure where a person is gradually exposed (through imagination or in real life) to a hierarchy of anxiety-provoking stimuli. This is done in the context of maintaining a state of calm through deep muscle relaxation or by other relaxation procedures. The advantage of SD is that it can be used for people with LD who may not have the ability to use the skills of imagination. Here, people can be exposed to anxiety-provoking stimuli in vivo (in real-life contexts). Pleasurable activities, such as eating or drinking or being with a favourite person, can be used instead of the relaxation procedure, which may enable the person to remain in a state of calm while being exposed to the anxiety-provoking stimuli. Individuals can also carry out SD by themselves – known as systematic self-desensitization. This form of SD can be used to treat problematic fears, such as fear of flying.

Lindsay and his colleagues (1988) describe the development of a group anxiety management treatment incorporating training and exposure treatments for dog phobia with people with LD. The treatment procedures have several components, including increased contact with dogs; changing dogs as treatment progresses; graded exposure to dogs, eliciting anxiety from an early stage in the programme; modelling reasonable reactions to dogs; encouraging individuals to have control over dogs; and promoting generalization of coping behaviours. The procedures are illustrated by the cases of two women who were assessed on overall ratings of fear, the number of positive approaches to a dog, the number of negative reactions to a dog, and self-assessments of anxiety. Both women responded to treatment. The study suggests that the exposure treatments may be a successful means of helping people with LD overcome their phobic anxiety.

The principles of SD can be applied in health promotion and behaviour change programmes in a number of settings.

2.2 Relaxation training

Relaxation training is used for anxiety management, and its methods range from progressive muscle relaxation, where several muscle groups are individually tensed and relaxed, to imagery-based procedures, yoga and meditation. Benson and Havercamp (1999) suggest that relaxation training can be a primary intervention technique for managing generalized anxiety or part of a treatment package. Relaxation techniques such as progressive relaxation, developed by Jacobson ([1929] 1938), and abbreviated progressive relaxation (relaxing several muscles groups at the same time) (Bernstein and Borkovec, 1973) have been used with people with LD.

Lindsay et al. (1989) explored anxiety treatments for adults who have moderate and severe LD by undertaking a study based on the simplification of a technique called progressive relaxation. The authors identified the problems of previous studies in which anxiety is measured indirectly – for example, through a decrease in hyperactivity – and attempted to overcome this by using direct measures of anxiety and relaxation before treatment, during treatment and after treatment had finished. Fifty people with moderate and severe LD (IQ 30–55) were randomly allocated to five groups: individual behavioural relaxation training, individual abbreviated progressive relaxation training, group behavioural relaxation training, group abbreviated progressive relaxation, and a control group. Anxiety measures were taken in accordance with the behavioural anxiety scale. Treatment lasted for twelve sessions for all interventions; for subjects seen individually each session lasted between 30 and 45 minutes, and for those seen in groups between 60 and 95 minutes. The study demonstrated that, in the short term, group behavioural relaxation training is better than individual sessions in the management of anxiety. It would be of further interest to explore whether this intervention proves useful for managing anxiety in the longer term and whether regular sessions would be required to sustain the improvement.

2.3 Modelling

Modelling or observational learning is based on social learning theory and involves an individual observing a peer who is performing the behaviour appropriately. Modelling is widely used in our daily interactions and behaviours, and parents use it to teach language and skills to their children. This is a useful technique for teaching people with LD to manage problems such as stress, anxiety and fear. Modelling can be used with people with LD in one-to-one individual interaction or in a group context. What is essential is for the person to observe a peer showing acceptable/culturally appropriate behaviours in dealing with situations or as a response to stress/anxiety. A systematic procedure should be followed in the use of modelling – i.e., the setting, individual or group sessions, types of acceptable behaviours to be observed, and the necessary instructions and guidance to be provided should be predetermined. Modelling can also be introduced through films and video clips, which is known as symbolic modelling (Bandura, 1986).

3 Cognitive approaches

Cognitive behavioural therapy originates from the works of Albert Ellis (1962), who formulated the Rational Emotive Therapy (RET), and Aaron Beck (1967a), who studied the cognitive factors associated with depression (see also chapter 12). According to Dobson and Dozois (2001), all cognitive behavioural therapies share three fundamental beliefs.

1   *Cognitive activity affects behaviour.* This is based on the belief that cognitive appraisals of events can affect the response to those events and that there is clinical value in modifying the content of such appraisals.
2   *Cognitive activity may be monitored and altered.* It is assumed that the therapist is able to have access to and is fully able to map cognitive activities, which can be altered.
3   *Desired behaviour change may be affected through cognitive change.* It is assumed that the behaviour change may be the result of overt reinforcement contingencies that can alter the behaviour and also the mediational influences on cognitive restructuring and behaviour change.

3.1 Cognitive behavioural therapy

The term 'cognitive behavioural therapy' (CBT) is used to describe a range of therapeutic models that share the same aims and characteristics. The key underlying assumptions of such approaches focus on:

- thoughts, images, perceptions and other cognitive mediating events that affect overt behaviour as well as emotions

- mediating conditions in a systematic, structured manner to facilitate the change in behaviour and emotions
- people as active learners, not just passive recipients of environmental influence; to some extent they create their own learning environment, and sometimes their specific learning histories result in cognitive dysfunction
- treatment goals centred around creating new adaptive learning opportunities to overcome cognitive dysfunctions and to produce positive changes for the person, which can be generalized and maintained outside the clinical setting
- the person as having an understanding of the intervention strategies and goals and participating in planning and defining these. (Stenfert Kroese, 1997)

Dagnan (2012) states that cognitive therapy poses major emotional, cognitive and intellectual challenges for people with LD. Hence it is important to have an assessment to identify the person's

- receptive and expressive language abilities to determine the complexity of language that will be safe to use
- ability to recognize emotions in themselves and others
- ability to understand how the events in their external world affect their internal emotions
- ability to understand the idea of 'cognition' and whether they are aware of what they 'say to themselves' in different situations.

Literature concerning the use of CBT for people with LD is scarce at present. Lindsay et al. (1997) highlight the key issues for the lack of adequate research in its application: (1) the notion that people with LD are devalued and of little interest to the research community; (2) the assumption that they do not have as stable or potent cognitions as those without learning disabilities, and as a result it will be difficult to conclude that any changes would be as a result of clinical manipulations; (3) the notion that the manifestation of mental illness in people with LD is the same as in those without LD may have obstructed the need for any focused research in this population. In addition, the inability to self-report may have led to the lack of adequate research using CBT models.

The evidence base regarding the application of CBT for treating anxiety-related illnesses in people with LD is limited. Lindsay and his colleagues (1997) propose an adapted model.

- *Setting an agenda*: Discussion with the client about the possible steps of the treatment in simple language and possibly with visual cues. Lindsay et al. suggest that this may allow clients to understand the various concepts involved and to organize the difficult materials in a systematic and simple way.
- *Isolating negative thoughts*: This can be a difficult phase for clients. Some people may be able to report negative thoughts through

therapeutic interviews. Role-play sessions can also help the client to expose the anxiety-provoking thoughts and feelings. Lindsay et al. suggest an interesting method of role reversal of the client and therapist. In this context, the client as therapist can ask what 'the client' is thinking, and the 'therapist' can then ask leading questions of 'the client'. The authors state that this method may be useful in revealing a clear picture of the nature of thoughts that may be important for the client.

- *Eliciting underlying symptoms*: This is done by identifying the themes across automatic thoughts, such as identifying the symptoms of sleeplessness, fear, panic attacks and other behavioural symptoms.
- *Testing the accuracy of cognitions*: Lindsay et al. suggest the use of simple and direct methods of checking out the accuracy of the cognitions. This may be done verbally, by reflecting the thoughts back to the client in a simple form, using humour and stories to check out its accuracy.
- *Generating alternative cognitions*: Lindsay et al. suggest that this is done by using the converse of negative thoughts. For example, if the client says, 'People are laughing at me when I'm standing at bus stop', the converse of the thought to be used here will be: 'No one is looking at me. No one is bothered about me.'
- *Monitoring thoughts and feelings*: This involves the use of simple tools such as cartoon representations of the emotion (happy, embarrassed, sad) to monitor thoughts and feelings.
- *Role-play*: Anxiety-provoking situations can be re-enacted using role-play to help the client to understand the relationship between their thoughts and anxiety-related feelings and behaviours.
- *Homework*: Lindsay et al. suggest setting homework (keeping records of thoughts, emotions and behaviours). They argue that this will help to monitor the extent of maladaptive thinking that has occurred during the week and to provide situations in which more adaptive responses can be practised.

Several reports have appeared on the assessment of depression in this client group, and there is a pressing need for more research into treatment of depression in people with LD. Two case studies by Lindsay and his colleagues (1993) of individuals with mild intellectual disability illustrate the clinical applications. All the elements of cognitive behavioural therapy for depression were maintained and simplified. Both participants were able to monitor their feelings of depression, and the frequency of suicidal thoughts was recorded. Individuals saw improvements in both cases on the Zung depression inventory and on the daily monitoring of depressive feelings. This is an encouraging approach to the treatment of depression and demands further exploration through larger-scale controlled studies.

In recent years cognitive behavioural techniques have been applied to psychotic symptoms with some reports of positive results. There is little in the literature to suggest that such techniques have been used to help people with LD who experience psychosis. Legget et al. (1997), however, attempt to explore whether teaching psychological strategies for managing auditory hallucinations in people with learning disabilities is effective. A case report describes the use of a cognitive behavioural strategy with a woman with mild learning disabilities. A number of benefits of the intervention are noted, including decreases in subjective distress and use of 'PRN' mediation (i.e., taken 'as required' or 'when needed' – from the Latin *pro re nata*), as well as improved mood and reported increases in the use of positive coping strategies and self-esteem.

Case Study 5.2:

Debi is twenty-three years of age with Down's syndrome who exhibits ritualistic behaviour and obsessions around personal cleanliness following use of the toilet. She lives at home and attends a day centre five days a week. However, she is missing the majority of sessions in the day centre because she may be in the toilet for up to three hours. This behaviour also results in her missing or delaying transport home.

Activity 5.2

How will you assess Debi's behaviour and needs?

What type interventions can you suggest and what is the rationale for these interventions?

3.2 Anger management

The manifestation of mental health disorder in people with LD may take the form of physical aggression towards others, destruction of property and verbal aggression. The aim of anger management training is to develop coping skills so that the individual is able to appraise the anger-provoking situations, process this information, and respond with socially appropriate and adaptive behaviour (Novaco, 1975). The key components of anger management training are (1) cognitive restructuring, (2) arousal reduction, and (3) behavioural skills training (Black et al., 1997).

Psychologists and some behaviour specialist nurses organize anger management groups or individual sessions for people with dual diagnosis and severe aggressive behaviour. Moore et al. (1997) describe the process of conducting a nine-week course on anger management with a group of people with LD. The nine sessions had a set pattern as indicated in table 5.1.

Anger management groups allow a person to:

- gain positive experiences from participation in a group
- develop an understanding of what anger is and how it affects us all

Table 5.1 Anger management course content
Session 1, Introductions: Familiarization with group, learning names, setting group rules – e.g., confidentiality.
Session 2, Starting to talk about feelings: Looking together in small groups at pictures of people displaying different emotions. Groups begin to identify emotions and to talk about the experience of these emotions.
Session 3, More about feelings: The 'I feel …' game: someone reads a statement about an event and each person in the small group talks about how the situation described might have made them feel; in the large group, individuals start to make connections between feelings and actions.
Session 4, Think about anger: What makes people angry? Demonstrate role-plays with the facilitators. Learn about the signs of anger in other people. Take individual photographs of each other smiling and looking angry.
Session 5, What we do with angry feelings: Brainstorm the functions of anger and how it is expressed. What can we do if other people are getting angry? Role-plays by facilitators with audience participation; group members join in with suggestions of what might make the situation better.
Session 6, Recognizing own anger and anger in others: Practise using the most popular techniques from session 5 role-plays between group members. Find out what works best for each person.
Session 7, Practising anger management: Make a video of how we deal with anger; everyone else has a chance to manage a situation where someone else is angry and to demonstrate a way of expressing their feelings.
Session 8, Practising anger management: More practice.
Session 9, Review of achievements: Share what has been learnt, talk about how people felt about the course.

Source: Adapted from Moore et al. (1997).

- learn tricks to help deal with feeling angry
- feel like an 'expert' instead of feeling out of control.

It is important that named nurses or key workers attend the anger management group along with the person with LD. This will allow them to:

- learn from participation in the group experience
- develop an understanding of what makes clients angry from the client's perspective
- learn what does and doesn't help.

The evidence base for anger management and its effectiveness in people with LD is growing. A component analysis (Benson, 1986) of a cognitive behavioural anger management programme was conducted with adults with LD attending vocational training. Self-control training was given in one of four groups: relaxation, self-instruction, problem-solving, or a combined anger management condition. The dependent measures included self-reports, ratings of videotaped role-plays, and supervisor ratings. The results revealed decreases in aggression responding over time and no significance between group differences. The study suggested that anger management training with 'mentally retarded' adults may be effective.

Rose et al. (2000) describe an evaluation of a group intervention for reducing inappropriately expressed anger (as aggression) in people with LD. Group intervention was compared to a non-treatment group consisting of people referred to the group but who had to wait to participate. A reduction in expressed anger and measured levels of depression occurred after treatment. Reductions in expressed anger were maintained at six and twelve months' follow-up. However, scores on the depression scale tended to increase on follow-up. While caution must be expressed when considering these results, group therapy shows promise for reducing inappropriately expressed anger in people with LD.

Lindsay et al. (1998) undertook a study of three individuals with LD who exhibited aggressive behaviour. The exploration of attitudes to anger and aggression included direct observation, self-recording of frequency of aggressive incidents, self-recording of feelings of aggression, provocation role-plays and provocation inventories. Treatment involved two forms of relaxation (brief relaxation therapy, known as BRT, and abbreviated progressive relaxation, known as APR), discussions and exercises on the understanding of emotion, and role-plays. The study, which was positively evaluated, suggests the need for tailor-made interventions based on comprehensive needs assessment.

A randomized controlled trial by Willner et al. (2002) examined the efficacy of a cognitive behavioural group for fourteen people with LD referred for anger management. Participants were randomly assigned to a treatment and a waiting list group. Treatment consisted of nine two-hour group sessions, using brainstorming role-play and homework. Among the topics addressed were the triggers that evoke anger, physiological and behavioural components of anger, cognitive and behavioural strategies to avoid the build-up of anger, coping with anger-provoking situations, and acceptable ways of displaying anger. The intervention was evaluated using two inventories of anger-provoking situations and was completed independently by both clients and carers. The treatment group improved on both client and carer ratings relative to their own pre-treatment scores and to the control group. The degree of improvement within treatment was strongly correlated with verbal IQ. The treatment group showed further improvement relative to their own pre-treatment scores at three-month follow-up.

In conclusion, this section shows that CBT approaches can be useful in working with people with LD and calls for more work by nurses using adapted models of CBT with such clients.

4 Psychodynamic approaches

Psychodynamic approaches focus on psychoanalysis, and psychotherapy is based on psychoanalytic approaches as proposed by Sigmund Freud (see chapter 1). Psychotherapy has been in use for well over a hundred years, but it still remains a complex procedure based on the skill of the therapist. Strupp (1978) describes it as an interpersonal process designed to bring about modifications of feelings, cognitions, attitudes and behaviour which have proven troublesome to the person now seeking help from a trained professional.

As psychodynamic approaches focus on the expression of thoughts and feelings using verbal language, its application to people with LD is a professionally challenging option. The works of Waitman and Conboy-Hill (1992), Sinason (1992), Hollins (2001) and de Groef and Heinemann (1999) provide us the insight into the application of psychotherapy for people with LD.

Rather than concentrating primarily on changing symptoms, psychodynamic approaches focus on bringing about more radical changes in the personality or resolution of unconscious conflicts. The relationship between the patient and the therapist is an important part of therapy, and this is seen as a vehicle for change in the patient. In the psychodynamic approach, depression stems from the relationship with parents or from early childhood experiences. It is suggested that an 'injury' may be caused by the relationship with the mother due to separation, loss, abandonment, or lack of emotional responses. The child may learn to internalize and be dependent on the mother figure and, as he or she grows up, becomes overly dependent on significant other people such as paid carers. Guthrie and her colleagues (1998) suggest that the real or unresolved conflict over dependency and hatred, and the aggressive impulses, are directed at the self and experienced as depression.

Hollins (2003) comments that a common assumption is that the intellectual impairment of the client will prevent them from 'meaningful, emotional engagement'. She further states that part of the assessment interview for dynamic psychotherapy should include an honest appraisal by the therapist of his or her own feelings and reactions to the client with learning disabilities. The difficulty of establishing a therapeutic dialogue in the presence of communication problems has been seen as a barrier to people with LD having access to, or making effective use of, psychotherapy. However, art therapists and those in related disciplines have a long history of working through means of expression other than speech (RCP, 2004).

People in distress generally have the option of using their own personal resources to cope or of turning to others for support, advice and other forms of help – traditionally family, friends, community members, doctors or priests. A person with LD may have limited personal resources to cope with ordinary life stresses and may not have the ability to ask others for help because of limited communication or lack of adequate support. Traditional treatments for psychological problems in people with LD have tended towards behavioural management, skills training and medication. Over the past fifteen years, there has been a small but growing interest in extending the application of psychotherapeutic interventions to cover people with learning disabilities. Psychotherapy has been demonstrated to be an effective form of treatment for people with psychological problems. However, there is considerable resistance to attempts to generalize these findings to those with LD.

Case studies published in the last two decades have provided evidence for the benefit of various psychotherapeutic approaches with people with LD. However, there are only a few outcome studies.

Frankish (1992) reports the findings of psychodynamic therapy with a six-year-old child with LD with behaviour problems in a one-to-one therapeutic setting. Beail and Warden (1996) present some preliminary outcome data on nine men and one woman (eighteen to forty-nine age range). The reasons for referral were aggressive behaviour (four people), sexually inappropriate behaviour (three people) and psychotic/bizarre behaviour (three people). This study used specific outcome measures and reported significant reductions in psychological symptoms as well as an increase in self-esteem.

Beail (1998) reports an outcome study of individual psychoanalytical therapy provided in normal clinical practice for twenty-five men with intellectual disabilities who were referred for behaviour problems. Twenty of the participants completed treatment. In almost all cases the problem behaviour was eliminated, and this was maintained at six months' follow-up.

A meta-analysis of studies relating to psychotherapy with people with LD conducted by Prout and Nowak-Drabik (2003) reported a wide range of designs, types of interventions and participants involved. The overall analysis indicates that psychotherapy with people with LD produced a moderate amount of change and is moderately effective or beneficial.

Due to the emphasis of using spoken language as a medium of interaction in psychotherapy, its application with people with learning disabilities was ignored for a number of years. A report from the Royal College of Psychiatrists on psychotherapy and LD (RCP, 2004) suggests the need for psychotherapy to focus not only on mental health and emotional difficulties but also on issues of impairment, disability and handicap. This report suggests that current provision of psychotherapy for clients with LD in the UK ranges from highly specialized services, providing individual and group psychoanalytic therapy, through to individuals or groups of clinicians who facilitate psychotherapeutic understanding in the day-to-day work of carers, professionals and support staff. The report further states that 'some of the more specialist expertise needed for effective psychotherapy for people with learning disabilities will be in establishing a productive treatment alliance through the development of an effective "language" and therapeutic context.' The process of assessment may be more prolonged and will involve more people than generic services. Specific issues may require more attention, such as consent or the practicalities of therapy. Adaptation and flexibility of therapeutic approach is essential; this may often stretch or conflict with some of the common and traditional tenets of psychotherapy. The importance of working with the whole system around an individual is highlighted. The application of psychotherapy for people with LD requires modifications, and the evidence base needs to emerge with practice examples and research studies looking at the process and outcomes of therapy.

Summary

▶ The application of psychological approaches in teaching new skills and behaviour and interventions for promoting emotional wellbeing form the bulk of the therapeutic practice of learning disability nurses.

▶ The evidence base of the various psychosocial interventions is limited and there is a need for more evaluation of the various approaches.

▶ There is an urgent need for the development of practice-based evidence models that may help to highlight the factors contributing to the long-term sustainability of these interventions.

▶ Nurses are in a good position to develop behavioural, cognitive and psychotherapeutic interventions for people with LD.

5

Question for discussion

1 Consider the different strategies that can be used by adult nurses when an individual with learning disabilities is admitted to an acute hospital.

Further reading

Emerson, E., and Enfield, S. (2011) *Challenging Behaviour*. 3rd edn, Cambridge: Cambridge University Press.

Lloyd, J., and Clayton, P. (2014) *Cognitive Analytic Therapy for People with Intellectual Disabilities and their Carers*. London: Jessica Kingsley.

Raghavan, R. (2012) *Anxiety and Depression in People with Intellectual Disabilities: Advances in Interventions*. Brighton: Pavilion.

Claire Surr

KEY ISSUES IN THIS CHAPTER:

▶ Why it is important for nurses to have dementia care-related knowledge and skills
▶ How dementia can affect adults of all ages
▶ The application of a biopsychosocial model to dementia care

BY THE END OF THIS CHAPTER YOU SHOULD:

▶ have an understanding of dementia as a syndrome
▶ be able to discuss the person-centred model of dementia care and its application to adults living with the condition
▶ have a range of strategies for supporting the psychological needs of people with dementia.

1 Introduction

Improving the quality of care for people with dementia is a global priority (WHO/ADI 2012). Dementia is a major cause of disability in older people, and the number of people with the condition in the UK is estimated to reach 950,000 by 2021. Around one-third of those with dementia reside in care homes (Knapp et al., 2007) and over 80 per cent of care home residents are estimated to have dementia (Alzheimer's Society, 2013). More than one-quarter of hospital beds are occupied by people with dementia, with 97 per cent of nurses reporting they work regularly with people with the condition (Alzheimer's Society, 2009). Dementia is therefore a condition that almost every nurse will come across during their working career. However, current quality of care for people with dementia is a concern. Recent government reports (DoH 2009; 2012) set out key targets for major improvements in dementia care and research in England, which include a health and social care workforce that is informed and effective in supporting people with dementia. It is, therefore, imperative that nurses have an in-depth understanding of the needs of people living with dementia. However, the majority of nurses say working with people with dementia is challenging (Alzheimer's Society, 2009) and, in a national audit, over two-thirds reported they had not been provided with sufficient training and development in care of this patient group (RCP, 2011). This chapter will examine how nurses can better understand and meet the holistic and often complex needs of people with dementia.

2 What is dementia?

The term 'dementia' is used to describe a number of different disease processes, all of which have common symptoms that involve a decline in memory, reasoning, communication and daily living skills (Knapp et al., 2007). The most common sub-types of dementia are Alzheimer's disease (50–75%), vascular dementia (20–30%), Lewy body dementia (<5%), and fronto-temporal dementia (5–10%) (Prince, Albanese, et al., 2014). The underlying brain disease in each form of dementia is different. For example, in Alzheimer's disease, amyloid plaques and neurofibrillary tangles are present, often alongside loss of neurons, white matter and synapses (Reitz et al., 2011), whereas, in vascular dementia, arterial brain lesions are present (Korczyn et al., 2012). While many people with dementia have mixed pathologies of Alzheimer's disease with vascular or Lewy body dementia, mixed pathologies are currently underdiagnosed (Prince, Albanese, et al., 2014). Although dementia can affect people of any age, Alzheimer's disease and vascular dementia occur most frequently in older people.

Dementia is a progressive condition, leading to increasing cognitive impairment and dependence. The disease processes associated with dementia cause brain cells to die, damage the blood vessels and blood flow to areas of the brain, or affect the functioning of nerve cells. The symptoms are similar to those found in other conditions which cause cognitive problems, including depression, delirium, medication side effects and alcohol misuse. Therefore, it is important that these treatable causes are ruled out both in the diagnostic process and if cognition worsens. There is currently no cure for any form of dementia. There are medicines available which may slow the progress of the disease, but they are not suitable for use with all types of dementia and may cause adverse side effects (Birks, 2006).

2.1 Younger people and dementia

While dementia is most common in older people, with 7.1 per cent of those (around 850,000) over the age of sixty-five in the UK estimated to have the condition, there are currently over 40,000 people under the age of sixty-five who have been diagnosed (Prince, Knapp, et al., 2014). The prevalence of different sub-types of dementia is different in younger people, with around one-third having Alzheimer's disease, 20 per cent vascular dementia, 12 per cent fronto-temporal dementia and 10 per cent alcohol-related dementia (Korsakoff's syndrome) and dementia with Lewy bodies. Younger people have a particular set of issues and support needs, including being more likely to be in work, having a spouse or partner who works, having dependent children, having more financial commitments, being likely to have fewer physical health problems, and being more likely to continue or wish to continue sexual intimacy in relationships. Existing services are often not tailored to meet the needs of younger people with dementia, who often have to access support through older people's services. A lack of appropriate service provision can leave people feeling marginalized and less able to cope with the condition (Clemerson et al., 2014). Research also indicates that younger onset dementia has an average lifetime duration of 3.4 years longer than for older people, meaning the stress and burden of caring is likely to be higher in carers of this group (Svanberg et al., 2011). Therefore, younger people with dementia and their families have additional unique needs that nurses need to be aware of in the provision of care to this group.

3 Models of dementia

The biomedical model and biopsychosocial model of health and care have been discussed in chapters 1 and 2 of this text. This chapter will examine their application in the context of dementia.

3.1 The biomedical model

The biomedical model remains a dominant discourse of dementia today. It views the disease process within the brain as responsible for all the impairments and behaviours seen in people with the condition. However, the lack of effective medical treatments to prevent or cure dementia means the biomedical model has often struggled to provide practice with effective solutions for the treatment and care of sufferers. Consider case study 6.1.

> **Case Study 6.1:**
>
> Anne came alone by ambulance to the A&E department of Northborough General Hospital following a fall. A neighbour had found her on the ground in her front garden. Anne has moderate Alzheimer's disease and has a suspected fractured neck of the femur. Staff in A&E have been trying to get a case and medical history from her, but she is very upset and agitated, and they have had little success in getting answers from her. Following a difficult visit to X-ray, where staff had to use restraints in order to get a clear image of her hip, she is now shouting out, 'Help me, help me', and, 'Susan', over and over again, and staff are unable to quieten her down. She hit a nurse who was trying to help her into a hospital gown.

6

> **Activity 6.1**
>
> Which of Anne's actions/inactions/behaviours do you think can be clearly attributed to her Alzheimer's disease? Which actions/inactions/behaviours may not be related to her having Alzheimer's disease?
>
> What other explanations might there be for some of Anne's actions or behaviours? What more might you need to know?

Behaviours like Anne's, such as agitation, aggression, delusions, hallucinations, depression, anxiety, apathy, disinhibition and irritability, often called 'behavioural and psychological symptoms of dementia' (BPSD) (Cummings et al., 1994), 'neuropsychiatric symptoms' or 'challenging behaviours', are reported to be one of the most challenging aspects of caring for a person with dementia. From a biomedical perspective, these behaviours are seen as inevitable symptoms of the disease process that need to be managed, usually pharmacologically. Commonly, antipsychotic medications have been used as the first line of treatment; however, these have limited effects and have been linked to increased risk of strokes and excess deaths (Banerjee, 2009). A reduction in their use is a governmental priority (APPGD, 2008).

In the case study, only Anne's reduced ability to provide a medical history has a clear direct relationship to her dementia. However, her ability to answer questions may be further impaired by a range of factors, including pain, stress and the speed and manner in which the questions have been asked. Anne's Alzheimer's disease means she is likely to experience difficulties in processing information, in making sense of her current situation, and with short-term memory. This can lead to increased confusion and fear in an unfamiliar environment. Pain from her injury is also likely to cause agitation (Husebo et al., 2011). Difficulties she may have in understanding why she is being undressed by a stranger might have led to Anne hitting out when having her clothing removed.

Therefore, by taking a more holistic view, Anne's current feelings appear most likely to be causing her behaviours/actions. It is apparent that the standard biomedical model can offer only part of the picture. Therefore, a number of critiques of traditional biomedical understandings of dementia have been offered and, from these, a range of alternative approaches outlined which emphasize the importance of psychosocial aspects. One of the most prominent theories is person-centred care.

4 Person-centred dementia care

The person-centred approach to dementia was popularized in the 1990s (see, for example, Kitwood and Bredin, 1992; Ebrahim et al., 1993; Kitwood, 1997) and has become a term that is synonymous with providing good quality dementia care through a biopsychosocial perspective. A contemporary definition of person-centred care utilized in a range of key publications (for example, NICE/SCIE, 2006) is Brooker's (2004) definition, known as the VIPS model:

- Valuing each person regardless of age or cognitive ability
- recognizing the uniqueness of each person and treating him/her as an Individual
- taking time to find out how things look and feel from each person's Perspective
- providing a positive Social psychology around a person.

Kitwood (1993) developed a theory of the experience of living with dementia, which underpinned the delivery of person-centred care. To do this he used the following 'equation' of interrelated factors, which is also often called the enriched model of dementia:

$$D = NI + P + B + H + SP$$

where

D – the presentation of dementia in any one person – is influenced by:

NI – neurological impairment

P – personality

B – biography, or life history

H – health

SP – social psychology (or the social environment surrounding a person).

The remainder of this chapter will examine each element of the enriched model in more detail.

4.1 Neurological impairment

At a simplistic level, each part of the brain is responsible, generally speaking, for different functions, although in reality most functions involve complex networks which cross over several brain areas. Each type of dementia has a different pattern of disease within the brain. For example, in Alzheimer's disease, as the condition progresses, damage is global throughout the brain, and so there is usually deterioration of many abilities. Early in the disease process, though, cognitive deficits may be limited to very specific abilities. In vascular dementia the damage may occur in very specific areas of the brain, so the person may notice deficits in some functioning and none in others. The progress of vascular dementia is usually less gradual than that of Alzheimer's disease and often more step-wise. Figure 6.1 and table 6.1 outline the main areas of the brain and the functions they serve.

6

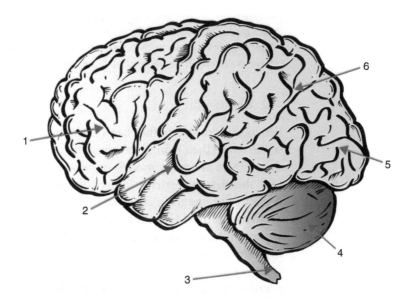

Figure 6.1 The brain and its functions

Table 6.1 Functions of parts of the brain		
Part of brain	**Key on figure 6.1**	**Function**
Frontal lobe	1	Planning, judgement, decision-making, feelings/emotions
Temporal lobe	2	Memory, knowledge, understanding, language and communciation
Parietal lobe	3	Bodily awareness, finer movement, skilled actions
Brain stem	4	Swallowing, breathing, heartbeat, basic life functions
Occipital lobe	5	Perception and vision
Cerebellum	6	Balance, posture and basic movement

While dementia is a condition that causes significant disabilities, impairment of abilities in one area does not indicate the person is incapable of other aspects of life. An unsupportive physical and social environment can highlight impairments rather than reinforce remaining abilities, and this can lead people with dementia to experience an unnecessary loss of independence.

It can be helpful to consider people living with dementia as having a disability (Bartlett, 2000) in order to develop approaches around reducing the impact of neurological impairment. The social model of disability (Oliver, 1990) moves from a biological focus to an examination of the society in which disabled people live and are contextualized (Parr and Butler, 1999). It asserts that a person is disabled not by their impairment but by society and the physical and social world it creates. Therefore, a person with dementia may be less disabled in an environment where large, clear signage containing pictures and words supports way-finding, where picture menus support choice at mealtimes, or where staff provide appropriate prompts to enhance independence in activities of daily living.

Activity 6.2

Referring back to case study 6.1, what might the hospital and staff have done to support Anne better during her visit to A&E?

4.2 Personality

Personality consists in the characteristics and ways individuals behave, which reflect their manner of adjusting to or coping with their environment. There are many models of personality. However, psychological trait theories are perhaps utilized the most within a health context. A trait is an enduring characteristic of personality, which underpins behaviour (Stuart-Hamilton, 1994). Traits such as gregariousness or shyness, for example, seem to have roots in both biology (nature) and learning (nurture) (Walker et al., 2012).

Some of the best-known theories have sought to place traits within a number of predisposing factors. Probably the most commonly used is the five-factor model of personality (Costa and McCrae 1992):

- extraversion – sociability, assertiveness
- neuroticism – anxiety/worry, moodiness
- agreeableness – trust, altruism
- conscientiousness – thoughtfulness, organization
- openness – imagination, insight.

Each factor is a continuum along which every individual will fall. Higher or lower degrees of certain factors may suggest greater or lesser abilities to cope and adapt in certain situations. For example, a person with dementia with a high degree of extraversion may be more likely to cope better with a move into residential care or a stay in hospital than someone with low extraversion. Throughout our lifespan we may utilize psychological strategies to work with or adapt to particular traits, so, while a person may have an underlying trait of shyness, they may have developed strategies for overcoming this in social situations. However, the ability of a person with dementia to apply these psychological strategies and cope as effectively in difficult situations may be reduced. Therefore, personality may provide us with clues about the potential coping strategies and mechanisms of dementia sufferers.

Some studies have found an association between personality dimensions and likelihood of people with dementia expressing certain behaviours, including a relationship between previous neuroticism and anxiety and previous agreeableness and agitation and irritability. However, previous studies on personality and behaviour lack a robust sample size and exhibit methodological weaknesses (Rouch et al., 2014), and therefore the relationship of personality to behaviour in someone with dementia is likely to be more complex than a simple linear correlation. Nevertheless, it is useful, when nursing a person with dementia, to take into account how previous personality may relate to present behaviours.

Personality change is thought to occur to some degree across the life course (Helmes et al., 2013). However, significant personality change may occur in people with dementia, and this is a particular feature of fronto-temporal dementia (FTD). One particular form of FTD, the behavioural variant (bvFTD), can cause the person to make sexual or inappropriate remarks, lack empathy, and display socially embarrassing behaviours (Piguet et al., 2011). The person with FTD usually has little insight into their personality and behaviour changes, and this can make supporting them and their family particularly complex for nurses.

6

Activity 6.3

Referring back to case study 6.1, how might the hospital and staff have better understood and worked with Anne's personality to support her during her visit to A&E?

Personality is not the only predictor of how people cope and adjust. The next section will consider another important factor, life history.

4.3 Biography/life history

How people with dementia act and react in the present is closely linked to their life history. People may form associations between things occurring in the present day and their experiences of the past. If dementia causes the boundaries of past and present to become blurred, then a person's ability to contextualize experiences becomes more difficult. As shorter-term memories also fail, the past can become clearer than the present and may be drawn upon more often and more easily to explain and understand the present. This is sometimes described as people 'living in the past' or 'returning to childhood'. However, it is not an accurate picture of the processes that are occurring.

Many people with dementia will have experienced traumatic life events, such as war, displacement and bereavements. Often the physical and social environment within institutional care settings can trigger recall of traumatic memories, which may lead to activation of strong emotions. The person may or may not be able to explain why they feel this way, and it can be difficult for carers to understand if they have no knowledge of a person's life history. For others, however, their current situation or surroundings will trigger positive memories. People may re-enact past work or other roles. For example, Bert, who was an electrician, may remove light switches from walls, or Helen, who used to be a nurse, may assist other residents and like to spend time in the manager's office. This can either be effectively supported by staff as a means to enhancing wellbeing or it can be viewed as 'problematic' and requiring management. The latter approach can often result in distressed reactions from the person with dementia.

An approach that is often unhelpfully used with people with dementia is reality orientation, which traditionally involves reorienting a person to the present. While prompts within an environment can be helpful in supporting sufferers to stay orientated to place, date and time, this is often extended to an approach of always correcting them, which can lead to distress and anger, as carers are constantly challenging the reality of the individual. Often what is important in recall of memories is not the factual content but the emotions behind it. For example, a person may say that people keep coming into their house and taking their possessions. This may not be factually true, but it may reflect their way of expressing an underlying feeling of being lost and unsafe. A more positive approach can therefore be to validate the underlying emotions and to try to understand the triggers for the feelings.

Activity 6.4

How would you feel if you went to A&E and were told you needed to be admitted? You know you have to pick your children up from school, but the hospital staff say it is fine and not to worry. You can't make any phone calls and have no one with you.

Would anyone be able to convince you that you do not have children to collect? Would staff saying your children are grown up and, therefore, do not need collecting from school help you feel better?

4.4 Health

People with dementia are at increased risk of experiencing physical health problems and delirium (NICE/SCIE, 2006). However, because of their impairments, their ability to understand and communicate ill health may be reduced. Therefore, nurses need to be extra vigilant in assessing for and treating physical health problems. This can be something as simple as ensuring the person has their glasses, hearing and walking aids, in order to support communication and independence, through to identifying more serious health problems.

A number of physical and mental health problems can cause dementia-like symptoms, including depression and delirium. These illnesses should therefore be excluded before it is concluded a person's confusion may be due to dementia. Delirium and depression can also occur alongside dementia. A sudden increase in confusion may indicate delirium and low mood and reduced interest may indicate depression. Physical health problems, too, can cause some of the behaviours that may be experienced by people with dementia. For example, being in pain may cause a person to become agitated or withdrawn. Nurses should never attribute behaviours to a person's dementia and should always look for potential underlying physical as well as emotional and environmental causes.

People with dementia are at risk of dehydration and weight loss. Nurses need to assess an individual's ability to eat and drink and should ensure appropriate support is provided to enable them to feed themselves as independently as possible but also to maintain good nutritional status and hydration. This may mean providing one-to-one support at mealtimes. Swallowing problems can occur as a person's dementia progresses. Speech and language therapists can provide specialist swallowing assessments and advice and support on appropriate diets and approaches to eating and drinking.

Physical health needs require specialist consideration when a person has dementia. Those with the condition are susceptible to all the illnesses associated with older age and when they are unwell are usually less able to communicate with those who care for them. Therefore, nurses need to use their observation and assessment skills in supporting the health needs of dementia patients.

4.5 Social psychology

Social psychology relates to the physical and social environment and relationships that surround a person with dementia. In order to understand how this impacts on the individual, Kitwood and Bredin (1992) proposed five psychological needs which may be supported or undermined by their social psychology:

- identity
- attachment
- comfort
- occupation
- inclusion.

4.5.1 Identity

Identity relates to having a sense of who you are and also the feeling that others recognize and understand you as a person. It is supported by a connectedness to one's past life and experiences (Brooker and Surr, 2005). Identity is an inherently social structure which arises out of social experience, thus existing only through our relationships with others (Surr, 2006).

As outlined in chapter 4, sense of identity is managed through a process of creating biographical narratives that position new memories and experiences in the context of the past, thus supporting an integrated sense of self. What is created is not a factual account of our life but our own interpretation of events (Neimeyer and Metzler, 1994).

Having dementia creates some difficulties with regard to maintaining a sense of identity, particularly where ability to recall the past and create narratives that assimilate new life events becomes impaired. Therefore, as memories fade for people with dementia, the retention of a person's life story by others, in order to support identity, becomes increasingly important. Thus, nurses need to know about a person's life history and use it effectively to support both practice and the person's identity.

4.5.2 Attachment

Attachment means any behaviours that attempt to gain or retain closeness, either emotional or physical, to a desired other (proximity-seeking behaviours), particularly evident during periods of loss or ill health (Browne and Shlosberg, 2005). Attachment behaviours stem from emotional bonds formed during infancy (Bowlby, 1953). Three attachment styles have been identified (Browne and Shlosberg, 2005):

- *secure* – confidence that an attachment figure will be available when needed and the ability to seek attachment figures when required
- *avoidant* – the tendency to maintain emotional distance and to mistrust others
- *anxious-ambivalent* – a constant fear of abandonment and the need for the continued presence of an attachment figure to feel secure.

Attachment theories have been applied to understanding the needs and behaviours of people with dementia. Miesen (1993) examined what he called 'parent fixation', where dementia sufferers act as if their parents are still alive. He challenged the standard biomedical view that these were delusions and hallucinations symptomatic of dementia, arguing that parent fixation is the expression of a need to feel safe and secure in an environment that is failing to meet those needs. Attachment behaviours may include asking for parents, expressing a desire to go home, calling out, and constantly seeking reassurance.

Nurses need to be aware of the attachment needs of people with dementia and how these may be expressed and to have individualized strategies for meeting them, such as talking to the person, holding their hand, or making available attachment objects such as dolls.

4.5.3 Comfort

Comfort in the context of person-centred care is defined as each person's need for closeness, security and soothing of emotional or physical pain (Kitwood, 1997). Within nursing theory, comfort is defined as the striving for relief from stressful healthcare situations, for which holistic approaches are required (Kolcaba, 1994). Every individual will have their own preferred ways of feeling comforted. For some, this may be through physical closeness and touch, while others may prefer talking and comforting words.

As discussed earlier, behaviours displayed by people with dementia are often labelled as 'challenging' or symptomatic of the disease when they may be an expression of an unmet need. Nurses need to conduct thorough, holistic assessments of people who exhibit distressed behaviours in order to understand their underlying cause, which may be rooted in physical, psychological, spiritual, social or environmental discomfort.

4.5.4 Occupation

Occupation is being involved in the process of life in a way that is personally significant or meaningful and which draws on a person's remaining abilities (Kitwood, 1997). A meaningful activity is an occupation that is seen as significant by the person. Vernooij-Dassen (2007) highlights how activities permit expression and connection with others, but also how living with dementia reduces the capacity to perform activities and to communicate, and so the ability to engage proactively in activities may be reduced or lost. Meaningful activities can provide pleasure and enhance wellbeing. People with dementia report finding most meaning in activities that support their psychological and social needs (Harmer and Orrell, 2008). Activities considered as meaningful can range from work-related occupations to household duties, leisure and hobbies, and social encounters.

As a person's dementia progresses, their ability to initiate engagement in meaningful activity will be reduced, as may their ability to remain engaged independently, and so it becomes important that those providing care support the individual to initiate engagement and to continue to participate in meaningful activities. With creativity and commitment from staff, opportunities for meaningful activity can be provided in any type of care environment.

4.5.5 Inclusion

Inclusion involves a sense of belonging in the context of individual relationships and in wider society. It is not just about being in the presence of others but about feeling welcome and part of a social group. A major barrier to inclusion experienced by people with dementia is stigma, which Goffman (1963) described as the effects of being positioned as a member of a socially undesirable group.

The stigma associated with a diagnosis of dementia is one of the factors that prevents people from seeking help and an early diagnosis (Koch et al., 2010). Older people report fear of developing dementia and of feeling uncomfortable in interacting with friends or relatives who have the condition (Corner and Bond, 2004). The stigma associated with dementia can also vary according to cultural and social background. For example, cultural perceptions and knowledge of dementia and beliefs about caregiving and familial responsibilities can prevent people from asking for help and support (Sun et al., 2012). The effects of stigma may cause those with dementia to feel shame and embarrassment (Kitwood and Bredin, 1992) or a sense of loss of social identity (Sabat, 2001); to worry about how other people will react towards them (O'Sullivan et al., 2014); to experience social isolation (Lockeridge and Simpson, 2013); or be subject to discriminatory treatment or restricted access to health services.

Nurses therefore need to adopt non-stigmatizing, non-discriminatory and non-exclusionary approaches to support sufferers. People with dementia may also need extra help to feel included, particularly in social situations – for example, by being included in conversations and discussions about their care – when they may be less able to initiate and maintain social contact.

In summary, these five psychological needs offer ways of understanding the psychosocial frameworks that are needed to underpin good quality dementia care. The next section will examine further practical ways in which nurses can support or undermine any or all of a person's psychological needs in how they interact with a patient with dementia.

5 Malignant social psychology and positive person work

Malignant social psychology (MSP) usually occurs unintentionally in everyday care when psychological needs are not met. Positive person work (PPW) is the opposite and reflects person-centred approaches that support psychological needs (Kitwood, 1997). MSP and PPW have been operationalized into seventeen observable types of each interaction, called personal detractions and personal enhancers, respectively (table 6.2), within the Dementia Care Mapping™ (DCM™) tool (Bradford Dementia Group, 2005). DCM™ is an observational tool set within a practice development process whose aim is to capture the experience of formal care from the perspective of the dementia sufferer. The observations are then fed back to care staff to develop person-centred action plans for improving care. After a period of implementation, the cycle is repeated to monitor progress and develop further actions (Brooker and Surr, 2005).

Table 6.2 List of personal detractions and enhancers

PD type	Description	PE type	Description
Intimidation	Making a participant fearful by using spoken threats or physical power	Warmth	Demonstrating genuine affection, care and concern for the participant
Withholding	Refusing to give attention when requested or to meet an evident need	Holding	Providing safety, security and comfort to a participant
Outpacing	Providing information at a rate too fast for a participant to understand	Relaxed pace	Recognizing the importance of helping to create a relaxed atmosphere
Infantilization	Treating a participant in a patronizing way as if they were a small child	Respect	Treating the participant as valued and recognizing their experience and age
Labelling	Using a label as the main way to describe or relate to someone	Acceptance	Entering into a relationship based on an attitude of acceptance
Disparagement	Telling a participant that they are incompetent, useless or worthless	Celebration	Recognizing, supporting and taking delight in the participant's skills and achievements
Accusation	Blaming the participant for things they have done or have not been able to do	Acknowledgement	Recognizing the participant as unique and valuing them as an individual
Treachery	Using trickery or deception to distract or manipulate a participant	Genuineness	Being honest and open with the participant in a way that is sensitive to their needs and feelings
Invalidation	Failing to acknowledge the reality of a participant	Validation	Recognizing and supporting the reality of the participant
Disempowerment	Not allowing a participant to use the abilities that they do have	Empowerment	Assisting the participant to discover or employ their abilities and skills
Imposition	Forcing a participant to do something or denying them choice	Facilitation	Assessing the level of support required and providing it

6

Table 6.2 (continued)			
PD type	**Description**	**PE type**	**Description**
Disruption	Interfering with something a participant is doing, breaking their 'frame of reference'	**Enabling**	Recognizing and encouraging a participant's engagement
Objectification	Treating a participant as if they were a lump of dead matter or an object	**Collaboration**	Treating the participant as a full and equal partner in what is happening
Stigmatization	Treating a participant as if they were a diseased object or an outcast	**Recognition**	Recognizing the participant's uniqueness, with an open attitude
Ignoring	Carrying on in the presence of a participant as if they are not there	**Including**	Enabling the participant to be and feel included, physically and psychologically
Banishment	Sending the participant away, excluding them, physically or psychologically	**Belonging**	Providing a sense of acceptance in a particular setting
Mockery	Making fun of a participant and making jokes at their expense	**Fun**	Using and responding to the use of fun and humour

Source: Bradford Dementia Group (2005), reproduced with kind permission from the University of Bradford.

Now consider case study 6.2

Case Study 6.2:

Anne moved into residential care four weeks ago after being discharged from hospital. Since then Anne has not slept in her bed and instead naps throughout the day and night in a chair in the hallway. When her key worker said that, if she didn't sleep in her own bed soon, she may have to go back into hospital, Anne swore at her. Anne often tries to leave the building when visitors arrive. She frequently fills her pillow case with her clothes and belongings and carries this round – staff call her 'The Hobo' – and she recently hit a member of staff who took the pillow case off her. At mealtimes staff feed Anne because she takes a long time to eat her food and it becomes cold before she has finished.

A few days ago student nurse Beth found Anne crying by the locked door to the care home, saying that her cats will die if she doesn't get home to them. Beth gave Anne a hug and told her that her cats were safe as they had moved in with her niece. She said she expected Anne must miss them and asked Anne to tell her about them. Anne became calmer after talking about her pets. Yesterday Beth brought in a cuddly toy cat to show Anne. Since then Anne has had the cat with her at all times, and she slept in her bed with the toy cat for most of the night.

Activity 6.5

What personal detractions have occurred in the example in case study 6.2 and what impact have they had on Anne? What personal enhancers have occurred in the case example and what impact have they had on Anne?

Which psychological needs are being supported and undermined? What else might the care home do to support Anne?

How might Anne's experience and care and support needs be different if she is aged sixty-one as opposed to eighty-five?

Summary

▶ Dementia is a condition that causes significant disability in adulthood and later life and impairs a person's ability to adapt and adjust. An individual with dementia needs extra support, and therefore the skills needed to provide good dementia care are central to good nursing care.

▶ Person-centred dementia care is recognized best practice. It acknowledges that providing good care for those with dementia is complex and requires nurses to address people's biopsychosocial needs.

▶ Nurses should ensure care they deliver to dementia sufferers supports their need for comfort, identity, occupation, attachment and inclusion.

Questions for discussion

1 Considering each element of the enriched model of dementia, identify ways that nurses can provide, within their own clinical setting, a social and physical environment that is supportive to people living with dementia.
2 What approaches might nurses use to help them find out more about the life history of a patient with dementia for whom they are caring?
3 How can nurses involve the family and friends of dementia sufferers in supporting the delivery of person-centred care?

Further reading

Alzheimer's Research UK, brain tour: www.alzheimersresearchuk.org/brain-tour/.
An online interactive tour of the brain and its functions.

Alzheimer's Society, factsheets: www.alzheimers.org.uk/site/scripts/az_home.php.

A range of research-informed factsheets on topics related to dementia written in an accessible style.

Brooker, D. (2007) *Person-Centred Dementia Care: Making Services Better.* London: Jessica Kingsley.
This book provides an overview of person-centred dementia care and a person-centred organizational audit tool.

Downs, M., and Bowers, B. (eds) (2014) *Excellence in Dementia Care: Research into Practice.* 2nd edn, Maidenhead: Open University Press.
This volume includes a range of research-informed chapters on a variety of contemporary dementia-related topics.

Kitwood, T. (1997) *Dementia Reconsidered.* Buckingham: Open University Press.
This is a seminal text on dementia. It reflects the culmination of Kitwood's work on person-centred dementia care.

Nursing Those
in Pain

James Jackson

KEY ISSUES IN THIS CHAPTER:

▶ Why is the ability to feel pain essential?
▶ The physiology and motivation aspects of pain
▶ Gender differences and coping strategies
▶ Treatment and pain management

BY THE END OF THIS CHAPTER YOU WILL BE ABLE TO:

▶ appreciate the motivational importance of pain in our daily lives
▶ discuss how mood and personality can moderate the pain sensation
▶ explain why different people will feel the same pain in different ways
▶ critically consider strategies used to cope with pain and why some are more effective
▶ appreciate the role of nurses in reducing patient anxiety.

---

1 What is pain? Why do we need it?

What is pain? What purpose does it serve? The International Association for the Study of Pain (IASP) describes it as being 'an unpleasant sensory and emotional experience associated with actual or potential tissue damage, or described in the terms of such damage' (Bonica, 1979). Three decades on, this remains the IASP definition of choice. It has never been bettered, as it considers both physical and emotional aspects together and states that pain is unpleasant. The last phrase, '*in terms of such damage*', allows us to consider cases where pain exists but there is no actual injury. This last category is known as *neuropathic pain* and can occur because the nerves themselves are damaged. NICE (2014) suggests the most common causes of neuropathic pain include diabetes and multiple sclerosis.

So pain is unpleasant, but why is it subjective? Imagine being tickled in playful manner by your brother/sister, and then imagine being tickled in the same way by a known serial killer. Each would be physiologically similar but would invoke very different emotions. Pain is just the same. It is our individual and unique interpretation of a sensation, based on our mood and personal appraisal. This makes pain a very individual thing. Unfortunately, this makes pain a challenge to measure.

There are many standard methods of pain assessment to consider (see figures 7.1 to 7.3).

The visual analogue scale (figure 7.1) asks patients to make a single mark on the line. A VAS is often 100 mm in length, and, to score, you simply use a ruler to measure how many millimeters along the scale the mark lies.

The numerical/descriptive scale (figure 7.2) gives the patient two choices as to how to respond. The higher numbers indicate more self-reported pain.

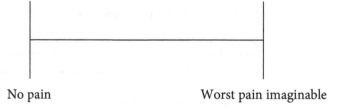

Figure 7.1 Visual analogue scale (VAS)   No pain   Worst pain imaginable

1	2	3	4	5	6	7	8	9	10
No pain	Mild pain		Moderate pain		Severe pain		Very severe pain		Worst pain

Figure 7.2 Numerical/descriptive scale

Wong-Baker FACES® Pain Rating Scale

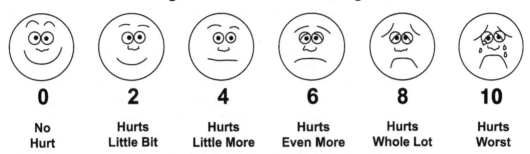

0	2	4	6	8	10
No Hurt	Hurts Little Bit	Hurts Little More	Hurts Even More	Hurts Whole Lot	Hurts Worst

©1983 Wong-Baker FACES® Foundation. www.WongBakerFACES.org
Used with permission. Originally published in *Whaley & Wong's Nursing Care of Infants and Children*. ©Elsevier Inc.

Figure 7.3 The Wong–Baker FACES scale (WBS)

If you are using the Wong–Baker FACES pain rating scale (figure 7.3), you must explain to the patient that each face represents someone who may be in pain. Face 0 seems to be unaffected and as such he/she would seem to be in no pain. Face 1 represents someone who may hurt just a little, face 2 a little more, and so on. As you may imagine, the WBS has found use in paediatrics, and it is worth stressing to children that someone does not have to crying to be in a lot of pain. Garra et al. (2010) confirm the WBS to be valid when measuring chronic pain in children and also suggest that the VAS has 'an excellent correlation in older children with acute pain' (2010: 53). Note that, when using any of the above, after time has passed and treatment has been implemented, it is important to ask the patient to complete the same scale for a second time. Has their score reduced? If so, then we may be able to assume that their pain management strategy has had some effect.

For a more challenging scenario, imagine situations where the patient is unable effectively to communicate that they are in pain – e.g., patients with limited knowledge of English or patients recovering from a serious stroke. Cunningham, McClean and Kelly (2010) looked at the assessment and management of pain in care homes and reported that, while pain is 'a universal experience' (2010: 29), recognition of pain in dementia patients is often lacking, with far-reaching consequences for the individual. The authors submit that, if you have to make a pain diagnosis in non-communicative individuals, there are six different things you can observe: body language, changes in activity patterns/routines, changes in interpersonal interactions, facial expression, negative vocalization, and changes in mental state (e.g., increased irritability and depression). Rapid advances in neuroimaging are suggesting that, in the future, it may be possible to measure physiological change in the patient, even if communication is not possible (e.g., Brown et al., 2011). Brown and his colleagues took sixteen participants and applied both painful and non-painful thermal stimuli to their forearms. By monitoring whole-brain activity, they were able to distinguish between painful and non-painful stimuli with an 81 per cent success rate. It is clearly early days, but there is an increasing movement in the literature away from self-report, the current 'gold standard for pain assessment' (ibid.: 1). Such efforts are worth making because the subjective and personal experience of pain renders self-reporting problematic and open to bias. For example, a depressed patient may report more pain than another patient. Are they actually in more pain, or is their subjective appraisal being affected by their depression? Imagine a patient complaining about a headache or chronic back pain, both conditions that cause distress but come with no visible physical symptoms. If you ask them to describe it, they may say their head is 'throbbing' or that it is 'seven out of ten'. But what do they mean by that? Is it the same sort of sensation that *you* would describe as 'seven out of ten'? Is their 'seven' your 'four'? Very quickly, there is risk of reduced understanding between nurse and patient while you evaluate their condition.

Case Study 7.1:

Lynne is a 69-year-old woman and sole carer for her older husband, aged seventy-eight, who is partially blind and suffering from signs of early dementia. For over a decade, Lynne has had fibromyalgia – 'a long term condition that causes pain all over the body' (www.nhs.uk/Conditions/Fibromyalgia/Pages/Introduction.aspx) and has suffered consistent pain and extreme fatigue. With her husband now needing constant care, she is no longer complaining of her own pain and is instead focusing on his needs. For example, she has struggled to get about for many years, rarely walking very far so as to avoid further pain in her legs. Now, with her husband unable to go to the shops for her, she shops without complaint.

Activity 7.1

What is going on here? Has Lynne's fibromyalgia improved? Is she merely gritting her teeth and going to the shops because there is no one else there to do it for her? Or, wrapped up in caring for her husband of forty years, is she distracted to the point where she is now less aware of her own pain? Let us imagine that Lynne is offered respite care by her local authority. Will the reduced responsibility offer her much needed rest, or will it grant her extra time to focus on her own worries and her chronic pain condition? If the latter, what are the consequences?

Now we are thinking in terms of self-appraisal, let us choose some words that describe pain. These are generally words with negative connotations, such as 'agony', 'distress' or 'unrelenting'. Each hammers home the emotional consequences of pain, and each reflects an innate desire to avoid pain whenever possible – or to diminish it – whether this is by withdrawing our hand or favouring our other leg, etc. Pain is unpleasant, and that is why it is useful to us. Pain is detected and signals sent to the brain by way of specialized pain receptors known as nociceptors (the term comes from our word 'noxious'). Thus, nociception is the process by which the brain is made aware of pain and then acts to reduce injury or further tissue damage. In the case of a burnt finger, we can study how pain receptors recognize a sudden increase in temperature, how this information is signalled to the brain, and how the brain responds by moving muscles to withdraw the injured hand. We can even note the changes in blood pressure and oxygen intake to help respond to the emergency. Yet there is also unpleasantness, and this motivates us to change our behaviour, both now and in the future.

Imagine a little boy on his first birthday. He is sitting in his high chair, and out comes a cake with a candle on top. The lights have been switched off, and he is in awe of this flickering flame in front of him. Before anyone can stop him, he reaches out to grab the candle. It burns him, and he starts to cry. Sensibly enough, the human brain is wired up to remember moments of intense emotion, and this little boy learns quite quickly – and remembers for life – that candle flames are painful and that he should never do that again. Noel et al. (2012) invited 110 children to undergo a cold pressor task (CPT). Here the children were asked to immerse their hand – up to the wrist – in cold water (10°C) for several minutes. They could remove their hand at any time if it became too uncomfortable or too painful to leave it in (the process was ethical since participants had control over the stimulus). Furthermore, the 10°C was significantly higher than the 2°C to 6°C used in adult CPT studies (e.g., Master et al., 2009). Two weeks later, the children were asked to recall the experiment and rate how painful the task had been. After two more weeks, they repeated the experiment. The main finding was that their repeat performance was more closely related to their recollection (two weeks previously) than their first performance (four weeks previously). In other words, it is not experience that determines future pain but the memory of that experience, and the children with the most negative memories went on to develop the greatest expectations of future pain. On repeating the task, they were naturally more wary of the cold water and, because they were focusing all their attention on their hand, the same pain seemed worse. Such findings are critically important if we are to consider patients undergoing a series of operations or painful treatments. Appreciation of the patient mindset between one intervention and the next can allow nurses to mitigate patient anxiety and alleviate future biases towards expectancy of pain.

So far we have confirmed that pain is nasty and that memories of past pain help you plan against future pain. To further understand the role of pain in our lives, let us consider those rare instances where individuals cannot feel pain at all. One such condition is congenital insensitivity to pain (CIP), a rare genetic condition affecting one in 2 million people. At first glance this sounds like a blessing: no distress, no need for painkillers, and no long-term aches or niggling hurts. The sufferer feels pressure but lacks the unpleasantness that goes with it. Cervero (2012) relates the story of a footballer with CIP unable to feel pain but able to appreciate the severity of tackles made against him. After a harsh tackle, this man was not above pretending to be in pain in the hope of receiving a free kick. This is important. Pain has two basic components: intensity/location (i.e., where and how severe) and motivational unpleasantness (i.e., a horrible feeling driving you towards the reduction of pain). People suffering from CIP have the first but not the second. There are many single case studies (n = 1) in the literature describing individual CIP sufferers. For example, Ma and Turner (2012) recount treatment of a healthy two-year-old boy who would bite down hard on his tongue and lips. He even self-extracted one of his own teeth! Similarly, Cox et al. (2006) mustered six individuals with injuries to their lips and their tongues – often severe enough to require plastic surgery. In two cases, the entire forward third of the tongue had been bitten off. All these injuries occurred in the first four years of life, before the children were old enough to consider logically the consequences of their actions. Cox and his colleagues also describe a young street performer (with CIP) who would run knives through his arms and walk across burning coals for money. This young man died after jumping off a roof, obliviously walking home on broken legs, and then later succumbing to blood poisoning. Pain is a vital warning system, and our ability to detect tissue damage and the parallel desire to prevent or limit such damage is vital to our wellbeing and our very survival. Pain is essential.

2 The circuitry of pain

At the most basic level, pain signals are carried up the spinal cord to the brain, informing us of tissue damage. When such damage occurs – or if the nociceptor itself is destroyed – pain receptors leak an acidic cocktail of chemicals into the surrounding area. This 'inflammatory soup' contains many different chemicals which sensitize and antagonize neighbouring cells (e.g., De Felipe et al., 2006). This makes neighbouring nociceptors more likely to fire. You can see this in action when you cut your finger. It is not just the damaged area that is sore but the surrounding area as well. The purpose of this is to convince you to keep the damaged area sheltered and out of use by making it more sensitive to pain. This is known as hyperalgesia, and sunburn is a good example. Here, the whole area will throb and will require soothing creams and lotions. Even worse, perfectly normal sensations are now perceived as being painful (Gustorff et al., 2013). Even a shirt sleeve worn over the affected area now hurts because nearby nociceptors have been chemically encouraged to fire. This is known as 'allodynia' – meaning 'other pain'. Note that hyperalgesia and allodynia are subtly different. The former increases the intensity of pain already present (i.e., pain receptors fire more often) whereas the latter conveys further pain (i.e., other pain receptors firing when they shouldn't). This side effect of sunburn tends to peak 24 to 36 hours after onset and often lasts more than 96 hours (four days). It motivates us to protect and shelter the damaged area, giving it time to heal.

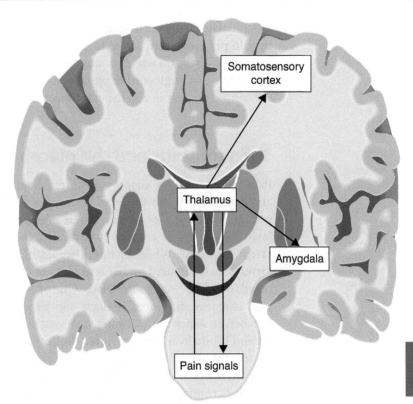

Figure 7.4 Pain pathways: one leads to the somatosensory cortex (location/intensity) and the other leads to the amygdala (motivational unpleasantness).

7

When nociceptors fire in the presence of noxious stimuli, these signals are transmitted to a region at the very centre of the brain known as the thalamus. Think of the thalamus as a junction box which gathers up sensory information before projecting it up to more specialized areas for processing. Pain signals end up in the somatosensory cortex – which processes touch – and it is here that we note where the pain is coming from (Peyron et al., 1999) and how bad the damage may be (Aziz and Ahmad, 2006). This is shown in figure 7.4 – note the second pathway branching off towards another region known as the amygdala – an area of the brain critical to emotion and motivation.

As stated, pain has two components: (1) awareness of where pain is coming from and how intense it is; and (2) emotional unpleasantness – that all-important motivational drive to encourage action. The latter is driven by activity in the amygdala, a region critically important to the processing of emotion, fear-conditioning and motivation (Phelps and LeDoux, 2005), and it has been shown to play a role in pain modulation (Neugebauer et al., 2004). In other words, it can enhance pain sensations (hyperalgesia) and/or reduce them (hypoalgesia). The latter is particularly interesting, as there are many occasions in which more stress results in better pain tolerance (e.g., Rhudy and Meagher, 2000). This link between the amygdala and pain intensity is well evidenced but not fully understood. For example, Bonaz et al. (2002) monitored brain activity in twelve patients with irritable bowel syndrome (IBS), inflating latex balloons to induce rectal pain. They found that changes in pain perception are linked to changes in amygdala activity. This is important. That pain signal coming from your cut finger or scalded foot is altered – is strengthened or weakened – by your brain, dependent on the context you are in and the emotions that you feel.

3 Endorphins and the placebo effect

Pain comes in many shapes and forms. Sometimes it is debilitating and sometimes it can be coped with more readily, even by the same person on different occasions. An excellent example is the pain suffered by soldiers in combat. It is sudden and shocking – but, to an extent, expected. While an injury would never be anything to look forward to, the injured soldier is likely to be evacuated – particularly in this day and age – to a safer place. One of the first people to compare pain tolerance in injured civilians and wounded soldiers was Henry Beecher, an American anaesthetist serving as a battlefront medic in the Second World War. He discovered that, for injuries of similar severity, 80 per cent of civilians would request morphine while only 30 per cent of soldiers would do so (Beecher, 1956). During one battle, with many casualties coming in, he ran out of morphine. With no effective pain-killers available, he acted out of desperation and lied to the soldiers in his care, infusing them with a saline solution while telling them it was morphine; 40 per cent of these deceived soldiers reported a reduction in pain severity. After the war, Henry Beecher would go on to investigate the 'placebo effect', claiming that 35 per cent of patients gain relief from placebos. Nowadays, it is recognized that he made some methodological mistakes (e.g., Kienle and Kiene, 1997), but his work is still considered ground-breaking and the starting point for placebo research.

Increasing scientific evidence in support of the placebo effect shows just how readily the mind is able to overrule signals from damaged tissue elsewhere. This is a fundamental aspect of the biopsychosocial model discussed in chapter 2. Meissner (2011) describes a healthy male participant being told he would receive a hypotensive drug to reduce blood pressure before instead receiving a harmless placebo. Over the next half hour, blood pressure was seen to drop 13 mmHg – falling from 113 mmHg to 100 mmHg. One theory is expectancy – the idea that, if you are given a pill and are explicitly told 'this pill will lower your blood pressure', it is somehow possible to activate normally inaccessible areas of the brain that control blood pressure. More believably perhaps, Flaten et al. (2011) suggest it is the reduction in negative emotion which makes treatments effective. For example, you have a nasty headache so you take an aspirin. You are now less anxious because you know your pain will disappear relatively soon or, at the very least, be much reduced. Flaten and his colleagues suggest it is this reduction in anxiety that makes a sugar-coated placebo as effective as real medication. Hyland (2011) goes further, suggesting that placebo effects can go beyond short-term symptomatic relief and that it may be possible to achieve long-term placebo responses through a good relationship with your GP/doctor. This highlights the important role nurses play in the effective management of pain.

Multiple publications suggest that pain management practices 'fall short of ideal' (Twycross, 2008: 3205) when the patients are children. Worryingly, it has been reported that nurses have a tendency to assume – incorrectly – that some pain is to be expected during a hospital stay (e.g., Woodgate and Kristjanson, 1996). It is also known that nurses can distance themselves from young patients in order to cope best with a challenging and emotional environment (Nagy, 1999). Furthermore, nursing students are expected to behave professionally when interacting with patients in pain. Put all this together, and it would seem that many nurses avoid verbal interaction with children in their care, particularly when the parents are on site, on account of the sometimes distressing nature of the role. Twycross reported that all nurses involved in her study rated communication with children about their pain as being 'highly critical' to the task at hand (2008: 3212) but 35 per cent of nurses – in an admittedly small sample – were not observed communicating with children at any point during multiple shifts (two to four shifts each on average).

7

Case Study 7.2:

Student nurse Beth is currently working on a children's ward helping to care for children recovering from surgery and suffering post-operative pain. Because of the sometimes distressing nature of such a challenging yet rewarding role, it could be tempting for a student nurse to maintain a professional detachment. Beth does not want to do this and wishes to support both children and parents at a difficult time.

Activity 7.2

Is such a stance correct, and does it have therapeutic value?

For many years it has been suggested that the placebo effect somehow encourages secretion of the body's own natural painkilling chemicals – endorphins. Endorphins are opiates from the same molecular family as morphine and heroin. Morphine is an effective painkiller simply because it is a turbo-charged variant of your own endorphins. Anything encouraging you to release endorphins increases your tolerance to pain by inhibiting incoming pain signals. Endorphins are produced in the hypothalamus in response to stress (see chapter 9), and this activity is initiated by the amygdala (Nakamura et al., 2013). Unfortunately, endorphins are challenging to measure – they do not cross the blood–brain barrier and they do not show up in blood samples

(Dunbar, 2012). Instead, you have either to extract a sample directly from the spine – a procedure not without risk – or to use radioactive dyes and expensive brain-scanning techniques. Laughter – however pleasant – places stress on the respiratory system so it elicits endorphin release. Admittedly, laugher may not sound stressful, but it involves a lot of breathing out without much breathing in. It is exhausting as a lot of muscles are used, and over an extended period of time it can even be painful. Dunbar et al. (2012) made use of this, confirming that live comedy performances increase pain thresholds whereas live dramas do not. Janssen and Arntz (2001) came up with a similar finding when they used electrical stimulation to evoke pain before and after novice parachute jumps. Under normal conditions, after their first ever parachute jump, volunteers (n = 12) tolerated bigger shocks than beforehand. However, a second group (n = 12) received a naloxone injection before the jump and did not report any improvement in pain tolerance afterwards. In order to appreciate this, we need to know what naloxone is. Naloxone is a well-known opioid antagonist used to counter heroin or morphine overdoses (Coffin and Sullivan, 2013). This means that naloxone binds more effectively to opiate receptors than opiates do (see figure 7.5). It pushes them out of the way and renders them ineffective.

A classic example is reported by Levine, Gordon and Fields (1978), who studied recovery from tooth extractions under local anaesthetic. Participants given painkillers or placebos three hours after extraction reported less pain. However, when injected with naloxone 60 minutes later (four hours after extraction), the placebos stopped working. Furthermore, many people find acupuncture to be an effective analgesic – i.e., it alleviates pain. It works because acupuncture is enough of a stressor to encourage endorphin release. In addition, we know that, if you inject people with naloxone, you can render acupuncture ineffective (Mayer et al., 1977). This last paper has been taken as proof that

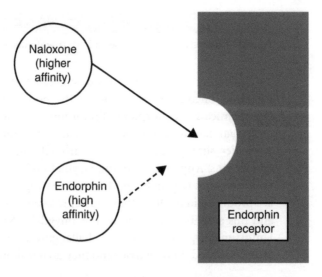

Figure 7.5 Illustrating the affinity between naloxone and opiate receptors

acupuncture has scientific merit – i.e., we know of the mechanism and we can block it – yet it also shows the importance of endorphins. Heavy exercise, and even anticipation of heavy exercise, encourages endorphin release, and this is the basis of 'runner's high'. This occurs when people exercise strenuously, even if not actually running (Boecker et al., 2008). It can be problematic, as heavy endorphin release increases the risk of exercise-related injury – i.e., joints put under excessive stress by an unwitting runner receiving no warning aches. Furthermore, when a woman gives birth she secretes lots of endorphins, making natural labour less traumatic for both mother and child (the baby is not yet able to produce endorphins in sufficient quantities). A mother not producing more endorphins in the run-up to giving birth is associated with requests for additional pain medication during labour (Dabo et al., 2010).

4 Gender differences and coping strategies

We can treat painful conditions with a myriad of pharmacological options. Drugs exist that target compounds within 'inflammatory soup', and painkilling drugs such as morphine act like artificial endorphins. But non-pharmacological methods can also be effective. It seems true, though controversial, that men have a higher pain threshold than women, particularly in the presence of others. It is commonly stated that men could never cope with the pain of pregnancy, but Ruau et al. (2012) studied 72,000 medical records and confirmed across multiple conditions that women repeatedly self-report more pain in every condition. In a systematic review of ten years of pain research, Racine et al. (2012a) considered 122 separate studies and concluded that women have significantly reduced tolerance to thermal pain (i.e., cold and heat) and when pressure is applied to tender areas of the body. No differences were found for chemical pain (e.g., chilli in the eye) or internal pain. Women are also more likely to develop chronic visceral disorders (e.g., pelvic and intestinal pains), even if the reasons are not fully understood. One theory is that women differ from men in some basic gastrointestinal functions (Hudson et al., 1989). Furthermore, while women are more likely to report headaches, back pain, arthritis and a host of other chronic pain conditions (Riley et al., 1998), they also have greater biological complexity (i.e., the menstrual cycle), and this makes it much more difficult to unpick gender differences in pain tolerance. In a second systematic analysis of biopsychosocial factors (e.g., hormonal differences and coping styles), Racine et al. (2012b) considered 129 further studies and stated that physiology alone was not consistently able to explain gender differences in pain tolerance. Let us move away from the outdated idea that women are somehow less physiologically robust. Recent research suggests that women naturally tend towards less effective coping strategies (Keogh and Herdenfeldt, 2002), and it is these tendencies which result in their reporting more pain than men.

So what are the better coping strategies? Both Jackson et al. (2005) and Thompson et al. (2008) agree that men are more likely to ignore/deny pain whereas women reinterpret it. Jackson and his colleagues ran several variations on the cold pressor task (CPT), confirming that men do better overall, but, when specific coping strategies were suggested, female performance exceeded male performance. This suggests that training can mitigate male advantages. Nevertheless, women are more prone to catastrophizing, a process where the individual over-attends, paying so much attention to a threat that it becomes all-consuming. Women typically score higher than men on scales measuring catastrophization (D'Eon et al., 2004).

Activity 7.3

Which coping style is likely to be most effective: one denying the existence of pain or one where pain is accepted but imagined as being easier to tolerate? How can you go about encouraging the former without being dismissive of the patient?

---

5 Treatment

Effective pain intervention must focus on how patients interpret pain signals. As ever, the emotional aspect is critical. In the right state of mind or under helpful conditions, individuals are more able to cope. An excellent concept to promote is self-efficacy, the ability to control a situation (see chapter 4). Clearly, if you are badly hurt, control is limited, but it helps reduce anxiety if you can exert control in some small way (Bandura et al., 1987). The best example is patient-controlled analgesia (PCA), which incorporates any method where patients can administer their own pain relief. In hospitals, this tends to refer to an infusion pump delivering pre-programmed amounts of intravenous analgesic when the patient presses a button. It has numerous advantages over requests for nurses to dispense painkillers on demand or at set times of day. By definition, the patient has control, and PCA has become an effective technique managing post-operative pain. PCA plus opioids are more effective than opioids alone, and patients do not use more medication than in conventional methods. Furthermore, patients prefer PCA, and there are fewer side effects provided patients and medical staff have clear instruction (Walder et al., 2001). It is easy to see why PCA is effective. Firstly, patients suffering side effects from their medication can space it out to suit their needs, and PCA can also mitigate inadequate pain relief. For example, if you receive medication every three hours, it is likely that pain levels will begin to creep up after two-and-a-half hours. Partly, this could be due to the medication wearing off and, partly, there will always be anxiety – however attentive medical staff are – that the next dose will be late. If patients can medicate themselves, anxiety is reduced.

Buhagiar et al. (2013: 465) state that 'disregard of individual variability is a chief contributor to inadequate pain relief'. Pain is subjective, as seen, and hypervigilance, general anxiety and depression all influence the pain sensation. Yet the biopsychosocial model has three components, and we should consider the third – social factors. Fillingim et al. (2002) report that men perform better at pain tasks with an element of competition. A study by Master et al. (2009) also illustrates the importance of social considerations. The authors took twenty-five women with long-term partners (more than six months together) and asked them to put their left hand behind an opaque curtain so that an unseen experimenter could apply thermal stimulation to their forearm. This occurred under several different conditions, including holding a squeeze ball in their right hand or viewing a photograph of a chair. In only two conditions did the women report less pain, and these were when they were viewing a photograph of their partner or when they were holding his hand, even when he was hidden behind another opaque curtain. It was concluded that seeing or touching loved ones provides memories of being loved and supported. Master and her colleagues recommended that bringing photographs of loved ones to painful procedures should be encouraged, particularly if loved ones cannot be there in person. Importantly, since loved ones may vary in their ability to provide effective and timely support, it was even suggested that photographs may be a better option than the real thing! Another CPT-based example is that of Brown et al. (2003). Here, undergraduate students immersed their hand in 2°C water alone, with a friend, or in the presence of a stranger. In accompanied scenarios, supporters were asked either to engage the participant in conversation (active support) or not to speak or make eye contact (passive support). Participants reported less pain regardless of condition. It was only important that someone was there. Finally, Essex and Pickett (2008) used data from the Millennium Cohort Study to investigate childbirth in women forced to give birth by themselves – either those who chose to be unaccompanied during labour or those with no companion available. Mothers unaccompanied at birth were significantly more likely to need an epidural.

7

6 Conclusion

In this chapter we have seen how essential pain is. In addition, we have seen how the brain interprets pain and how vital human appraisal and context is to that process. The brain can stimulate release of natural opiates (endorphins) to take the edge off pain – from a nursing point of view, this last point is quite relevant. How can people be best cared for to promote pain tolerance? Stress/fear can temporarily increase tolerance of pain but increased anxiety and catastrophization can make it worse. Why are fear and anxiety so different? A good paper is by Rhudy and Meagher (2000: 65), who define fear as an 'immediate alarm reaction to present threat' while anxiety is a 'future-orientated' emotion leading to heightened vigilance that focuses attention on possible threats. Fear and stress lead to opiate release and are akin to the Hollywood cliché where the hero fights off the bad guys, only to discover afterwards that they were wounded all along. Increasing stress is not encouraged (see chapter 9), but anything that reduces patient anxiety is a weapon that can be used to mitigate pain. A final paper is by Ulrich (1984), who looked at the effect of natural views – i.e., trees seen though a hospital window – versus a brown brick wall. Patients with tree views had shorter post-operative stays, required less analgesic (painkilling) mediation, and had fewer negative evaluative comments from nursing staff.

Summary

- ▶ Pain is important to our survival. It motivates us to withdraw when in danger.
- ▶ There are two components to pain: a 'where/how intense' component and an emotional 'subjective' component. The latter can be manipulated.
- ▶ Men tend to have greater tolerance to pain, thought to be because of their reduced tendency to catastrophize (though many men do and many women don't).
- ▶ Anxiety reduction and the presence of social support, even if in the form of a stranger (i.e., an unknown nurse), can assist pain management.

Questions for discussion

1 Consider the pain rating scales described above (figures 7.1 to 7.3). Can you provide an example for when each would be appropriate?
2 Could it ever be ethical for a doctor to prescribe a placebo? Be aware that trust is a vital aspect of the relationship between health professional and patient.
3 Why would men be less likely to report pain in a competitive/ sporting environment?

Further reading

Cervero, F. (2012) *Understanding Pain: Exploring the Perception of Pain.* Cambridge, MA: MIT Press.
Using decades of research experience, Cervero comprehensively explores the mechanisms of pain.

Vanessa Taylor and Beverley Norris

7

KEY ISSUES IN THIS CHAPTER:

▶ Grief reactions to loss associated with the end of life from the perspective of:
  • the patient
  • the family
  • the healthcare professionals
▶ The role of social support in end of life care
▶ The role of the nurse in providing end of life care

BY THE END OF THIS CHAPTER YOU SHOULD BE ABLE TO:

▶ identify the range of losses experienced by people throughout their life course which can influence their responses when facing loss at the end of life
▶ explore some traditional and contemporary theories of grief
▶ examine the concept of social support, identifying its significance to those receiving end of life care
▶ consider how to integrate the theories of grief and social support into your practice to support patients and families facing loss
▶ identify the support needs of healthcare professionals providing end of life care.

1 Introduction

Palliative care, as defined by the World Health Organization, integrates the physical, psychological and spiritual aspects of patient care and offers a support system to help patients with terminal illnesses live as actively as possible. Palliative care within the last twelve months of life is regarded as end of life care. This concerns both people whose death is imminent, expected within a few hours or days, and those with:

- advanced, progressive, incurable conditions
- general frailty and coexisting conditions that mean they are expected to die within twelve months
- existing conditions if there is a risk of dying from a sudden acute crisis
- life-threatening acute conditions caused by sudden catastrophic events (NCPC, 2011).

While it is acknowledged that some people will benefit from palliative care before this time, this chapter focuses on end of life care.

In the United Kingdom, approximately 500,000 people die every year (ONS, 2013). Dying and death occur in almost all areas of health and social care practice (NELCIN, 2013). Working with dying and grieving people can be demanding. Each patient and family has particular needs and, regardless of their illness or care setting, is deserving of expert care. Some, but not all, people with end of life care needs will require the involvement of specialist palliative services. For many, end of life care will be provided by their usual healthcare professionals. Currently, palliative care is delivered at three levels: (1) palliative care approach (2), general palliative care and (3) specialist palliative care (Gamondi et al., 2013a). The first two levels are delivered by the usual professionals, integrating palliative care philosophy and methods in normal settings. In contrast, the last is provided by multi-professional teams specializing in the provision of care to patients and their families whose needs are highly complex. These models of service delivery require all health professionals to have, as a minimum, education in the philosophy, principles and practice of palliative care (Gamondi et al., 2013a, 2013b).

1.1 The context of end of life care

The promotion of high quality end of life care, with equity of access to services, is core to UK-wide health policies (DoH, 2008a; DHSSPS, 2010; NHS Scotland, 2011; Welsh Government, 2013). In 2008, the Department of Health in England published its *End of Life Care Strategy*, which stated that: 'implementation of the Strategy will make a step change in access to high quality care for all people approaching the end of life. This should be irrespective of age, gender, ethnicity, religious belief, disability, sexual orientation, diagnosis or socioeconomic deprivation' (DoH, 2008a: 2).

The *End of Life Care Strategy* outlines a six-step pathway and identifies the support and services that people should be able to access during the course of their illness:

Step 1 Discussions as the end of life approaches
Step 2 Assessment, care planning and review
Step 3 Coordination of care for individual patients
Step 4 Delivery of high-quality services in different settings
Step 5 Care in the last days of life
Step 6 Care after death.

Activity 8.1

Reflect on the support and services available to, and accessed by, one of your patients with end of life care needs and their family. To what extent were the six steps achieved?

For patients in the last year of life, the gradual loss of the ability to perform personal aspects of self-care, the anticipation of pain and other physical discomfort, and the deterioration in physical appearance and functioning may all contribute to a heightened sense of vulnerability. Individual factors may affect the degree to which patients find such needs tolerable or threatening and the extent to which they can accept support and cope with the transition to end of life care and death (Tan et al., 2005). The support, care and information required by the patient, their family and caregivers, both during the illness and into bereavement, are integral to the end of life care pathway (DoH, 2008a) and will be explored throughout the chapter in relation to case study 8.1.

8

Case Study 8.1:

Beth is a student nurse working in the community with her mentor, Sue. Sue and Beth are visiting Geoff, a patient with cancer of the prostate. On previous visits Geoff and his wife, Joyce, have discussed the future with Sue and the GP and are aware that, due to the advanced nature of his cancer, Geoff is likely to be in the last year of his life. When discussing his preferences for care, Geoff expressed a wish to be cared for and die at home if possible. He is being looked after by Joyce, supported by health professionals and a small group of close friends. The couple have a son, Steve, who lives over 200 miles away, and, though he tries to visit as often as he can, his work and other family commitments make this difficult so his contact with his parents has been through daily telephone conversations. However, Steve has managed to organize a visit and had arrived at his parent's home the previous evening.

> **Case Study 8.1 (continued)**
>
> During the visit, Beth noticed that Joyce appeared tense and looked more tired than on previous occasions. It transpired that the family had experienced a difficult night. Geoff had been in pain and Steve had wanted to call an ambulance, as he believed his father needed to be admitted to hospital. Joyce had followed the advice she had previously been given by Sue about what to do if Geoff experienced pain and gave him an extra dose of oral morphine. This eventually reduced the pain. However, Geoff was not as comfortable as he had been, and Joyce was beginning to doubt her ability to care for him at home.

> **Activity 8.2**
>
> Consider the scenario of Geoff, Joyce and Steve. Identify actual and potential losses that, individually, they might be experiencing.

2 Understanding loss

Conceptually, within healthcare, loss is usually associated with dying, death and bereavement. However, loss is part of everyday living and will also be a constant encounter for professionals (Machin, 2009). For nurses to support patients, families and their colleagues effectively, and reconcile the emotional impact associated with personal loss, it is valuable to have an understanding of the concept of loss. Machin (2009) describes three dimensions of loss.

1 *Developmental loss and change* throughout life – for example, attending school for the first time, leaving home or getting married. Influenced by social relationships and support, successful management of these experiences of separation and loss can provide a rehearsal for more emotionally significant losses.
2 *Circumstantial losses* are described as unpredictable and often produce profound distress. Examples are separation/divorce, loss of employment, retirement, diagnosis of a life-limiting illness, and a move from home to nursing/residential care.
3 *Invisible grief and undervalued people* represent the third dimension of loss. Machin (2009) describes 'disenfranchised grief' involving people in socially 'unacceptable' or unacknowledged relationships; those experiencing stigmatized loss such as suicide; and those experiencing 'hidden' loss from miscarriage, stillbirth, abortion or infertility.

When thinking about the actual and potential losses Geoff, Joyce and Steve may be experiencing, you might have identified, for Geoff, the loss of his health, the potential loss of his employment and a change to his role(s) within the family. Ultimately, Geoff is also responding to his own death. Joyce may be experiencing the loss of her role as wife as she focuses on caring for Geoff at home, as well as the loss of her husband. Steve may be reacting to news of his father's loss of health related to the cancer diagnosis as well as the potential loss of his parent. We know very little about the nature of past and current relationships between Geoff, Joyce and Steve, in particular whether they were close or disengaged, caring or dismissive. Each will react and respond to their losses in different ways and will require different types of support to meet their needs during this period and, for Joyce and Steve, their bereavement following Geoff's death. To aid understanding of the diversity of responses and behaviours of those coping with loss, and to facilitate their care, grief theories have been developed using a rich variety of psychological and sociological approaches, including attachment theory. The theories discussed below can help deepen understanding, enabling nurses to engage confidently with those experiencing loss and to deal effectively with their needs and distress.

2.1 Theoretical perspectives

The wealth of grief theories that have been developed supports Walter's (1997) view that grief is more complex than any one model can provide. Freud, in his paper 'Mourning and melancholia' ([1915] 1957), discussed the concept of 'grief work', which he described as a psychological process that a person has to complete in order to move on and form new relationships (Silverman, 2005). 'Traditional theories' of grief, including those from Kübler-Ross (1969), Parkes (1972) and Worden (2010), support the need for 'grief work'.

2.1.1 Stages of grief

Elizabeth Kübler-Ross (1969) studied the experience of dying patients. By listening to them telling their stories, she proposed that those facing death coped with their loss as a process with five distinct stages (table 8.1). While the theory has received criticism for the rigidity of the stages, Kübler-Ross did acknowledge that these stages may last for varying lengths of time, may replace each other or may exist concurrently. Her work also promoted the importance of talking with patients about the terminal stages of their illness, as emphasized in Step 1 of the six-step pathway on p. 118.

2.1.2 Phases of grief

Through his extensive work with the bereaved, Parkes (1972) developed a theory describing four phases of grief (table 8.1). While the phases appear to be similar to the stages identified by Kübler-Ross, these reflect research with bereaved adults rather than dying people. The four phases explain the transition of bereaved people from

Table 8.1 Summary of grief theories		
Kübler-Ross (1969)	**Parkes (1972, 1986)**	**Worden (2010)**
1 Denial and isolation	1 Period of numbness	1 To accept the reality of the loss
2 Anger	2 Yearning	2 To process the pain of grief
3 Bargaining	3 Disorganization and despair	3 To adjust to a world without the deceased
4 Depression	4 Reorganized behaviour	
5 Acceptance		4 To find an enduring connection with the deceased in the midst of embarking on a new life

'incomprehension and denial, through a distressed state of confrontation with reality and, finally, to some form of resolution'.

The stage and phase theories of grief should be regarded as descriptive, not prescriptive, guidelines. Indeed, Parkes and Prigerson (2010) explained that the 'phases of grief' provide too rigid a framework and, given the variation from one person to another in the characteristics and duration of their grief, should no longer be used.

2.1.3 Tasks of mourning

William J. Worden developed a different theory, describing grief as a process and not a state. He suggested that people need to work through their reactions in order to make a complete adjustment. In Worden's tasks of mourning, grief is considered to consist of four overlapping tasks, requiring the bereaved person to work through the emotional pain of their loss while at the same time adjusting to changes in their circumstances, roles, status and identity. The tasks are complete when they have integrated the loss into their life and let go of emotional attachments to the deceased, enabling them to invest in the present and the future. Worden's description of the process of grief supports Freud's idea of grief work and, as with Parkes, draws on attachment theory to 'provide a way for practitioners to conceptualise the tendency in human beings to create strong affectional bonds with others and a way to understand the strong emotional reaction that occurs when those bonds are threatened or broken' (Worden 2010: 13).

Attachment theory (Bowlby, 1980) is a developmental approach to understanding the formation and maintenance of relationships related to a person's felt security. Bowlby observed that, when they feel threatened or upset, children seek security in the form of a reliable adult who symbolizes safety and security. A pattern of attachment is established in childhood in which the presence of threat or danger causes an individual to seek out protection from people perceived to offer safety. Different attachment styles are described, including secure, anxious and avoidant. Attachment behaviours are thought to be 'activated' in times of stress or ambiguity or when there is a perceived or real threat.

Although attachment theory has been widely applied to parent–child relationships, it has been highly influential in the study of grief and bereavement, highlighting how the patterns of attachment established in the early years may influence a person's future attachments and predict their response to loss and bereavement. Differences in attachment styles affect a person's health-seeking behaviour and their capacity to be soothed by, or accept help from, healthcare professionals. In end of life care, the dynamics between health professionals and the people they care for are thought to be influenced by attachment patterns that are played out in the relationship between patient and professional (Tan et al., 2005). Patients or family members, for example, who may be perceived by health professionals as overly dependent or demanding, may be feeling anxious, vulnerable or abandoned. Their behaviour may represent an anxiously attached individual who is frightened that they will be abandoned, and who is testing out the responsiveness of their carers by frequently ringing the bell or repeated requests for reassurance from the professionals providing their care. Similarly, a person who has experienced early stress, trauma and insecure attachment may find grieving more difficult than someone who had a secure early attachment.

The relationship that patients develop with a health professional depends not only on their attachment style but also upon the contributions from other professionals and family caregivers. In end of life care, however, an understanding of attachment theory may help practitioners to be aware of the specific needs and sensitivities of their patients and be more successful in forming therapeutic relationships that are experienced as supportive (Tan et al., 2005).

8

Activity 8.3

After accessing relevant sources, including the references at the end of this chapter, briefly describe each of the stages, phases and tasks of mourning identified in table 8.1.

In contrast to the traditional theories of grief outlined above, contemporary theories challenge the idea of 'grief work' as an emotional pathway to overcoming loss. They acknowledge the highly individualistic grieving processes and expressions of it influenced by cognitive, social and cultural dimensions (Machin, 2009).

2.1.4 Dual process model of grief

Stroebe and Schut (1999) offer a significant advance in our understanding of grief work. They outline a dynamic theory of grief which gives equal recognition to the cognitive and social adaptation to loss. Their 'dual process model' describes how a person has to cope with the experience of loss alongside other changes that result from that loss. The person is exposed to two types of stressor – those that are loss-orientated and those that are restoration-orientated. Loss orientation focuses on emotions and experiences of what has been lost and may be associated with the 'grief work' identified by phase and task theories above. Stressors that are restoration orientated focus on events associated with ongoing life and the need to adapt to new challenges on account of changed social circumstances. Restoration orientation, therefore, acknowledges the social perspective of the changes that result after loss, including adjusting to new roles, undertaking new tasks and developing new relationships.

While previous theories centred on loss, Stroebe and Schut (1999) recognize that both expressing and managing feelings are important. The dual process model introduced a new concept, that of oscillation between coping behaviours. Grief is viewed as a dynamic process in which the authors propose that people can, at times, confront and, at times, avoid the stressors in either orientation and so oscillate from thoughts that concentrate on the loss object to thoughts that focus on what is happening to them. The process of oscillation is how a person manages to survive the pain of loss but also manages to reintegrate into life as they grieve. While still close to the loss experience, a person may remain mainly in loss orientation but, over time, may spend more time in restoration orientation. The process of oscillation emphasizes the model's flexibility, avoiding a focus on a 'normal pattern of grief' and enabling a myriad of responses. The degree of oscillation is individual and determined both by the circumstances of the loss and by the person's personality and cultural background (Stroebe and Shut 2010).

The theories of grief outlined above suggest that those experiencing loss need to engage with and work through it, so that life can be reordered and meaningful again. Practitioners may be familiar with the stage/phase theories in identifying cognitive, social and emotional factors. Worden's tasks of mourning give a framework to guide the bereaved in their grief work, while the dual process model demonstrates the need for the bereaved to deal with secondary stresses as well as the primary loss, with time away from both. It is also important to recognize that the bereaved do not need to forget and leave the deceased behind, but can integrate them into their future lives by means of a continuing bond (Klass et al., 1996).

The continuum of emotion focused and restoration-orientated approaches offered by these theories provide health professionals with a way to acknowledge individual responses to loss and the requirement for nurses to tailor their support to the individual response rather than to any professionally prescribed expectation. Most research has been on the individual. However, understanding the family dynamic is also important in identifying possible tensions between members and assessing how they may influence or be influenced by others, as well as understanding what the loss or death means to each member. Each bereaved person is unique and will deal with a significant loss/death in their own way; therefore there is no single right or wrong way to grieve. The challenge that faces practitioners is to find what helps their patients best. No single theory of grieving is recommended, as all have various components that may be helpful.

Activity 8.4

Reflect back on the case study of Geoff and his family. How might theories of loss, grief and attachment help Sue and Beth make sense of this situation?

As highlighted above, many theories focus on the grief of individuals. Frequently, however, the losses experienced during end of life care and death affect a whole family. Family members, including children, can influence and be influenced by others, and the losses and death may mean different things to each person. As families like Geoff, Joyce and Steve face Geoff's life-limiting illness, they may experience vulnerability in response to a number of threats, among them threats to independence, security, control and life. Feeling vulnerable may make people regress to patterns of behaviour associated with childhood as they seek reassurance and security from 'attachment figures', which may take in the healthcare professionals caring for Geoff. Certain factors either inhibit or enhance a family's grief. Families in which there are fragile relationships, secrets and divergent beliefs may have more difficulty in adjusting, whereas families who have frequent contact and encourage each member to share their feelings may find it easier.

Knowledge of theories of loss and grief can be useful when caring for families, as long as they are not applied in a prescriptive manner. For example, there may be evidence of denial, anger, despair or acceptance in the response of family members. The phase or stage representations of grief outlined in table 8.1 can offer some insight into these responses. Beth and Sue may notice differences in coping styles between individual family members or even with the same individual at different points in time, reflecting Stroebe and Schut's (1999) dual process model. Facilitating the person to express their emotions may be the most effective way of helping them at times, while instrumental support could be the priority on other occasions.

The significance of family members' experience and their perception of the care delivered to their loved one at the end of life cannot be overestimated. The strength of feelings of bereaved relatives about poor quality care was influential in bringing about the public inquiry into the Mid Staffordshire NHS Foundation Trust (2013) and a review of the use of the Liverpool Care Pathway (DoH, 2013). An understanding of the needs of the patient, of those close to the patient, and of the interventions that will offer optimum support is essential to providing a satisfactory standard of end of life care.

3 Social support

People coping with loss may need help and support from others. This may take different forms and be provided by different people, including those in the individual's social network and health and social care professionals. There is considerable research identifying that social support assists people to adjust to the stresses of illness, when experiencing loss and during bereavement (Benkel et al., 2009). Assistance may be tangible, such as financial aid, or intangible, such as emotional help.

Four characteristics of social support are identified (Stewart, 1993).

- *Emotional support* involves the provision of care, empathy, love and trust. It is described as the most important attribute by which support is communicated to others.
- *Instrumental support* involves the provision of tangible goods, services or aid such as financial assistance or the undertaking of specific tasks such as shopping and helping with physical care.
- *Informational support* is defined as the information provided to a person during times of stress for the purposes of aiding problem-solving and decision-making.
- *Appraisal, or affirmational, support* involves communicating information or affirming the appropriateness of acts or statements made by a person.

Each element of social support enables the exchange of reciprocal caring actions to enhance health and wellbeing. Reviews suggest that social support has direct, indirect and interactive effects on a person's physical and mental health. The wellbeing benefits include fulfilling basic social needs and enhancing social integration. A 'buffering' effect has also been proposed in which the tendency of stressful events to produce emotional distress is diminished with the perception of social support and enhanced coping abilities (Cohen and Wills, 1985).

Among conditions for social support are an individual's social network, their embeddedness within the network and the social climate. Social supportive behaviours cannot occur without a structure of people (network) with the quality of connectedness (embeddedness) required to generate an atmosphere of helpfulness and protection (social climate) (Langford et al., 1997). Geoff, Joyce and Steve, like others facing the end of their life or providing terminal care, may, therefore, require different types of support to be provided by their social network of family, friends and health professionals.

Activity 8.5

Considering the case study at the start of the chapter, what different types of support might Beth and Sue offer Geoff, Joyce and Steve?

3.1 Supporting the patient facing the end of life

A nurse caring for any patient should use effective communication and assessment skills to meet the needs of an individual, rather than adopting a 'one size fits all' approach. This is particularly important in end of life care, when physical, psychological, social and spiritual issues can all arise and impact upon one another. All aspects of life can be affected. Physical deterioration can result in a reduced ability to fulfil roles within the family or society, leading to many different types of loss (Strada, 2013). Progressive physical deterioration and the increased dependency needs that emerge during a terminal illness may lead to a crisis of attachment. In some individuals, having to rely on others may trigger fears of dependency and contribute to a wish to end their life. The better the nurse understands the world of a patient, including what and who is important to them and their usual support systems and coping strategies, the more likely it is the nurse will be able to provide appropriate support. However, it needs to be remembered that this is a time when both the patient and those close to them are trying to orientate themselves and find ways to cope and find meaning in a changed landscape.

As discussed above, knowledge of the range of theories, including loss, attachment and grief, can be helpful and offer insight into how a patient responds to the various losses they are experiencing. We have considered the possible changes and losses that Geoff is facing: it is likely that he has lost some independence, because we know he requires his wife to care for him. This may signify a change in their relationship if Geoff had previously considered it to be his role to look after his wife. There is much we do not know, such as Geoff's relationship with Joyce and Steve and how he spent his time before his illness. Did he work or spend time on hobbies? How have these activities been affected? Is it possible for Geoff to use the same coping strategies or to rely on the same people who have supported him in the past? The answers to these questions would form a valuable part of the nursing assessment and may help Beth and Sue both to attend to Geoff's specific needs and sensitivities and to be more successful in forming a therapeutic relationship that is experienced as supportive. Perhaps most significantly, we know that Geoff is aware that he is facing the end of his life, probably within the year. As with anything, people will respond differently to such news, but NICE (2004b) acknowledges that high levels of psychological distress and uncertainty are more likely to be experienced at times when the prospect of facing up to death may be brought more clearly into focus, such as when someone is diagnosed with a life-limiting illness or when their illness has advanced to the point that the healthcare team believes they are in the final year of life. It is recommended that assessment of needs at such key points should be a minimum requirement of the healthcare team in relation to psychological support.

It may seem obvious that facing the end of life would be distressing, but it is useful for the nurse to consider in more detail the possible sources of this distress. The patient may experience fear or anxiety about the actual process of dying. Faull and Taplin (2012) highlight the impact of an individual's previous exposure to the death of others. Anxiety may stem from a belief that dying always involves pain or other distressing symptoms if this reflects what the patient has seen or heard in the past. In this respect, knowledge of the patient's previous exposure to death and dying is valuable. If Geoff was experiencing such anxiety, it is possible that some fears could be allayed if he was given the opportunity to express and discuss them with a health professional. A good knowledge of symptom management would be useful in such a discussion, but the information can be given later if a nurse does not possess this knowledge. The use of active empathic listening skills to allow Geoff to express his concerns would be the initial important step towards the possible relief of some distress.

Allowing and encouraging patients to express their concerns and responding with empathy can be helpful in several ways. It may facilitate a beneficial emotional release for the patient and help them gain a better understanding of their own thoughts and feelings, as well as help the nurse plan individualized care. It is likely that a patient faced with the prospect of dying will have concerns beyond the physical effects of their illness. Vanistendael (2007) draws attention to three existential questions that those at the end of life may be contemplating:

- What meaning does my life have?
- What does it mean for me that at one point I shall have to let everything go?
- What holds and supports me at this time in life when everything is slipping out of my hands?

Vanistendael suggests that positive concepts such as hope and meaning might emerge from what might appear an overwhelmingly negative situation, bringing a new openness to what is important in life and a potentially positive aspect to the experience. For example, when considering the above questions, a patient may develop clarity about who or what is important to them and, as a result, foster hope regarding how they would like to spend whatever time remains.

Most of us prefer to have some control over our own destiny, and anxiety may result from a fear of losing control at the end of life. The need to empower those receiving end of life care has received increasing recognition. Following a review of the literature on psycho-spiritual wellbeing in patients with advanced disease, Lin and Bauer-Wu (2003) conclude that a sense of empowerment and confidence has a positive influence. The *End of Life Care Strategy* (DoH, 2008a) places great emphasis on facilitating choice regarding care, including the opportunity for patients to be looked after at home. The strategy recommends initiatives such as the Gold Standards Framework and the Preferred Priorities for Care document to facilitate discussions allowing patients to make informed choices, which are then communicated to the relevant people and agencies with the aim of providing a coordinated approach to care. The initiation of such discussions as part of end of life care require effective communication skills from the healthcare professional but, handled sensitively, may help the patient to establish preferences and priorities not only for their care but also for how and with whom they might want to spend the limited time they have remaining.

3.2 Supporting the family

The quality of the relationship between the nurse and the family of those facing the end of life can be significant in terms of quality of life for the patient but also for the family. Öhlén et al. (2007) argue that relatives may have a simultaneous need for support in caring for their dying family member and support in maintaining their own wellbeing during this period. The aims of palliative and end of life care identified above include providing support for family members in their own right (DoH 2008a). An understanding of common stressors for families at this time and of possible supportive interventions will help nurses provide appropriate care.

Evidence suggests that the quality of the patient's experience, as perceived by the family, impacts upon the quality of the family's experience (ONS, 2013). Concerns for the patient – any unpleasant or distressing symptoms experienced, such as pain, fatigue, poor appetite, dry mouth, vomiting, constipation, confusion, hallucinations or depression (Andershed, 2006) – constitute a major source of stress for relatives. This can be accompanied by a sense of helplessness associated with being unable to relieve such symptoms, with the progression of the illness, and with difficulties accessing services (Perreault et al., 2004).

Caring for a relative at the end of life has been shown to involve increased burden and responsibility, which can result in loss of income, time, control and achievement of aspirations for the family member involved (Andershed, 2006). Despite these difficulties there is evidence indicating positive aspects for caring for a relative in such circumstances. These tend to be associated with feelings of having coped and demonstrated an inner strength despite the hardships. For some it has been shown that there are benefits around being able to care and demonstrate love for their dying relative, resulting in enhanced closeness and giving meaning to their final time together (Hudson, 2004).

Öhlén et al. (2007) highlight that this is often a time of great uncertainty when relatives face existential issues and are confronted with mortality, perhaps for the first time. Andershed and Ternestedt (2001) examined relatives' involvement in palliative care and developed the concepts of 'involvement in the light' and 'involvement in the dark'.

Involvement in the light is characterized by a family member being well informed (informational support), having a relationship with staff that is based on trust and confidence (affirmational and emotional support), and experiencing involvement that they find meaningful (instrumental and emotional support). Involvement in the dark is characterized by family members who do not think they are well informed or acknowledged by staff and feel isolated. As a result, they feel unsupported in their attempts to support the patient. Relatives who lack other forms of social support and have little time to adapt because of the rapid trajectory of the illness were found to be more at risk of being 'in the dark', but Andershed and Ternestedt suggest that, even when this is the case, the attitude of professional carers can make the difference between involvement in the light and involvement in the dark. They promote a humanistic attitude 'characterised by respect, openness, sincerity, confirmation and connection' (2001: 560). It is important in cases where less confident relatives may experience difficulty asking questions that nurses take the initiative in assessing information needs rather than simply waiting for questions to be asked. A confirmatory, supportive attitude from staff can build confidence and help family members be involved in a manner that is meaningful to them.

It is evident in the case study that the pain experienced by Geoff resulted in distress and anxiety for both his wife and his son. Given that psycho-social factors have an impact upon the experience of pain, it is quite possible that his family's anxiety served to worsen Geoff's pain, creating a vicious circle of distress. Steve's feelings of helplessness may have been intensified by his not being familiar with the situation. Steve had just arrived at his parents' home and was probably in need of information regarding what to expect and how pain could be managed. Joyce was informed and knowledgeable in her approach to easing Geoff's pain, but, when faced with Steve's doubts, may have needed affirmational support to reassure her she was doing the right thing. During their visit, Beth and Sue would be in a good position to help this family by using effective communication skills, empathy, and professional knowledge to meet their needs.

For Joyce and Steve, support will also be important following Geoff's death. At this time, the social network provides most support for the bereaved (Benkel et al., 2009). Specialized expertise from professionals is needed most during the period close to the death and is complementary, required when the social network is lacking or not able to meet the individual needs of the bereaved. Having these social resources available to cope with stressful life events, alongside personal resourcefulness and a positive life perspective, is described as highly influential in shaping whether the grieving process will be met with resilience or vulnerability (Machin, 2009). Where internal resources or resilience, to manage the emotional, social and practical aspects of the loss situation, and external sources of support are inadequate, the bereaved may be vulnerable to depression (Relf et al., 2008). These findings highlight the benefits of professionals assessing the social support needs and network of the bereaved to develop strategies for providing optimal assistance (Benkel et al., 2009).

3.3 Supporting the healthcare professional

Activity 8.6

As health professionals and members of a multi-professional team, what impact might providing end of life care have on Beth, Sue and other team members? Consider what help they might require to deliver end of life care to Geoff and support to Joyce and Steve.

When confronted with dying and death, healthcare professionals may also experience the grief reactions discussed above. Research by Papadatou (2001) revealed that the reactions of professionals can fluctuate between 'experiencing' and 'avoiding' feelings of grief. The 'experience' of grief may include the range of emotional, cognitive, behavioural and physical responses already identified. In contrast, 'avoidance' of the loss experience may involve suppression of feelings, humanizing the dead patient, de-humanizing the dying patient, and distraction through engaging in clinical duties. Similarities with Stroebe and Schut's (1999) dual process model are acknowledged. While fluctuation is described as healthy and adaptive, enabling the professional to give meaning to dying and the death of each patient and integrate these losses into their life and daily work, complications have been identified when there is a persistent lack of fluctuation resulting in burnout (Papadatou, 2001).

Burnout can arise when personal feelings and reactions are repeatedly ignored or suppressed (Wrenn et al., 1999). Three common symptoms which characterize burnout are identified at the individual professional and/or healthcare team level when caring for dying people and their families:

- a deep sense of emotional exhaustion manifested by low energy, chronic fatigue and feeling drained by work, accompanied by low self-esteem, depression, anger and resentment towards patients, colleagues and oneself
- a distant and depersonalized approach towards patients and families who are treated as 'cases' and their needs disregarded; attention may be focused on the physical needs of the patient or on avoiding the patient
- a sense of decreased efficacy and lack of accomplishments characterized by feelings of helplessness and demoralization.

Burnout may also be expressed through absenteeism, greater staff turnover, increased clinical errors, physical symptoms and team conflict.

In a seminal review of occupational stress in hospice and palliative care, Vachon (1995) identified that there had been less staff stress and burnout than among professionals in other settings. Early recognition of the potential stress inherent in palliative care and the development of organizational and personal coping strategies to deal with the stressors were identified as a contributing factor. However, staff in hospice/palliative care experienced increased stress when mechanisms such as social support, involvement in work and decision-making, and a realistic workload were not available. Vachon concluded that the stress that exists in palliative care is due largely to organizational and societal issues, although personal variables, including length of experience, professional qualifications, personal values, personality and social support, were also influential. More recently, Tan et al. (2005) suggested that the attachment style of the clinician may play a role in the kind of relationships that develop with those requiring end of life care. For example, the attachment style of the clinician may contribute to the extent to which there is a mutual avoidance of emotion-laden concerns or difficulty establishing appropriate boundaries in the caregiving relationship. Tan and her colleagues suggest that awareness of their own attachment histories and relational needs may help professional caregivers to reflect on their own contributions to their relationship with patients and to become more sensitively attuned to them. It is, therefore, essential that nurses are equipped with the knowledge, skills, self-awareness and attitudes they need to care for patients who are dying, because almost all will, at some point, care for dying patients (Riley, 2008).

In addition, Machin (2009) emphasizes the importance of professional support through collaborative teamworking and supervision, alongside a balance of relationships and activities outside work, to enable practitioners to function with resilience. Resilience involves protective processes which help to counteract stressful and adverse impact of end of life care and contribute to effective outcomes (Papadatou, 2006).

Four forms of mutual support between healthcare professionals mitigate the increased stress caused by exposure to end of life care (Papadatou et al., 1998). These are identified by the International Work Group on Death, Dying and Bereavement as relevant to all professional caregivers involved in dying, death and bereavement care (Papadatou 2006):

1 *informational support* – awareness of the factors pertinent to the caregiving role
2 *clinical/practical support* – collaborative teamworking which is mindful of the individual carer's needs
3 *emotional support* – team, unit and department recognition of the impact of working with loss and providing opportunities for personal debriefing and/or time-out for staff

4   *meaning making support* – debriefing and reflection on practice to facilitate the team to develop shared meaning about their work with loss and grief.

Beth, Sue and the members of the multi-professional team will all need to recognize their personal issues and feelings related to dying and death. Developing self-awareness and a personal philosophy are identified as important for care providers to understand their attitudes about dying and their own death (Wrenn et al., 1999). For Beth and Sue, this will involve identifying their values, beliefs and goals and the philosophy of palliative/end of life care. Developing their knowledge and competence during pre-registration programmes and through continuing professional opportunities will enhance their understanding and contribution to the delivery of the palliative care approach and general palliative care. The National End of Life Care Programme (2009) published its 'Common core competences and principles for health and social care workers working with adults at the end of life' and, more recently, the European Association of Palliative Care (Gamondi, 2013a, 2013b) detailed ten core competencies for all health and social care professionals to guide their development to deliver end of life care (table 8.2).

Table 8.2 EAPC levels and core competencies in palliative care	
EAPC agreed levels of education for professionals involved in palliative care	**EAPC ten core competencies in palliative care**
Palliative care approach General palliative care Specialist palliative care Achieved through: • continuing professional development • undergraduate pre-registration • undergraduate post-registration • postgraduate study	1 Apply core constituents of palliative care in the setting where patients and families are based
	2 Enhance physical comfort throughout patients' disease trajectories
	3 Meet patients' psychological needs
	4 Meet patients' social needs
	5 Meet patients' spiritual needs
	6 Respond to the needs of the family carers in relation to short-, medium- and long-term patient care goals
	7 Respond to the challenges of clinical and ethical decision-making in palliative care
	8 Practise comprehensive care co-ordination and interdisciplinary teamwork across all settings where palliative care is offered
	9 Develop interpersonal and communication skills appropriate to palliative care
	10 Practise self-awareness and undergo continuing professional development

Source: Gamondi et al. (2013a, 2013b).

Team, organizational and environmental culture are all identified as determining expectations and defining the context by which professional caregivers will respond to end of life and bereavement situations (Papadatou, 2006). As a team member, and being aware of the national policy, Beth will contribute to the delivery of a shared philosophy and common goal for Geoff's end of life care and bereavement support for his family.

Summary

▶ End of life care involves an appreciation of the range of losses experienced by the patient, their families and carers, both during the patient's illness and after their death.
▶ Effective communication skills used by nurses to facilitate exploration of the preferences and priorities for life and care can empower those facing death.
▶ Theories of loss, grief and social support can provide a useful insight into the reactions and responses of individuals, their families and carers to end of life care, but it should be recognized that individual responses will vary.
▶ End of life care is provided, for many, by the patient's usual healthcare professional. Developing personal and professional knowledge and the skills associated for such care, alongside a supportive team and organizational culture, is identified as determining expectations and sustaining professional caregivers.

Questions for discussion

1 What are the opportunities and challenges your team and service face in implementing the *End of Life Care Strategy*? How might the challenges be overcome to meet the range of social support needs of patients requiring end of life care and their families?
2 How are the support needs of professional colleagues recognized and how might support of staff providing palliative and end of life care in your service be enhanced?

Further reading

General Medical Council (2010) *Treatment and Care towards the End of Life: Good Practice in Decision Making*, www.gmc-uk.org/End_of_life. pdf_32486688.pdf.
Providing treatment and care towards the end of life often involves decisions that are clinically complex and emotionally distressing; some decisions may involve ethical dilemmas and uncertainties about the law that further

complicate the decision-making process. While aimed at doctors, this guidance provides a framework to support addressing the issues in a way that meets individual patients' needs.

Price, B. (2003) Mapping the social support networks of patients, *Cancer Nursing Practice* 2(5): 31–6.
Provides practical guidance for using social support network mapping to identify the potential support needs of those facing loss.

Relf, M., Machin, L., and Archer, N. (2008) *Guidance for Bereavement Needs Assessment in Palliative Care*. London: Help the Hospices; www.londonhp. nhs.uk/wp-content/uploads/2011/03/Bereavement-needs-assessment-guide. pdf.
This guidance brings together theory and research focused on individuals' coping responses and provides a practical assessment approach to help professionals recognize resilience and vulnerability in the bereaved.

8

Part III
Mental Health in the Nursing Environment

CONTENTS

Dealing with mental health issues, be they seemingly minor issues such as stress and anxiety or major ones – for example, patients who appear to be hallucinating or hearing voices or who are under the influence of drugs or alcohol – is part of a nurse's working life. Part III begins with a chapter on stress. Although it is not a mental health disorder in itself, a period of prolonged or intense stress can affect both body and mind. The relationship between a person's mental state and the immune response is explored, with particular focus on the effects of stress on the immune system – how it initially enhances it but ultimately shuts it down. Cancer, as both a disease and a stressor, is considered in relation to the power of 'fighting spirit' in resisting disease. Throughout, the chapter emphasizes the part nurses can play in reducing patient stress and the effect this has on successful treatment.

Chapter 10 examines the nature, diagnosis and treatment of anxiety and depression, two mental health conditions commonly encountered in healthcare settings. Such conditions can have a significant impact upon the quality of the lives of individuals and the people around them. Using the biopsychosocial model, the chapter examines the nature, theories and treatment of anxiety and mood disorders in order to inform effective nursing practice.

The final chapter in this section discusses altered mental states, such as hallucinations and delusions often arising from psychosis. Core psychological theories that can account for these altered states are examined and the evidence base evaluated. For example, the chapter explores and evaluates the contribution cognitive psychology has made in accounting for the complex phenomenology of the unusual experiences of psychosis. It concludes by looking at the relationship between mental health and substance misuse.

Stress and Illness

James Jackson

KEY ISSUES IN THIS CHAPTER:

▶ The human immune system (i.e., antibodies and white blood cells)
▶ The stress response (adrenaline and cortisol)
▶ The relationship between stress and illness (psychoneuroimmunology)
▶ The effects of chronic stress on cancer progression and longevity
▶ The moderating effects of personality on illness progression

BY THE END OF THIS CHAPTER YOU SHOULD BE ABLE TO:

▶ define stress and appreciate the importance of cognitive appraisal
▶ understand the basis of the immune system
▶ appreciate the relationship between the immune system and stress hormones, particularly the reasons why stress hormones blunt our immune response
▶ see how suffering a chronic illness (e.g., cancer) can be a stressor all of its own, further hindering recovery
▶ appreciate the importance of personality type and how patient mindset is a critical factor in the treatment of illness.

1 Introduction

Stress and illness have a very close relationship. In essence, stress increases your chances of succumbing to illness and, importantly, ensures you are less able to fight off that illness quickly. It is a double effect. As this chapter progresses, we will see how mindset can affect the immune system and, correspondingly, how chronic stress results in poorer physical and mental health.

We will begin with two examples. The first was documented by a physician – John Noble MacKenzie – in the late nineteenth century (cited in Vits et al., 2011). MacKenzie was treating a woman with a severe allergic reaction to roses. He had an artificial rose in his office and was surprised when the patient arrived and, on sight, manifested an allergic reaction to the artificial rose. She had not realized it was fake and responded physiologically as if it were real. The second example is a study by Futterman et al. (1994) involving fourteen male actors with at least one year's acting experience, all of whom were trained in the method acting technique. Here, actors relive their own memories in order to gain understanding of the characters they play. They were asked to read a 100-word briefing and then, after some preparation time, improvise a realistic scene. Among scenarios to act out were being distressed after failing an audition; celebrating the news of their new starring role with friends; and making up and reading out a 'neutral' article from a magazine. Before and after each session, the actors had their immunological readiness tested (i.e., how effectively could they fight off disease at that moment). It was found that preparing for a negative scene by drawing on personal memories of audition failure reduced their white blood cell counts and their immune responsiveness and left them vulnerable to infection and disease. Correspondingly, drawing on past success to prepare for a positive scene increased white blood cell count and heightened immune responsiveness.

2 Stress, immunity and psychoneuroimmunology

The biopsychosocial model suggests that psychological and biological systems are interconnected. This presumed interdependence led to a new field of research – psychoneuroimmunology. Psychoneuroimmunology is the interdisciplinary study of the relationship between stress and immune function. An example is provided by Kiecolt-Glaser et al. (1995), who considered the stress of caring for a relative with Alzheimer's disease. Both carers and comparable controls were given a 3.5 mm punch biopsy wound. Wound healing took significantly longer in caregivers, and their white blood cells were found to be significantly less effective (e.g., they produced fewer chemicals when stimulated). In essence, then, the simple existence of psychoneuroim-munology is validation of the biopsychosocial model (Trilling, 2000).

So is stress as a challenge to be faced just the response that the body makes – for example, a heart beating faster and with more force – or, as Lazarus (1999) states, does it also include the person, their personality and their environment? We will assume that Lazarus was correct, and that stress is that moment when the individual realizes that the resources they have are not sufficient to meet the demands of the situation. As such, all good models of stress – including the theory of cognitive appraisal (Lazarus and Folkman, 1984) – recognize its subjective nature. When we encounter a challenge, we assess it. Are we in control? Are we in trouble? Can we cope? Our individual personalities come to the fore. For example, an individual with high self-esteem is more likely to believe they have the skills needed to cope with a given situation, and so is less likely to perceive a situation as stressful. The earlier examples (see Futterman et al., 1994) support the biopsychosocial model (see chapters 1 and 2) in that mindset and mood can moderate the ability of the body to challenge disease and illness.

Since stress and immune function are intertwined, we must also, briefly, consider how the immune system works. Essentially, it uses two different strategies in the battle against disease.

1   *Cell-mediated immunity* is the most aggressive and most readily understandable method by which the body fights off disease. Here, white blood cells (known as leukocytes) act in similar fashion to single-celled algae. They seek out invaders, make physical contact and then engulf them. In addition, leukocytes will target our own cells if they have been taken over by viruses, and they will destroy these as well.

2   *Humoral immunity* involves the synthesis and release of proteins known as antibodies (Ab). These may also be referred to as immunoglobulins (Ig), though the terms are interchangeable. Each antibody is shaped like a letter 'Y', and their purpose is to latch onto invading bacteria and viruses by way of the two arms of the 'Y'. Cells are not perfectly smooth and have proteins jutting up from their surfaces that allow the cell to be recognized. These shapes – known as antigens (antibody generators) – allow the immune system to distinguish cells that belong to the body from cells which do not (i.e., invaders). When found, antigens promote synthesis of new antibodies designed to bind with them (Hahm and Bhunia, 2006). These may 'tag' the cell to mark it for engulfment or, if the antigen is somehow important to the invader, the antibody can bind to it, rendering the invader harmless (see figure 9.1). Many specific antibodies pass from mother to baby via the placenta and from breast milk (Jackson and Nazar, 2006). Any antibodies formed by the mother when she fought off disease can pass across, boosting the baby's ability to fight off similar infections in future.

9

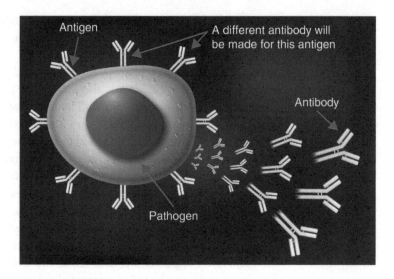

Figure 9.1 Antibodies binding to an invading pathogen

Imagine you have recently been infected by pathogen X. If you have come across this illness before or acquired resistance from your mother, you will carry copies of an antibody able to bind to the invader on first contact. All you need to do is produce this antibody in large numbers and the pathogen is defeated long before it could make you ill. However, if you do not have this 'silver bullet', you will fall ill as the disease bypasses ineffectual defences and takes hold. As you feel worse, your body is striving to produce a useful antibody. When it finally produces one that works, you churn it out in large numbers and the pathogen is finally overwhelmed. You will then store a small number of these antibodies away in your bone marrow to be brought out later if needed. The next battle against pathogen X will be won more quickly. For example, adults catch fewer colds than children because they have been exposed to more of them and have built up stronger immunities over their lifetime (Fashner et al., 2012).

There are two different classes of cell in the immune system: B-cells and T-cells. Both originate in the bone marrow but, while B-cells stay there until needed (B for bone), T-cells migrate to the thymus (T for thymus). The thymus is *not* to be confused with the thyroid gland, which is something else. B-cells produce antibodies and T-cells are the leukocytes which engulf invaders. In addition, there are natural killer (NK) leukocytes that seek out mutating (cancerous?) cells and destroy them (Terunuma et al., 2008).

3 The stress response

In England between 1881 and 1890 the mortality rate for children under the age of one was 142 per 1,000 births. In 2010, the infant mortality rate in England and Wales for children under the age of one was four per 1,000 (Thompson et al., 2012: 16). The exact reasons are unclear, but it is thought that mass vaccinations, the development of antibiotics, improved sanitation, and advances in prenatal and postnatal care have all had an effect. Furthermore, the leading causes of death have changed dramatically. Most deaths in 1908 would be preventable today, but back then, with no acquired immunity, infectious and parasitic diseases accounted for a fifth of all deaths, a third of which occurred in the under-fives. Measles took 50,000 lives, tuberculosis and whooping cough killed 40,000 each, and diarrhoea and dysentery together claimed the lives of a further 100,000 (ibid.: 21). This sea change means that, while only 1 per cent of those individuals born in 1908 would reach the age of 100, we may expect that, across the UK, one-third of children born in 2012 will live to see 2112. In addition, cancers were rare in 1908, accounting for only 6 per cent of all deaths, and heart disease was not even seen as a significant cause of death. In 2010, cancer and heart disease were the cause of 55 per cent of all deaths in England and Wales (ibid.: 22).

What is this telling us? Effectively, we no longer succumb rapidly to virulent disease shortly after birth. Many more of us now live long enough to face other threats to our health and, as we grow older, our bodies are less able to cope with stress. For example, Ritvanen et al. (2007) studied teachers in Finland, comparing older teachers (mean age fifty-four) with younger teachers (mean age thirty-one). It was found that both provided similar blood samples at work, yet the older teachers had significantly more cortisol (a stress hormone) in their blood after work and at weekends. It was concluded that the older teachers suffered from an inability to recover quickly from occupational stress. It is this reduced ability to bounce back from stress that provides a foundation for modern health issues. Stress hormones such as cortisol (see box 9.1) come from a family of steroid hormones known as glucocorticoids. Their purpose is to mobilize sugars (i.e. glucose) in the face of danger, providing the metabolic fuel for escape. They are short-term aids to our survival, and our ancestors either escaped danger (stressor over) or succumbed (stressor over). The system is not good in the face of long-term chronic stress, and, worse, human beings have the capacity to worry about problems that either have not yet happened or may never happen. While an animal is sated when it has a full stomach, only a human being can worry on a full stomach about where the next meal will come from (particularly in times of famine). If you lie awake at night worrying about unpaid bills, your body is still priming you to fight or flee, and stress hormones continue to be released while this stressor is ongoing. These hormones will go so far as to shut down long-term projects such as reproductive capacity (e.g., Negro-Vilar, 1993), and, yes, your immune system (e.g., Cupps and Fauci, 1982). But why? Simply put, if you are in mortal danger – or if your body believes you to be in danger – why withhold valuable resources to maintain your immune system when you may need those resources now? For an excellent entry-level read, I would suggest *Why Zebras Don't Get Ulcers* (Sapolsky, 2004).

9

What are these stress hormones, and where do they come from? When the individual is under stress, it leads to a change in activity level in the amygdala. This is a critical region for processing emotions, particularly negative emotions such as fear. When a threat is perceived, the amygdala orders activity in the hypothalamic–pituitary–adrenal axis – commonly referred to as the HPA axis. This initiates a chemical cascade that results in hormones travelling to the adrenal glands. Adrenaline is then secreted rapidly to prepare the body for action (e.g., Cannon, cited in Breedlove et al., 2010). You can tell when adrenaline is released, as blood is transferred away from the stomach (which lurches) and the skin (which pales) and towards the muscles of the arms and legs – this is the 'fight or flight' response. Cortisol is less famous but is released from the adrenal glands within two minutes of the stressor beginning, though it can take up to fifteen minutes for cortisol secretion to reach its peak. This is the critical chemical, though it is well worth noting that there is a dramatic variation in how much cortisol people release and how long it remains in circulation (e.g., Clow, 2004). However, we generally assume two hours. Unlike adrenaline, which can be released in response to positive (i.e., exciting) as well as negative (i.e., scary) events, cortisol is a useful measure of stress. It is vital to our survival and regulates our energy reserves, but constant, repeated stress leads to real problems. Long-term conditions (e.g., depression) can lead to changes in the HPA axis. Indeed, *any* change in the normal working of the HPA axis has health consequences. This is one reason why chronic stressors can be detrimental to physical and mental health.

> **Box 9.1 Key stress response (hpa axis) terminology**
>
> *Adrenaline* (aka epinephrine) – a stress hormone produced in the adrenal gland to prepare the body for action. It encourages the liver and the muscles to release sugar (glucose) to power us to safety. It is a short-term chemical and production is shut down as soon as the stressor is over.
>
> *Cortisol* – also produced in the adrenal gland. It is released fairly slowly but remains in the body for up to two hours post-stressor. It has significant effects on the immune system, rendering this less effective in the fight against disease/illness.
>
> *Hormones* – chemicals that travel through the blood to affect organs elsewhere.
>
> *Hypothalamic pituitary adrenal (HPA) axis* – when a threat is recognized, the hypothalamus (in the brain) orders the release of further chemicals from the pituitary gland (also in the brain). These travel to the adrenal glands (above the kidney), ordering the release of adrenaline and cortisol.

4 Stress and illness

Cortisol has powerful immunosuppressive properties (Cupps and Fauci, 1982). Initially, this does not make sense – times of stress may lead to increased likelihood of injury and, while modern day stressors may include mortgage payments and bad traffic, our evolutionary past prepared us for a dangerous world. Stress (and cortisol secretion) should be expected to boost our immune system at such times. If we are injured, antibodies and leukocytes should be available to rush to the point of injury and instantly overwhelm possible invasion – perhaps some bacteria living in soil trapped beneath the claw of our prehistoric attacker? If stress begets cortisol and cortisol inhibits the immune system, why do we weaken ourselves when we are most at risk of injury?

As it turns out, there is a boost to the immune system at the start of a stressor (Croiset et al., 1987). During the first thirty minutes (stress onset), immune cells pour into the bloodstream to bring the fight to infections before they gain a foothold. So far, so good, but we must realize that the fundamental role of the immune system is to recognize what is 'self' and what isn't. Furthermore, if our immune system can operate at a higher level, why doesn't it always do so? The answer is that this is too costly and too risky. For example, when our anti-cancer (NK) cells are most active, they may attack healthy cells as well as malfunctioning ones. An overactive immune system can lead to conditions such as Type 1 diabetes, where insulin-producing cells are attacked, and multiple sclerosis (MS), where the neurons are attacked in similar fashion. A hyperactive immune system is a risk in itself.

Conditions resulting from attacks from your own immune system are known as autoimmune diseases. The standard treatment for these conditions is to put the patient on steroids (e.g., Tomiyama et al., 2011). Cortisol is a steroid and, as such, will supress this hyperactivity. T-cells provide a good example. Earlier we saw how T-cells are created in the bone marrow and migrate to the thymus gland. When T-cells are available in large numbers, the thymus is sizable, and when we are under sustained stress, the thymus is smaller. Since the 1950s, it has been known that autopsies allow pathologists to observe the thymus of the deceased and to discern if the individual had been under significant stress when alive. One striking example is given by Tanegashima et al. (1999), who compared cases of suspected child abuse with an age-matched control (23 months old) obtained from unsuccessful cardiac surgery. Thymus T-cell numbers were significantly reduced in the former, and the researchers suggested that thymus size 'might be used as an index of stress in cases of child abuse/neglect' (1999: 55). Lill-Elghanian et al. (2002) reported that cortisol induces cell death (apoptosis) in T-cells and B-cells, effectively ordering the self-destruction of immune cells before they become a trigger-happy risk. There is further support from Stein, Keller and Schleifer (1985), who found fewer T-cells and B-cells in depressed patients, and from Heiser et al. (2000), who found a similar situation in sleep disorder patients. Being depressed is stressful, and being unable to sleep is also stressful. Cortisol supresses immune function, resulting in individuals being more vulnerable to disease and less able to combat that disease. In the case studied by Heiser and his colleagues, it is worth noting that, when normal sleep patterns were restored, immune function returned to normal.

Before we move on, it is worth mentioning a chemical called dehydroepiandrosterone (DHEA). Note the 'epi' in the name: this signifies that DHEA is secreted from the adrenal glands in the same way as adrenaline. Multiple studies (e.g., Sacco et al., 2002) have suggested that this chemical enhances the immune system. DHEA is 'maximal' around the age of twenty before levels reduce in later life. This has important implications for nurses and other medical staff, particularly since cortisol levels do not decline with age (Orentreich et al., 1992). As we age, we lose this DHEA 'boost', but we continue to secrete cortisol when stressed. Butcher et al. (2005) looked at thirty-five men (>65 years) recovering from hip fractures. Thirteen developed further infection, and all of them had particularly high cortisol/DHEA ratios (i.e., lots of cortisol due to stress of injury, but low DHEA levels due to age). Injury in later life is far more likely to lead to infection and complication. From a nursing point of view, it is vitally important to be aware that older patients heal more slowly and, while they do so, are uniquely vulnerable to further infection. If infected, they are less likely to be able to beat that infection rapidly, if at all.

Case Study 9.1:

Student nurse Beth is on placement in a geriatric ward. A widower, 81-year-old Max, has been admitted with a suspected fractured hip after falling at home. When this was confirmed, it was decided that Max would have a hemiarthroplasty, a procedure where the head of the femur is replaced with a false prosthesis. The aim of the procedure is to get the patient up and walking quickly, especially important in an older person. If Max is moving, risks of complication are reduced. Can you think of any other reasons as to why he needs to be up and out of hospital quickly?

---

5 Stress and cancer

Jemal, Ward and Thun (2010) show that death rates are falling in the four major cancers – bowel, female breast, lung and prostate – but cancer is still capable of being a serious and terminal condition. The body has naturally occurring immune cells which seek out proto-tumorous cells, but we now know that, in the presence of chronic stress, they are reduced in number and prone to self-destruction. Now imagine being told that you have cancer, and think about your emotional response. Perrin et al. (2006) report that the most common responses of women with abnormal smear test results are shock, fear, self-blame, powerlessness and anger, and that is not even considering the understandable increase in anxiety about their future and the future of others in their care (Baze et al., 2008; this paper is interesting since the main author – Christine Baze – relates her personal battle against cervical cancer). In the same vein, Andersen, Anderson and deProsse (1989b) published a longitudinal study investigating 'psychological outcomes' in women about to be treated for survivable cervical cancer, a second group with a more benign condition, and a control group (no cancer). Unsurprisingly, receiving a positive cancer diagnosis results in distress: both clinical depression and clinical anxiety are common, often with accompanying confusion – cancer patients often forget instructions or attend appointments at the wrong hospital or on the wrong day, for example.

We have already seen that stress makes it more probable for cancerous tumours to be missed, but, once they have taken root, stress levels continue to be a factor. Earlier in the chapter, it was stated that a prime function of cortisol is to mobilize sugars, cells releasing glucose into the bloodstream to be sent to the muscles. Unfortunately, cancerous tumour cells replicate at tremendous rates. They require vast amounts of energy to do this and so promote angiogenesis – secreting chemicals which encourage growth of blood vessels towards the tumour (e.g., Wang et al., 2010). They are also very good at absorbing glucose from blood to support their high growth rates (Gillies et al., 2008). Thus, growing tumours benefit both from an increased blood supply and from increased glucose levels, particularly during times of chronic stress (e.g., following a cancer diagnosis).

Cohen et al. (2012) suggest that depth of depression and perceived stress determine cancer survival rates. As such, to help sufferers improve their chances of survival, a worthy aim is to reduce the depression and stress suffered – while recognizing that cancer diagnoses will always be stressful and depressing and there are limits as to what can realistically be done. One classic – and controversial – study is by Spiegel et al. (1989), who took eighty-six breast cancer sufferers and designed an intervention in the hope of reducing psychological distress. There was no other aim. Fifty cancer patients were placed in a treatment group attending weekly support meetings for a year alongside their routine care regime. The control group (n = 36) received standard care only. Ten years on, only three patients remained alive, as cancer survival rates were low in the 1970s. The researchers tracked the original participants through death records and discovered that participants attending the weekly support group survived a further thirty-seven months on average, while members of the control group – who received standard care for the time, but were not invited to make use of a weekly group – survived only an extra nineteen months. Spiegel eventually abandoned his research, considering it was unethical to deny support meetings to control groups. The extra time granted the treatment group was unexpected but has led to the medical establishment realizing that doctor and patient must face cancer together, and that the psychological wellbeing of the cancer sufferer is critical to successful treatment and/or increased longevity. However, we must be cautious; these findings were not always replicated because such studies are difficult to design and implement without being unethical. Can it be morally acceptable to deny some participants a treatment you believe is effective, even if your purpose is to test that effectiveness? Many people remain unconvinced. These arguments are highlighted in *Smile or Die* (2009) by Barbara Ehrenreich, herself a past cancer sufferer. She specifically warns against 'positive thinking' – particularly the belief that someone dying of cancer 'hasn't been positive enough'. Furthermore, a recent meta-analysis (Coyne et al., 2007) has been unable to evidence clear and positive effects of counselling. The authors cite numerous methodological issues.

Activity 9.1

It may yet be shown that treatment of anxiety and depression aids the longevity of the cancer sufferer. Research confirming negative effects of stress (i.e., more rapid tumour growth) is certainly flourishing. But, even if they do not improve cancer prognosis, cancer support groups must surely improve quality of life.

As a nurse working with cancer patients, could you start a support group? Who would you ask? Would your institution be supportive? What information could you provide for sufferers and who would you invite to speak? Construct a plan to make such a support group happen. Remember, the aim is not enforced happiness – it is stress and anxiety reduction.

---

6 Personality

Personality is critical to the fight against illness, as some personalities are more prone to stress and thus more prone to illness. For example, you could split people into 'proactive' or 'reactive' groups. What does this mean? Well, one study (Koolhaas et al., 1999) used lab rats in cages with the researchers deploying electrified prods so that they jutted in through the bars. Rats, being rats, would investigate these new objects and receive small electric shocks – nothing harmful, but something akin to a static shock and not very pleasant. Some rats would be 'proactive', take their bedding and bury the prod. 'Reactive' rats would retreat to the back of the cage and ignore the prod. Both strategies are viable, as both ensure no more shocks. However, the proactive rat has removed the problem and no longer displays signs of stress, while the reactive rat still has an electrified prod in their cage, and stress levels stay high. It is much the same with humans. Remember the biopsychosocial model (chapter 2). Mindset can affect illness progression within the body. We have already seen how excessive stress results in faster tumour growth, but can certain personalities cope better than others?

Let us stay with cancer. Nakaya et al. (2006) invited 1,052 Danish residents – all born in 1936 – to a 60-minute interview in 1975/6 to assess personality traits. Thirty years later, survival rates were investigated, and the study highlighted a link between neuroticism and risk of death from all causes, including cancer – a link found to be stronger in women than in men. Neuroticism is best thought of as the tendency to feel nervous and to worry, rather than feeling calm and safe. This prompts anxiety, depression, poor sleep quality, and so on. Negative mood states are inherently stressful and so will lead to illness, a fact evidenced by studies such as that by De Jong et al. (1999), which shows that high neuroticism leads to increased stress and immune system inhibition. Grov et al. (2009) – and many others – point out that individuals exhibiting high neuroticism are much more likely to over-report problems with their health, but also that such individuals approach their doctor much earlier if they believe themselves to be ill.

It has been known for many years that high blood pressure, inactivity, obesity and smoking are all rich indicators of future cardiovascular problems. Yet you can have all four and not suffer heart disease. Something else must be missing, and that something is personality type. Friedman and Rosenman (1974) came up with the concept of the coronary-prone (Type A) behaviour pattern, and their questionnaire classified people as a 'Type-A' or a 'Type-B' personality. Day et al. (2005) define Type As as being highly motivated, with a critical sense of time urgency. They are great achievers and they push themselves – often too hard – to reach challenging goals. For example, Type-A athletes rapidly return to training after injury (Korotkov et al., 2011), risking long-term, chronic injury problems. Day et al. define the typical Type B as being less ambitious and armed with an easy-going attitude to life. Friedman and Rosenman (1974) tracked more than 3,000 men over nine years; of the 257 who died during that period, 70 per cent were Type A. They concluded that Type As are more susceptible to stress. In short, Type As tend to success, but Type Bs live longer. Admittedly, this gives the sense that being Type A is somehow 'bad', but this isn't necessarily the case. There is a subset of Type-A individuals known as Type D – 'distressed'; these are Type As with an extra so-called toxic component – i.e., hostility towards others and a fear of disapproval (see figure 9.2). Note that, even though several papers (e.g., McKenna et al., 1999) have attempted to suggest a Type-C personality style ('C' for cancer-prone), support for this is limited.

Kupper and Denollet (2007) assessed Type-D personality through the DS-14 (Type-D Scale) questionnaire. The fourteen items include 'often talks to strangers' (they don't) and 'easily irritated' (they are).

Figure 9.2 Illustrating the different personality types

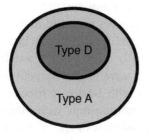
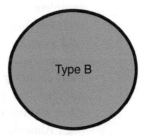

Actual numbers vary from study to study, with Bergvik et al. (2010) suggesting that 18 per cent of people are Type D, though the consensus seems to be consolidating around the 20 to 25 per cent mark. This is important, as Kupper and Denollet (2007) suggest that up to 52 per cent of cardiac patients are Type-D individuals. Type-D personalities are massively overrepresented in heart clinics. Having a certain personality means more day-to-day irritation and stress when dealing with others. Over a lifespan, this puts pressure on the heart and increases the risk of heart disease in later life. (The concept of personality types relating to health was also discussed in chapter 2.)

Case Study 9.2:

In her time on the ward, student nurse Beth has got to know Max quite well. He is a lively conversationalist, quite open and very cheerful. However, Beth learns that, apart from losing his wife some years ago, Max lives by himself; his only son lives some way away, with a family of his own, and is 'very busy'. At eighty-one years old, Max has outlived many of his long-term friends and, so far, has not received a visitor.

Considering what we have learnt, take stock of Max's personality and situation. Is he more likely to be a Type-A or a Type-B personality (or somewhere in between)? Are there factors likely to shield Max from the risk of further illness/infection while recovering on the ward (e.g., MSRA) or others which would make it more likely?

---

7 Conclusion

This chapter has covered a lot of ground, first explaining the immune system and the stress response and then the interaction between the two – the new-found field of psychoneuroimmunology. Stress results temporarily in a heightened immune response, but the cost of maintaining such vigilance is too high. Quickly, large numbers of natural killer cells would attack the 'self' as well as the 'non-self'. Stress hormones limit this risk by blunting the immune response, though, in the aftermath, this leaves us more vulnerable than before – succumbing to illness and taking longer to recover. Consider the major events in our lives – the bereavements, the uncertainties, the long hours and the looming deadlines. These really do leave us more vulnerable. One last example is from Cohen et al. (1998), who asked 276 participants to complete a life stressor interview and provide blood and urine samples to assess their stress levels before being inoculated with the common cold virus by way of nasal spray. Participants reporting month-long stressors were significantly more likely to catch a cold. Typically, the most enduring stressors were unemployment (or fear of job loss) and interpersonal problems with family or friends. Social stressors – i.e., stress stemming from relationships with others – are always potent (e.g., Almeida, 2005). Isolation in later life is also relevant, as people outlive friends and family. During your career it is likely that you will come across many older people who are much more vulnerable to disease and infection than they ever were before.

Summary

▶ The immune system defends the body by way of antibodies and white blood cells.
▶ The stress response results in the secretion of immunosuppressants (e.g., cortisol).
▶ Although the immune response is initially robust, the presence of cortisol reduces its effectiveness over time. This reduces the risk of a 'trigger-happy' immune system attacking the body's own cells.
▶ Personality and environment can moderate the ability of the body to withstand and recover from disease.

Questions for discussion

1 Is there such a thing as a 'wrong' personality type? Are some people, through no conscious choice of their own, more likely to become ill and be less able to recover from illness?
2 If such people do exist, what can nurses do to tackle the problem? Is face-to-face patient time an important consideration in swift and effective treatment?
3 Does a more challenging and difficult life – e.g., membership of an ethic minority group or low socio-economic status – lead to a greater likelihood of succumbing to illness?

9

Further reading

The following books are interesting and may enhance your understanding of the issues discussed here. The first chapter of Ehrenreich is particularly relevant, as it takes a critical viewpoint of 'positive psychology'. Sapolsky's volume is excellent, and he covers the stress literature in an enjoyable and amusing way.

Ehrenreich, B. (2009) *Smile or Die: How Positive Thinking Fooled America and the World*. London: Granta.

Sapolsky, R. 2004. *Why Zebras Don't Get Ulcers*. 3rd edn, New York: Henry Holt.

CHAPTER

10 Anxiety and Depression

Joe MacDonagh

CHAPTER CONTENTS

KEY ISSUES IN THIS CHAPTER:

▶ The nature of anxiety and depression
▶ How anxiety and depression affect people's lives
▶ Socio-cultural and environmental causes of anxiety and depression
▶ Nursing interventions for people with anxiety or depression

BY THE END OF THIS CHAPTER YOU SHOULD BE ABLE TO:

▶ describe generalized anxiety and panic disorders
▶ detail the main anxiety disorders and how they affect sufferers
▶ explain the biological, genetic and social causes of anxiety and depression
▶ outline some of the key nursing responses to those with anxiety or depression.

1 Introduction

In the course of your nursing work you will see patients and colleagues from different professional backgrounds with symptoms of anxiety and depression, as these occur across all backgrounds and in all walks of life. The focus on anxiety and depression in the media has led to ordinary people and well-known celebrities discussing their mental health issues publicly in a way not seen in previous generations, and many people are now keener to open up about their condition. So patients will want your support and advice as a nurse on possible treatments in coping with their anxiety or depression. These are particularly important, as they have a significant impact upon the quality of the lives of sufferers and of those around them. Nurses are well placed to understand anxiety and depression because they are privy to important social and personal details of a patient's life as well as their physical condition.

In this chapter we will examine the nature, theories and treatment of anxiety and depression in order to inform effective professional nursing practice. The chapter is divided according to anxiety and mood disorders.

Activity 10.1

So far, student nurse Beth has completed a number of nursing degree placements. One of her last was in a psychiatric setting, where adults of widely varying ages presented with a variety of challenging and chronic psychiatric disorders. Now she is back on a general surgical ward with patients of various ages and genders.

Before she began on this ward Beth discussed her last placement with the ward sister, who asked her what she had learnt from her experience and how the placement would inform her ongoing nursing practice. She asked Beth to reflect on how many of the psychiatric disorders she encountered may also be present in patients on this surgical ward and how they might affect different patients' care issues.

You may also have experience in some psychiatric or supported care settings, and a ward sister or charge nurse might ask you to consider the following questions. Based on your experience on different wards, how do you think psychological problems can cause or exacerbate physical illness? What influence do you think physical illness has on patients' psychological health? What would your answers be?

10

2 Anxiety disorders

All human beings feel anxious at some stage, but a minority experience anxiety on a chronic or continual basis, and this may have profound influences on their social and physical functioning. Such people may be made more anxious by being in hospital and away from their comfort zone, often their home, where they have developed anxiety coping mechanisms; it is important to be sensitive to whether a patient seems to be exhibiting a reasonable or heightened level of anxiety while being treated. In the absence of stated medication on their chart, it is important to observe for symptoms of anxiety.

- *Physiological* – the fight or flight response for stress, where heart rate is elevated and adrenaline is secreted. The body is reacting to a perceived threat, such as speaking in public, being in confined spaces or even seeing a spider. The extent of the threat is exaggerated and the anxiety response may continue when no threat is present.
- *Cognitive* – those who are anxious feel the worst is going to happen and they see problems when none actually exist. They have a heightened sense of alertness, or hypervigilance, to something happening.
- *Emotional* – people who are anxious are worried that something is going to happen, so they are fearful, restless and upset.
- *Behavioural* – faced with a perceived threat, a person may withdraw or defend (De Loos, 2001). This may involve aggression, as they feel under threat, and so their defence reaction is elevated.

All of the above symptoms apply to specific disorders, and it is important to remember that patients are acting unusually compared to others, as they are highly anxious about the ward surroundings plus their treatment outcome and what the latter will mean for their future social and physical functioning. In the first instance, patients should be informed about what they can expect from their hospital stay, which will help them not to be de-personalized or disempowered. We will look at further ways of helping patients below. For the purposes of this chapter, we will focus on two anxiety disorders which you may come across in your nursing career: generalized anxiety disorder and panic disorder.

2.1 Generalized anxiety disorder (GAD)

In addition to the symptoms above, those with GAD tend to worry chronically and extremely about both minor and major parts of their lives and feel that this worrying is uncontrollable; as many as 80 per cent of those with GAD may also have symptoms of depression (Bakish, 1999). This can profoundly inhibit their functioning, as much of their life is taken up trying to cope with this anxiety.

Women have significantly higher incidences of most anxiety disorders. These often occur with depression, which women also suffer from in higher numbers than men. Eaton et al. (2011), in the USA, found that there was a significant difference between both the GAD incidence in a national sample for females (5.8%) and males (3.1%) and for panic disorder in females (7.2%) and males (3.7%). They suggest this may be because women tend to 'report higher frequencies of some stressful life events than men do', and this is often coupled with environmental stressors, such as being poor and being a mother (Perry, 1996).

Case Study 10.1:

It all started years ago. I don't know when. I suppose it was after I lost my job and my confidence dried up. I wasn't able to provide for my family and I felt useless. Then I thought I was good at nothing and people would see this and I'd be found out. I went for a few job interviews but I was getting increasingly anxious before them. I'd sweat and sweat and would completely forget what I wanted to say in the interview, so I stopped applying for jobs. It didn't finish there, because I started getting wound up before family occasions and I would drink to calm my nerves, but that made it worse. So now I avoid anniversaries, birthdays and the rest of them. I'm starting to find going down to the shops difficult and I get my partner to buy as much as possible. I stay in watching TV a lot, which means I'm heavier than I've ever been and I'm starting to get out of breath when I climb the stairs. The last time I went to the GP she said she wanted me to come in for tests, because she said that she didn't like the fact that I was having chest pains, and that's why I'm here.

This was what one patient, Mike, said to student nurse Beth when she brought over his breakfast one morning. Patients often feel they can confide in nurses, and they may do so unexpectedly because they feel vulnerable or because that nurse has said or done something that suggests to the patient that they're more likely to understand what they are experiencing.

In this case Mike is describing how a general feeling of anxiety came to dominate his life, beginning with a perception that he had let down his family and leading to a feeling that he couldn't go out, which ultimately had an impact upon his health. The key issue for the care team will be to see how Mike's physical and psychological issues are interrelated and how they can be addressed. This may involve a combination of anxiety medication and a referral to a psychologist to help him to cope with each of his anxieties and how they relate to his overall anxiety. We will look at the possible medications and therapies available for GAD sufferers later in this chapter.

10

As seen in the case study above, GAD often has an impact upon all aspects of a sufferer's life. Its origin may be in a particular incident, or series of incidents, and then the inability to cope may be generalized. It may also have derived from the person's family, as anxiety may have genetic or behavioural origins. Either way, there are drug and behavioural treatments for this condition. These will be examined at the end of the next section, on panic disorder, on account of the similarities between the latter and GAD.

2.2 Panic disorder

Case Study 10.2:

Student nurse Beth was making a bed when she saw an older female patient, called Esther, leaning against a window sill looking distressed and peering around the ward wide-eyed, with an anxious expression on her face. Beth put down the sheet she was holding and went over to help Esther. As she did so, she saw that Esther was taking increasingly shallow breaths and was getting quite distressed. Beth called a fully trained nurse colleague over,

> **Case Study 10.2 (continued)**
>
> and they quickly established from her behaviour that Esther had had a panic attack. They helped her to sit down and reassured her that her breathing would go back to normal and that both of them were there to help her.
>
> Beth and her colleague are acting here as 'safe persons' (Sloan and Telch, 2002), which can be a very helpful way of assisting someone who is experiencing a panic attack, as the person is reassured by their physical presence and by expressions of comfort and support from people they perceive to be safe.
>
> When her breathing was deeper and more regular, Esther told Beth and her colleague that she had started having panic attacks after her first operation, for gallstones, as it went badly and she was in great pain.
>
> Then she started having these attacks every time she went to her GP, often in the waiting room. Now they were unpredictable, and she got upset at the thought of them happening to her in public places, so she tried to go out at night so others would not see her if she suffered an attack.
>
> Beth's colleague said to Esther that she would ask a psychologist to pop in to see her so that she could discuss her attacks and to examine the possibility of therapy when she was discharged. Before then she said she would give Esther some hospital leaflets and a book from the hospital library on anxiety and how best to manage it.

It is not always easy to tell when someone is having a panic attack, except as in the case study above when the person may be struggling to catch their breath, may be shaking and may be near to collapse or fainting. Panic attacks profoundly affect a patient's functioning and can be misinterpreted as a physical illness. If they are a common occurrence and do not seem to be provoked by anything in particular, and if people are worried about attacks so much that they change their behaviour, a diagnosis of panic disorder may be appropriate. This appears to be happening in case study 10.2, as the patient has had increasing attacks and is now changing the times she leaves her house. Panic disorder tends to be chronic once begun and is often co-morbid with GAD, depression and alcohol abuse (Craske and Waters, 2005). Nurses can provide the means for patients to discuss what they have experienced and thus can help patients to be aware of, and access, appropriate psychological and social support services.

2.3 Theories and treatments

In this section we will look at some approaches to the causes and treatment of anxiety.

2.3.1 Biological theory

This suggests that GAD has a biological cause. The GABA (gamma-aminobutyric acid) theory, for example, states that people with GAD have a deficiency in GABA, or in the number of GABA receptors – GABA being a neurotransmitter involved in the limbic system which affects behavioural, emotional and physiological responses to threat (Kalueff and Nutt, 2007). Those with this deficiency express anxious behaviour and feel general threats from their environment. We will see, below, that other researchers believe that such behaviours are being learnt from others, particularly one's family.

To address the biological deficiency which causes anxious behaviour, benzodiazepenes increase activity of gamma-aminobutyric acid (GABA). They are often prescribed only for short-term ease of anxiety symptoms as they can be addictive and have unwanted withdrawal symptoms, such as high levels of anxiety. Azapirones (Caycedo and Griez, 2001) reduce anxiety, have fewer side effects than benzodiazepenes, and are less likely to lead to dependency. Finally, some anti-depressants called selective serotonin reuptake inhibitors (SSRIs) have been shown to reduce anxiety and can be effective with some anxiety disorders (Nutt, 2001). Since they are often used with other anti-depressants, they are considered in greater detail in the section on depression below.

Anti-depressants are also highly effective in reducing panic attacks (Hollander and Simeon, 2008), which suggests that neurotransmitters are implicated in panic disorder and the diffuse, anticipatory anxiety that leads to panic attacks. Therefore, according to this approach, panic disorders have a biological basis. Suggested treatment involves benzodiazepenes, tricyclic anti-depressants or SSRIs.

2.3.2 Genetic theory

This suggests that those who are anxious have inherited their anxiety from their parents. In this respect, Noyes et al. (1987) suggest that those with GAD have a statistically higher chance of having relatives who also suffer from GAD. Another explanation for this could be that certain maladaptive behaviours are learnt in a family, rather than those behaviours being genetically inherited. This hypothesis, of familial influence upon anxiety, is examined further under the diathesis-stress theory below. Panic disorder may also run in families, and people whose parents or close relatives suffer from it are at heightened risk of having the condition themselves (Cavallini and Bellodi, 2005; Craske and Waters, 2005). This school of thought strongly emphasizes drug therapy as the treatment approach.

2.3.3 Cognitive theory

The cognitive theory suggests that those with GAD have maladaptive threat responses which predispose them to anxiety. These may be rigid and absolute and difficult to satisfy – e.g., 'I need to be alert at all times in hospital because prescription mistakes can be fatal.' In addition, people experiencing panic attacks may pay overly close attention to bodily sensations and may misinterpret them in a negative way. They may also engage in 'catastrophic' thinking or, if a patient, imagine the worst from their perceived symptoms. They may also worry about worrying, and so it may be important to help them cope, initially, with the effect of this worrying before attending to the root causes.

Cognitive behavioural therapy (CBT) (see chapter 12) helps people identify their automatic thoughts – of inability to cope in a social setting for example – and how these may lead them to become anxious or depressed. This approach enables the patient to develop coping mechanisms which help free them from high levels of anxiety and panic. CBT involves getting people with GAD or panic disorder to confront their anxieties by challenging and changing irrational thoughts.

CBT can be as effective as drug therapies and is more effective in preventing relapse (Borkovec et al., 2003), as those with anxiety can develop such coping strategies as relaxation and breathing techniques. If a panic disorder sufferer has a 'safe person' nearby, someone with whom they feel comfortable, they are less likely to experience emotional and physical symptoms of anxiety. Nurses may be able to fill this role when a patient experiences panic in hospital. Although this may lead to excessive 'checking in' by some patients (i.e., overly referring to the safe person such that they cannot function unless they do so), the safe person provides a basis from which patients can address their anxiety.

2.3.4 Diathesis-stress model

This model suggests that the cause of a mental disorder lies in a person's upbringing. For example, research (Ingram and Luxton, 2005) has found that, if a person is brought up in a family where they do not have strong bonds with one or both parents, and do not have a strong and supporting network of friends or relatives, then, if they experience adverse life experiences, they are more likely to develop a mental disorder – in this case, anxiety. Conversely, those who have strong parental bonds and well-developed social networks are more able to cope with life stressors and are less likely to develop mental disorders. Some also term this type of effective coping as 'resilience' and suggest that, the more resilient a person is, through having learnt resilience skills in their family, the more they are able to cope with life's difficulties.

Treatment under this model involves helping the person to develop their social network, their coping skills and their resilience in addressing stressful life events. It can also involve helping them to work with their family to address factors which caused, or prevented them coping with, life stressors. This treatment can involve the therapeutic interventions mentioned here and in other chapters (see particularly chapter 12 on CBT).

2.3.5 Socio-cultural influences: drift and social causation models

Other socio-cultural theories of mental disorders, applicable to both anxiety and mood disorders, are the 'drift' and the 'social causation' theories of mental illness (Hurst, 2012). The drift theory states that, because their illness influences their life chances, those who have mental disorders are more likely to move downwards in social class. This comes about because those from poorer social classes have less access to health services and so have poorer health outcomes.

The social causation theory, often taken as the opposite of the drift theory, says that those from less advantaged social classes are more likely to have (or be labelled as having) a mental illness and to find it harder to address. However, the theory also states that those suffering from mental disorders are from a lower social class to begin with, rather than finding themselves in that class by virtue of their illness, as the drift hypothesis suggests.

Whether you find the drift model or the social causation model to be more appropriate to a particular patient, proper health service supports will be more likely to help that person to address their issues and ensure they are better placed to prevent a reoccurrence.

2.4 Summary and evaluation

In this section on anxiety disorders we have examined a number of theories and treatments, ranging from the biological and genetic approaches to the cognitive and the social and socio-cultural approaches. In terms of treating anxiety disorders, cognitive behavioural therapy coupled with drug therapies can be effective in initially stabilizing the patient and providing them with concrete ways to address their condition (Craske and Waters, 2005).

3 Depression

According to Reber et al. (2004), depression is a 'mood state characterized by a sense of inadequacy, a feeling of despondency, a decrease in activity or reactivity, pessimism, sadness and related symptoms'.

Case Study 10.3:

One of the more chaotic, but enjoyable, training stints for student nurse Beth was on a maternity ward. The beaming mothers and proud fathers were initially emotional and worried but ultimately very grateful once their newborn baby was in their arms. The exception was Jenny, a woman in her mid-thirties, who was expecting her third child. Though her husband and family were regular visitors, she seemed to be muted in her responses to everyone. When Beth went into her room, Jenny would often be staring into

Case Study 10.3 (continued)

space, and it would take a minute or two for her to realize Beth was in the room. Once or twice Beth found Jenny weeping to herself.

Beth was so concerned about this that she told the ward sister what had happened and when. The ward sister said she remembered Jenny from when she had been in for her first two children. She said Jenny had suffered post-natal depression after her second child and that the depression had continued since then; her chart stated she was on anti-depressants. She said she would inform the resident psychiatrist and that Beth was to report any future symptoms, such as Jenny's ruminating behaviour (excessively going over things in her mind, shown by her seeming to be staring into space and being very distracted). The ward sister told Beth that, while a number of women suffer from post-natal depression, for some this could develop into a major depressive disorder. She also told Beth it was important for her to notice important indicators of depression, such as withdrawal, muted social behaviour and ruminating.

The British prime minister Winston Churchill referred to his depression as his 'black dog', and many well-known public figures have also suffered from depression, such as Diana, Princess of Wales, and the American actress Angelina Jolie. The journalist Rosemary McCabe wrote about her experience of trying to explain her depression to those around her:

> But how can you explain depression, despair and feelings of hopelessness to people who cannot – and will not – understand? But I am suffering, alongside many others. There is something fundamentally wrong with how I cope with stress, or with how I rationalise disappointment, or maybe just with how my brain manufactures serotonin … depression is something deeper, more insidious, that cannot always be expressed or explained. (McCabe, 2013)

What McCabe describes is part of depression, as are the feelings of sadness, of a sense of loss and of a sense of hopelessness about the future.

Depression involves disruptions in emotion, bodily function, behaviour and thought.

- *Emotional symptoms* These include 'anhedonia' – a loss of interest in, or not being able to feel, pleasure. There may also be a feeling of sadness and a sense of loss.
- *Physiological symptoms* Appetite is disrupted, with some people eating less and some eating more. While there may be extremes and other depression symptoms, there is a change from a patient's normal functioning. The change may involve, for example, the amount and type of food they normally eat. Both sleep and the sleep cycle are disrupted, which may involve early waking, sleeping less or sleeping more. Activity changes may include a depressed person moving more sluggishly, reacting more slowly, and being quieter in their speech and gestures, or they may be

the exact opposite – not being able to sit still, moving around, and fidgeting excessively with, for example, their hair, clothes or possessions. Exhaustion may be evident, with the depressed person complaining of constantly feeling tired.

- *Cognitive symptoms* Hopelessness, poor concentration, poor self-esteem, indecisiveness and inhibition of cognitive functioning are some of the main cognitive symptoms. In extreme cases, delusions and hallucinations occur.

In terms of depression symptoms and nursing practice, it is important to observe how the patient eats, sleeps, shows emotions, concentrates and performs tasks and to discuss any changes with their family. It will then be easier to understand how their social functioning has changed and how it may be addressed as part of their care plan (Melnyk and Fineout-Overholt, 2010).

3.1 Factors influencing depression

Diagnosis for depression is based on the severity of a patient's symptoms and for how long these continue. So, while many people cry and find it hard to eat or sleep normally after a significant negative life event, such as the death of a loved one, losing a job or undergoing a change in relationship status such as divorce, if this continues for a significant amount of time and inhibits work and social functioning, a diagnosis of depression may be appropriate (American Psychiatric Association, 2013).

Depression, if untreated, has profound consequences for people's physical health. It can make periods of stay longer for patients and make it difficult for them to overcome the physical disorder with which they present in hospital. Though depression may not be visible in the same way as a physical illness, it is just as important. Treating the condition holistically, in terms of a person's whole social functioning, will improve the chance of a successful care outcome.

3.1.1 Demographic factors

In terms of age, people between fifteen and twenty-four, those in early adulthood, are most likely to be diagnosed as clinically depressed (Rohde et al., 2013). Women are more likely to suffer depression than men, with a significant difference emerging from age thirteen onwards (Kessler, 2000; Nolen-Hoeksema, 2002), and are also at a heightened risk of depression after giving birth (Spinelli and Broudy, 2013). Eaton et al. (2011) suggest that 'one major theory to account for gender differences in depression involves the notion that women ruminate more frequently than men, focusing repetitively on their negative emotions and problems rather than engaging in more active problem solving.' This may be because women often occupy secondary and dependent places in society and in relationships; they suffer more from poverty, being in less powerful societal places (Nolen-Hoeksema, 2002), and from the social isolation of child-minding.

3.2 Theories and treatments: depression

There are three key theories and approaches to depression: biological, psychological and social.

3.2.1 Biological

The main biological theory is based on the number and efficiency of neurotransmitters in people suffering from depression. Those who favour the biological approach concentrate on the efficacy of anti-depressants acting on neurotransmitters – those chemical substances which regulate the transmission of signals across the synapses, or gaps, between neurons. The main neurotransmitters related to mood disorders are serotonin, norepinephrine and dopamine. The theories about their role include the lack of them, the lack of receptors for them, and their varying sensitivity at different times and in a person's differing mood states. Anti-depressants thus act in different ways on neurotransmitters to regulate a patient's mood.

All anti-depressants and their dosage must be appropriate for the mood disorder, based on the patient's feedback. Adjustment may be necessary if the patient feels that medication has not significantly improved their functioning or if the improvement in functioning is outweighed by side effects, which are pronounced for some people on certain anti-depressants (see box 10.1 for a list of the main anti-depressants).

Box 10.1 The main anti-depressants

Tricyclic anti-depressants: TRAs prevent the reuptake of the neurotransmitters norepinephrine and serotonin. The side effects can include excessive sweating, a dry mouth, blurred vision, sexual dysfunction, constipation and urinary retention. They can be fatal in overdose, which may be small multiples of the prescribed dose. Some patients may have to wait between one and two months for the drug to take effect.

Monoamine oxidase inhibitors (MAOIs): MAOIs prevent the MAO enzyme from causing the breakdown of neurotransmitters. Inhibiting this enzyme increases the amount of neurotransmitters in the synapses and so relieves depressive symptoms. They are as effective as tricyclics, but the side effects can include potentially fatal levels of high blood pressure if patients eat foods high in the amino acid tyramine, found in rich cheeses, chocolate, beer and red wine. Other side effects are similar to those with the TRAs, among them weight gain, liver damage and abnormally low blood pressure.

Selective serotonin reuptake inhibitors (SSRIs): SSRIs have a similar action to the TRAs but work in a different manner to prevent serotonin reuptake, which inhibits its effect. They begin acting within a few weeks for many

> **Box 10.1 (continued)**
>
> people, have less unpleasant side effects than other anti-depressants for some, are not usually fatal when taken in overdose, and are often used for other things such as anxiety disorders and problem eating. The side effects reported by some include feeling agitated, feeling unable to stop moving around, sexual dysfunction and indigestion. There have been reports of an increase in the risk of suicide for adolescents and the under twenty-fives on SSRIs.

Electro-convulsive therapy (ECT) is a controversial treatment (NICE, 2003). It involves sedating the patient, giving muscle relaxants and passing an electrical current through the brain. Proponents say it is successful with those who have not responded to drug therapies or who are severely catatonic – i.e., those who are very muted in their behaviour and who may whisper, if speaking at all, stare absently for long periods of time, and may occasionally hug themselves while rocking in the same spot and seem unresponsive to other therapies. Proponents say it is used carefully and only when other options have been exhausted. Those who oppose it say the memory loss it often induces is not acceptable and in some cases is permanent.

3.2.2 Psychological

In this section we will examine the behavioural (diathesis-stress and learned helplessness), cognitive and behavioural (CBT) and social (cohort effect) theories.

Behavioural: The diathesis-stress model we encountered in the anxiety section suggests that depression occurs because of negative life stressors coupled with a biological or genetic predisposition to depression and a poor parent–child attachment (MacDonagh, 2012), all occurring with a weak and unsupportive social network. Nurses can play an important role in a patient's care plan with observations and information they may receive from the patient about their social functioning. This can be used to help the patient in the long term to develop greater resilience and to address some of the reasons why they may not have a supportive network of family or friends.

Learned helplessness: If people face a constant stream of negative events and they feel they can do nothing about them, then they may feel helpless. Those in abusive or dysfunctional relationships may feel that, no matter what they do, they will suffer negative behaviour, so they feel helpless to do anything about it. Thus they 'learn' or generalize this helplessness to other situations, give up trying to resolve difficulties in their lives and slip into depression (Seligman, 1975). Peterson and Seligman (1984) reformulated the theory of helplessness to focus on how depressed people blame themselves for negative events, expect negative events in the future and feel they can't do anything about them.

Cognitive and behavioural: Aaron Beck is best known for his work in CBT (see chapter 12), but he also developed one of the most widely used scales for diagnosing depression: the Beck Depression Inventory (2008). He believed that those with depression make mistakes in how they view the world, often being incorrectly negative about themselves, the world and the future. Beck also believed that people with depression may exaggerate the negative in their lives and jump to conclusions based on little evidence. They may also overgeneralize a negative event to all possible and future events, seeing things in black and white terms, ignoring the positive, blaming themselves for things for which they were not responsible, and employing too many 'should' statements about things which are hard to achieve and about which they feel guilt and anger when they can't be achieved.

CBT is frequently represented as a means of identifying a client's triggers – those things which may make them automatically engage in types of behaviour which cause their depression to continue or a cycle of depression to begin.

3.2.3 Social theories

The cohort or group theory of depression suggests that there are different incidences of depression in different age groups. Kessler et al. (1994) present figures showing that younger age cohorts are significantly more likely to suffer from depression. Kessler (2000) suggests these figures show that 'there is a consistent trend for lifetime prevalence to be higher at all ages in successively younger cohorts … [meaning] that life-time major depression is becoming more common in recent cohorts', and that this may be due to older age groups, particularly those over the age of sixty, being more likely to have grown up in a time when closer communities provided greater social support. Conversely, younger age groups grew up in a time of significantly greater socio-cultural change and uncertainty, with traditional communities and familial structures changing rapidly, leading to less social support and therefore increased chance of depression. Furthermore, according to this theory, younger age cohorts tend to experience major depressive episodes earlier than those in older age cohorts. The greater, and earlier, incidence has implications for interventions with younger age groups, both in terms of public policy and in terms of providing treatment.

4 Conclusion

We have dealt with a great deal of information relating to anxiety and depression in this chapter. Resources and further reading, in addition to the references already cited, are mentioned below and will allow you to keep up to date with the latest research in this area. Both anxiety and depression can be chronic conditions, but recovery can be improved by an alert nurse who is sensitive to a patient's particular experience and how treatment may be tailored to address these issues.

Summary

▶ Anxiety disorders include generalised anxiety disorder and panic disorder.
▶ Anxiety disorders can be treated with benzodiazepenes, azaspirones and anti-depressants and talking therapies such as cognitive behavioural therapy (CBT).
▶ Depression is usually treated with drugs such as tricyclic anti-depressants, monoamine oxidase inhibitors or selective serotonin reuptake inhibitors and with cognitive behavioural therapy.

Questions for discussion

1 Suggest ways in which nurses can help patients to cope with their anxiety disorders and avoid future severe anxiety.
2 Consider how you would describe the benefits of CBT to a patient and how it would help them with their anxiety or depression.
3 How could you, as a nurse, explain to a patient the different types of anti-depressant medication and how these can help their depression?

Further Reading

Bentall, R. (2003) *Madness Explained*. London: Penguin.
An engaging, highly researched book challenging many psychology and psychiatry orthodoxies.

Rowe, D. (2003) *Depression: The Way out of Your Prison*. 3rd edn, London: Routledge.
A well-written self-help book on depression which could be recommended to sufferers.

Solomon, A. (2002) *The Noonday Demon: An Anatomy of Depression*. London: Vintage.
One of the most comprehensive books on the experience and treatment of depression, written by a sufferer.

Taylor, M. A., and Fink, M. (2006) *Melancholia*. Cambridge: Cambridge University Press.
Writing from a medical perspective, Taylor and Fink believe that melancholia is a more accurate term for depression, which is reflected in their diagnosis and treatment.

Yalom, I. D. (2006) *Momma and the Meaning of Life*. New York: Harper Perennial.
Excellent clinical short stories giving insights from a very famous psychotherapist.

10

The following online resources provide up-to-date and detailed material on psychology:

British Psychological Society blogspot: http://bps-research-digest.blogspot.ie/.

Blog of the (Aaron) Beck Institute: http://www.beckinstituteblog.org/.

The Mental Health Foundation: http://www.mentalhealth.org.uk/.

Altered Mental States

Steve Williams and Gabrielle Tracy McClelland

CHAPTER CONTENTS

KEY ISSUES IN THIS CHAPTER:

▶ Definitions and prominent features of psychosis
▶ Cognitive models underpinning psychosis
▶ Evidence-based cognitive behavioural therapy interventions in the treatment of psychosis
▶ Psychological theories of substance misuse and the impact of alcohol and substance misuse on psychological health
▶ Evidence-based interventions to support clients experiencing psychological difficulties due to alcohol and other drug misuse

BY THE END OF THIS CHAPTER YOU SHOULD BE ABLE TO:

▶ describe the main psychological theories and some of the features of cognitive behavioural therapy (CBT) for psychosis
▶ discuss the causes and manifestations of psychosis
▶ describe the causes and consequences associated with alcohol and other drug use
▶ describe the relevant factors associated with the assessment of alcohol and drug use.

1 Introduction

This chapter introduces and critically explores pyschosis. It outlines the definitions of relevant aspects of psychosis and discusses some of the implications and difficulties inherent in this. Major current psychological theories and models of psychosis and associated research are dealt with. The aetiology of psychosis is reviewed in the light of current accumulated evidence. Psychological interventions for psychosis and the relevant research evidence is overviewed. The role of drugs and alcohol in psychosis is then explored with attention to the role of the nurse and how this influences treatment. A series of interlinked case studies are provided to illustrate key points, highlight the potential role for the nurse, and stimulate the reader's reflective thinking.

2 What is psychosis?

Psychosis is a term strongly associated with schizophrenia. It is, however, a condition that can be found in a wide variety of health contexts. These include other mental health diagnoses, such as post-traumatic stress disorder, depression and bipolar affective disorder, as well as states of deprivation (e.g., sensory, sleep), drug-induced contexts and neurological conditions such as epilepsy and migraines. According to the Royal College of Psychiatrists (2012), psychosis happens 'when your thoughts are so disturbed that you lose touch with reality', signifying a severe underlying mental illness.

For nursing, psychosis is an umbrella term for a range of psychiatric diagnoses (e.g., bipolar affective disorder, delusional disorder, schizophrenia) that collectively form the 'severe mental illnesses' (SMI) (Ruggeri et al., 2000). According to the American Psychiatric Association, a person has an SMI 'when he or she has the following: a diagnosis of any non-organic psychosis; a duration of treatment of two years or more; [and] dysfunction, as measured by the Global Assessment of Functioning (GAF) scale' (cited in Ruggeri et al., 2000: 2). This historical distinction between types of psychoses attempted to differentiate between 'organic psychoses', where there is known organic brain damage, and 'functional psychoses', where there is an absence of this (Coltheart et al., 2011). This distinction assumed that cognitive deficits (i.e., qualitative shifts in the nature of thinking processes) for 'functional' psychoses were somehow not brain-based or neurological (Green and Harvey, 2014). This distinction has turned out to be fundamentally flawed, as is evident in the failure of neuropsychological testing to distinguish between cognitive deficits accompanying so-called functional (i.e., 'non-neurological') psychoses such as schizophrenia and those present in cases of head injury (ibid.). It also fails to reflect accurately the findings of neuroimaging studies that have uncovered significant differences in the appearance of brains in people with these diagnoses – e.g., the enlargement of the ventricles (Weinberger et al., 1979). There is currently a widespread consensus that psychosis has a strong biological component that, alongside other psychosocial factors (such as adverse life events, adverse environments, illicit drug use or periods of social isolation), contributes to a 'vulnerable predisposition' to psychosis (Garety et al., 2001).

'Recovery-based' nursing critiques of pathophysiological accounts of mental health difficulties have questioned the arbitrary nature of such definitions (Slade, 2009). For example, why should a person have to have two years' duration of treatment to meet the criteria of an SMI? Recovery, emerging from service-user/survivor accounts, emphasizes the value of living with and growing beyond distressing experiences (Deegan, 1988). This has become an alternative approach for understanding and thinking about working with 'mental illness' and calls for a shift in emphasis. In the traditional approach to working with mental illness, the central preoccupation is treatment of the symptoms and, as a result, wider contextual factors that can maintain difficulties can be sidelined (Williams, 2015).

The recovery approach does not call for the abandonment of treatment but, rather, for the recognition that it is just as important to address other aspects of the person's life. One example of this is that people with an SMI can often be prevented from working until their treatment has had a sufficient positive impact. Randomized trials of tailored supportive work programmes, however, have shown that people with an SMI show greater improvement in their condition when they are able to return to meaningful paid employment (Bond et al., 2001). Work is, of course, one of the ways in which we define ourselves and can foster the development of self-agency, positive self-regard and self-worth. The recovery approach emphasizes the need for services actively to support people in terms of their wider life goals that can help develop a valuable and meaningful life (Williams, 2015). Our case study of Jim will introduce aspects of the nature of psychosis and illustrate key aspects of both relevant theory and nursing practice.

11

Case Study 11.1: Introducing Jim

Jim (47) is troubled by voices saying he's 'special'. The television is talking to him about what he's doing. This has become more frequent over the last three months. To others he appears occasionally perplexed, sometimes distant, and troubled by something they cannot hear. His daughter Susan (21) has found him arguing loudly to empty space. He denies these things when questioned directly. His mood can change rapidly, but there are also long periods of relative stability. These mood changes can be a quick succession of tearful, distressed, angry, bemused and amused – in response to auditory experiences. Jim is becoming secretive and is collecting random newspaper articles.

2.1 Psychological accounts of psychosis

Psychosis encompasses a range of experiences and typically includes emotional changes and dysfunction in the cognitive processes of attention, perception or judgement. The most prominent signs of psychosis, particularly early on, are 'delusional beliefs' and 'hallucinations' (Garety et al., 2001).

Psychological accounts typically focus on these specific experiences, although some do seek to account for the entire diversity of experiences (Fletcher and Frith, 2009). Morrison (2001) proposes that the unusual experiences of psychosis, such as hearing voices that others cannot hear or seeing things that others cannot see, are examples of 'cognitive intrusion'. Intrusions are experiences (such as repetitive thoughts, images or impulses) that are unwanted and distressing and experienced as interrupting the person's ongoing mental activity. In Morrison's model, internal or external triggers result in an experience that is then misinterpreted as threatening the physical or psychological safety of the person. This leads to a negative mood (e.g., fear) and physiological arousal that, in turn, produces more unwanted experiences in a vicious cycle.

Morrison's 'intrusion model' thus seeks to account for 'delusions' and 'hallucinations' as experiences that are then misinterpreted in terms of what they mean. Jim hears, or perhaps mis-hears, the sounds from the television as saying something about him personally. He might then have thoughts seeking to interpret this, such as 'The telly is talking about me', 'I must be mad', 'Something bad is going to happen', that elicit strong feelings of fear. This in turn may trigger behaviours that are 'safety seeking' – for instance, 'hypervigilance'. Hypervigilance is a cognitive behavioural reaction to feeling threatened where the person becomes increasingly watchful for potential sources of threat. This may lead them to look out for potential evidence that confirms their distressing beliefs and at the same time prevent them from paying attention to information that disconfirms this belief (Morrison, 2001).

Delusions are false beliefs that are highly resistant to counter-evidence and are without factuality (McKay and Dennett, 2009). So it would be 'delusional' if you believed and acted as the company boss when you're actually the janitor. A crucial element in determining whether an idea is 'delusional' is if the belief lacks 'truth-value' (i.e., others do not share the belief and there is no supporting evidence that it is true). In addition, not being able to accept or seek out disproving evidence is an important factor in maintaining these kinds of belief. It's not unusual to have beliefs that others don't – consider UFOs, astrology and childhood fantasies. It is when these beliefs are also distressing and there is erratic or risky behaviour associated with them that they are more likely to be judged as 'psychotic'. So delusions, as in case study 11.2, are seen as arising from misinterpretation, with associated distress upon erroneous perceptual experiences.

> **Case Study 11.2: Jim becomes a member of the British monarchy**
>
> Student nurse Beth listens as Jim talks animatedly about how last week he saw his daughter Susan kneeling before him. He felt something momentous happen. On the television, mostly obscured by Susan's body, there was a news report on the royal family's new baby. Jim quietly recounts to Beth how he suddenly heard a voice say, 'Congratulations your highness'. He recalled noticing Susan was still kneeling and looking at him intently with wide eyes. He recalls a rush of thoughts and being left thinking – 'That must mean me. I must be a royal and that's why Susan is kneeling to me.' He looks at Beth anxiously to see what she makes of this.

Bentall et al.'s (1994) theory suggests a possible functional role for psychosis. For example, perhaps paranoia protects the person's self-esteem by reducing opportunities to realize the mismatch between idealized and actual self? (see also chapter 4.) This theory has developed from work on implicit (i.e., unconscious) self-representations that has found that people experiencing paranoia tend to show very slow reaction times when attempting to name the colour of low-self-esteem words in reaction time tasks, which indicates significant cognitive interference in processing self-concept-related stimuli. This kind of research into the thinking styles of people with psychosis demonstrates an 'external attribution' bias (Martin and Penn, 2002). With persecutory delusions, this so-called socio-cognitive bias increases the chance of persons blaming others rather than situations or themselves for negative outcomes. Socio-cognitive biases reflect a tendency to attribute ambivalent situations to others' possible hostile intentions and are hypothesized to reflect deficits in the abilities of individuals to understand other people's minds and intentions in particular (known also as a 'theory of mind' deficit). Another well-replicated difference between people with and without paranoia is found in 'jumping to conclusions' research (Garety et al., 1991). This latter study presented participants with containers of different coloured balls, blue and red, both with an 80 to 20 per cent mix. People with delusions are faster to choose which of the containers a sequence of balls has come from and feel more confident about their decisions even when mistaken (Bentall et al., 1991). These kinds of findings demonstrate that there are qualitative differences in the thinking strategies used by people with paranoia and suggest that, when working with people with delusional thinking, supporting them in how they consider and gather evidence about their beliefs about situations and others may prove beneficial.

Research on thinking styles has led to 'meta-cognitive training' interventions (MCT). The idea is that, if biases are implicated in developing psychosis, working with how people 'think about thinking' could help. Early results show a trend towards effectiveness, tolerance (i.e., the participants are able to cope with the demands of the intervention) and subjective improvement (by self-report) (Aghotor et al., 2010).

11

These micro-theories contrast with Frith's 'theory of mind' (ToM) deficit model (Corcoran and Frith, 2005, 1992). A ToM deficit is where there are problems with a person understanding and distinguishing between their own and (representations of) others' mental states. This is connected to a 'meta-representational' failure – that is, primary representations (thoughts or beliefs) are no longer linked up coherently to secondary representations (i.e., 'meta-cognitions' or thoughts about thoughts) (McCabe et al., 2005). For example, let's say in our case study scenario that Jim knows that the nurse wants him to take his medication on time. With a meta-representational error, Jim's experience shifts from recollecting that 'Beth told me to take my medication' to hearing a voice say, 'You must take your medication'.

2.2 The shifting aetiology (causal factors) of psychosis

Increasingly, a trauma-confusion account is gaining legitimacy as a valid aetiological component of psychosis. Read et al.'s (2005) landmark review of adverse childhood experiences and adult abuse implicate trauma with a mediating role in the development of psychosis. Typically, people with psychosis under-report abuse experiences (physical and sexual) (Dill et al., 1991) but tend to report reliably. Corroboration for childhood sexual abuse (CSA) was found in 74 and 82 per cent of cases, respectively, in studies by Herman and Schatzow (1987) and Read et al. (2003). This means that nurses should ask about and be prepared to work therapeutically with experiences of abuse during assessment and treatment. Such experiences are highly likely to result in a profound sense of loss – of trust in others, self-esteem and confidence – and an increased risk of subsequent difficulties in social and intimate relationships, mental health difficulties and attempted suicide (Cloitre et al., 2006). The trauma account of psychosis, while appealing, remains but one of a range of potential aetiological sources.

Recruiting participants to research studies into the role of abuse and trauma in the development of psychosis is difficult given the topic, low incidence, and complexity of experiences. What we know about abuse and psychosis is currently based on small and typically women-only participant samples. These studies are further flawed, having neglected to tease apart CSA versus childhood physical abuse (CPA) or to account for whether there was subsequent adult physical or sexual abuse (APA, ASA) in the life history (Read et al., 2003).

There is accumulating evidence from adoption studies (Tienari et al., 2004) and from the impact of environmental factors on genotype studies (e.g., cannabis and catechol-o-methyltransferaze; Caspi et al., 2005) that an underlying genetic susceptibility is a risk factor in psychosis. It is one of the most robust findings that a vulnerability to developing the condition diagnosed as schizophrenia is inheritable (Gottesman, 1991). This has emerged from adoption and twin studies, particularly of monozygotic twins, who share nearly 100 per cent of their genes. In Gottesman's review of family, twin and adoption studies conducted from 1916 to 1989 among twins where one has a diagnosis of schizophrenia, they found overall a 25 to 50 per cent probability that the other will develop the condition. In the same review, dizygotic twins and other siblings, who share on average only about half of their genes, had a 10 to 15 per cent probability of developing the condition of their sibling or twin.

These results are further supported by the finding that, the more distant the degree of genetic relatedness (i.e., first degree – parents, siblings – to second degree – grandparents, half-siblings, aunts and uncles), the more the risk of developing the condition is reduced. Historically, adoption studies have provided evidence that this inheritability is due primarily to genetic factors rather than to the shared environmental influence, by the finding that relatives of people with a diagnosis of schizophrenia continue to have a risk of developing the condition even when raised in healthy family environments. This has to some extent been challenged by more recent adoption studies, which have found that rates of psychoses are higher when the genetic vulnerability is associated with disruptive adoptive environments (Tienari et al., 2004).

Taken overall, the findings from behavioural genetic research indicate that psychoses such as schizophrenia involve multiple genes acting in concert and explain why, so far, attempts to identify a specific genetic locus of inheritability has met with failure (Kato et al., 2002). While it is relatively clear that inherited vulnerability increases the risk of developing psychosis, we remain unclear as to whether it is present in all cases and whether the predisposition is always expressed. Some cases could be explained solely by environmental risk factors. Given that the probability of developing the condition in monzygotic twins is not 100 per cent, this also suggests that some people with the vulnerability do not go on to develop psychosis. It is also possible that those who are genetically vulnerable, yet do not go on the develop the condition, are still able to pass on the vulnerability to their children. Indeed, this is borne out by findings that the rate of diagnosis of schizophrenia is elevated in the offspring of non-affected twins (Gottesman and Bertelsen, 1989).

11

Other potential sources of risk can be found in events that adversely effect the development of the foetus that could plausibly be sufficient to produce a vulnerability to psychosis. Obstetrical complications (OCs) that have an adverse effect on the foetal brain (e.g., pre-eclampsia and toxaemia), in addition to delivery complications that result in hypoxia (deprivation of oxygen to the foetus), are shown from numerous studies to be risk factors and have demonstrated that people with a diagnosis of schizophrenia are more likely to have a history of OCs (McNeil et al., 2000). There is also some compelling evidence that maternal infection is another source of environmental risk. This is evident in the increased risk of diagnosis of schizophrenia for individuals born shortly after flu epidemics or after being prenatally exposed to rubella (Murray et al., 1992; Brown et al., 2001). Exposure to infection during the second trimester may be the critical factor, as this is a vital time in foetal neurodevelopment.

A long-hypothesized theory of schizophrenia remains the much critiqued dopamine hypothesis. This hypothesis, in its current incarnation, seeks to link the gamut of risk factors (OCs, stress and trauma, drug use and genes) to increased dopaminergic functioning (Howes and Kapur, 2009). Dopamine is one of the core brain chemicals and is responsible for contributing to neural functioning in a wide variety of brain systems. That anti-psychotic medications are typically dopamine inhibitors that block (although not exclusively) the release and production of dopamine in the brain has been both the origin of the hypothesis and explanation for the efficacy of this class of medication. A major caveat has been that it is not possible to measure the levels of dopamine in the human brain directly. Neurochemical imaging techniques have been developed that measure dopamine levels indirectly by using radioactive labelling of the chemical precursors of dopamine. It is thus not possible to rule out other neurochemical contributions, particularly as the tracers being used may also bind to other receptors such as serotonin (ibid.). Nevertheless dopamine remains a strong aetiological factor because it is also implicated in the formation of delusions on account of its role in the processing of threat-related stimuli (Spitzer, 1995).

2.3 Cognitive psychological treatments of psychosis

As was previously discussed in section 2.1, Morrison (2001) proposed that hallucinations and delusions are kinds of intrusions and thus connected psychosis with anxiety and obsessive-compulsive disorders (OCD). OCD in particular is characterized by thoughts and compulsions that are evaluated as distressing and unwanted. Working with OCD using cognitive behavioural therapy (CBT) has drawn upon disorder-specific models such as that proposed by Wells (2000) and suggests that OCD models (among others) and psychological interventions used in their treatment could be fruitfully adapted to working with psychosis (see also chapter 12). CBT was developed by, Aaron Beck and hypothesizes that patterns of thinking are influenced by, and have an influence upon, actions, feelings and the situation (Beck, 1967a, 1967b). While it is an effective treatment for anxiety and depressive disorders (Hoffman and Smits, 2008), the efficacy of CBT for psychosis remains hotly disputed in the most recent round of systematic reviews (e.g., Lynch et al., 2010). It nonetheless remains the psychological treatment of choice for psychosis as recommended by NICE (2009a).

2.4 The efficacy of CBT for psychosis

In terms of efficacy, a recent review by Jones et al. (2012) showed no significant advantage for CBT over other forms of psychological therapies in reducing relapse. CBT was consistently shown to have an advantage in the longer term on measures of reducing affective distress. 'Meta-analyses' collect and summarize the statistical findings of previous bodies of research. Such reviews are unified only in agreeing on the need to improve study rigour (Lynch et al., 2010). Specific issues are the 'lack of blinding' and the 'lack of randomization' (Zimmerman et al., 2005). Lack of blinding is where the participant is not prevented from knowing whether or not they are in the group getting the experimental intervention. A lack of randomization critiques the procedure allocating participants to the conditions. If this is not done randomly, there is a chance that researchers are prone to bias by selecting participants that might be better suited to the intervention.

There are meta-analyses that, having collated and pooled all the statistical data from RCTs (randomised-controlled trials) on CBT, report 'moderate effectiveness' in reducing symptoms (Zimmerman et al., 2005). It is hard to be confident about such results because of the methodological shortcomings. Lynch et al.'s (2010) meta-analysis is the first to challenge the efficacy of CBT in reducing symptoms and concludes that, when issues of methodology and bias are accounted for, the effect size is, at best, only small and, at worst, becomes statistically insignificant.

Case Study 11.3: How Beth uses a CBT approach

Jim tells student nurse Beth about being royal. He looks anxiously to see what she makes of this. Beth listens intently to him and is careful to look interested and take his statement seriously. She is surprised but is careful not to laugh or try to ignore or bypass Jim's comment, as this would undermine their relationship. Cautiously, she says, 'So it sounds like you are telling me that you saw Susan kneeling and heard a voice from somewhere saying "Congratulations Your Highness"? Is that right Jim?' Here she is sticking to Jim's story and also remaining neutral to what the event means. She opens up the possibility of reinterpreting the 'voice'. Jim is reassured that he is being heard and taken seriously. He was worried she would just laugh at him.

'You seem worried about telling me this – I'm wondering what that's about?' Here Beth is reflecting on what she sees and is empathizing with Jim. 'I was worried that you might laugh at me or think I was crazy', says Jim. Beth goes on to explore in more detail what Jim's experience was. She questions him on how things seemed and felt beforehand and what evidence he bases his beliefs on. Later Beth has conversations about other beliefs where Jim recognizes that he has 'jumped to conclusions', so they can gently explore his convictions over time by looking at alternative explanations.

11

Qualitative research shows that therapy can enable alternative thinking about the meaning of experiences (Messari and Hallam, 2003). Messari and Hallam found that the majority of the participants in their study of client experience of CBT for psychosis reported that therapy was a form of learning about themselves and their experiences and exploring different ways of understanding things. A useful feature of this process was the impact of 'normalization' – learning that at times almost anybody can hear, see or believe things that others do not – for example, when people are highly stressed and/or sleep deprived. Another valued feature of CBT was the sense of collaboration with the therapist – as of two people working together to achieve the clients' goals (ibid.).

A further feature of CBT is the development of a shared 'case-formulation'. This is a personalized model to explain what is happening and suggests some of the triggers and factors involved (Grant et al., 2010). Pain et al. (2008) have found that having a CBT 'case-formulation' led to both positive and negative emotions and was not always seen by people with psychosis as beneficial. While some clients develop a sense of increased hope as a direct consequence of the formulation, others may experience pessimism. It is thus important to explore carefully whether the person may be drawing unintended assumptions from the formulation. They may, for example, wonder if their problems are too entrenched or powerful to change – particularly if the formulation points to the role of early life experiences (ibid.).

This section has introduced and explored psychosis with particular critical attention to the difficulties inherent in providing definitions of the presenting problems that sufficiently capture the highly individualized and diverse nature of psychosis. A review of the current state of empirical research in our understanding of the causes of psychosis has also been presented. This in turn has informed the development of cognitive behavioural therapy for psychosis. These aspects have been illustrated with case study examples to show some of their applications in clinical nursing practice. We will now turn to the role of drug and alcohol use and misuse with particular attention to psychosis.

3 Drug and alcohol use and mental health

Increasingly, nurses are likely to care for people experiencing psychological and physical health difficulties linked to drug and alcohol use. This is partly due to the high levels of drug and alcohol consumption in the UK but is also in response to people being identified as requiring help through drug and alcohol screening programmes in healthcare environments (although, notably, many do not seek support for drug and alcohol related issues, often because they do not feel that they have a problem or need help). Understanding the reasons why people use drugs and alcohol is complex, and there are a range of biological, psychological and sociological theories. Some of the psychological reasons for drug use may include a desire to relieve stress or to experience euphoria or a different state of mind (Hughes, 2009).

Mental health issues frequently accompany physical problems associated with drug and alcohol use; the relationship between them is complex, and often they are mutually reinforcing. For example, physical harms of drugs and alcohol, depending on the substance, can include problems related to toxicity and mortality, cardiovascular complications, dependence, and possible immunity related complications (Darke et al., 2008). An example of physical and psychological interactions can be the use of drugs or alcohol to self-medicate against the unpleasant effects of anxiety. Anxiety can be exacerbated when the sedating effect of the drug or alcohol begins to wear off and be enhanced by withdrawal experiences and interpretation of these. This can worsen anxiety and stimulate more prolonged and increased usage, creating a cycle of developing dependence. Drug and alcohol use may be a cause or a consequence of mental ill health and manifest in a variety of presentations. Symptoms may be mild and transient, such as low levels of anxiety, though a more severe and longer term mental health issue such as psychosis may be involved. Psychosis (as previously defined in sections 2 and 2.1) typically involves unusual beliefs without a basis in factuality (delusions) and seeing, hearing or feeling things that others do not (hallucinations). It is important to recognize that, while some drug and alcohol users may experience psychotic symptoms, these are a relatively rare consequence and may be due to underlying mental health issues that were previously present.

There are more than a thousand potent psychoactive drugs on the market, and the effects on the individual depend on a range of factors such as the amount, frequency, duration and route taken (Petersen and McBride, 2008). Drugs may be swallowed, injected, inhaled, smoked or taken rectally. The speed of absorption, the drug crossing the blood–brain barrier, physiological tolerance, and other personal factors, such as 'pre-drug use' and physiological and psychological health, also influence the effect on the user (DoH, 2011).

Psychoactive drugs tend to affect mood, sensory perception and cognitive functioning and are commonly taken with alcohol and other drugs, including prescribed drugs, which tends to result in more complex and unpredictable effects on the user. Individuals with existing mental health issues have a higher risk of substance misuse and psychological symptoms, depending on the drug used (Rasool, 2008). A further complication may be the use of several drugs simultaneously, often in conjunction with alcohol. Some people may experience a severe reaction such as a substance-induced psychosis, most commonly associated with cocaine, amphetamine and hallucinogens. Generally, a psychotic episode may occur either during drug intoxication or withdrawal, and the experience and symptoms will vary from person to person.

It is important to know which drugs have been used, as this influences treatment approaches and therapeutic interventions. While the clinical presentation of the patient may be similar for several drugs, the most reliable method to confirm the drugs actually taken is through urinalysis or testing blood, hair or oral fluid (DoH, 2007a). The most commonly used method in clinical practice is to test urine or oral fluid samples.

3.1 Alcohol and mental health

Alcohol and mental health problems are intrinsically linked. People with severe mental health problems are prone to use alcohol excessively, often to offset negative thoughts or feelings or to alleviate anxiety or low mood. Conversely, people who use alcohol excessively have an increased risk of experiencing such mental health difficulties as low mood or anxiety. The psychological symptoms associated with alcohol misuse depend partially on the amount and rate of consumption (Raistrick et al., 2006). Psychological symptoms during intoxication may include anxiety, depression and suicidal thoughts (Rasool, 2008). The harm potential escalates with an increase in alcohol consumption. Among other psychological symptoms sometimes associated with harmful alcohol use are hallucinations, delirium tremens and amnesia. Delirium tremens is a rare but very serious form of withdrawal delirium whose main features are increased confusion, changes in consciousness, persistent hallucinations and tremors, and it is also associated with increased heart rate, blood pressure and respiratory rate (DeBellis et al., 2005). Typically alcohol misuse affects mood and cognitive functioning and may manifest as depression, anxiety, impaired memory and, in severe cases, sensory perception (NICE, 2010).

Alcohol misuse can lead to increasing the risk of harm to self and others and the likelihood of seizures, accidents, respiratory arrest when sleeping, hypothermia, anger and violence (Rasool, 2008). Misuse is typically understood to be more than 2 to 3 units of alcohol a day regularly for women or 3 to 4 units for men. A standard unit is defined in the UK as a drink that contains 8 g of ethanol. Higher-risk drinking also includes binge drinking. This is characterized by drinking more than 6 units a day on at least one occasion in the past week for women and more than 8 units a day on at least one occasion in the past week for men, with associated dependence (DoH, 2007b). Alcohol dependence is characterized by craving, withdrawal symptoms, loss of control and tolerance, a progressive neglect of alternative interests, and a persistent use, despite evidence of harm and a narrowing of personal repertoire (taking the substance is more important than anything else) (Edwards et al., 2009).

3.2 How to recognize a person experiencing drug- or alcohol-induced psychosis

It is important that nurses are able to recognize when a person is experiencing mental health problems such as drug- or alcohol-induced psychosis and know how to respond. Focusing on the drug or alcohol use in isolation is unhelpful, as it offers a narrow perspective on the behaviour and potential favourable interventions. Zinberg (1986) suggested three changeable factors that need to be considered in terms of assessing drug use. These are the type of drug taken and the method of use, the person's mindset (attitude or substance use outcome expectancy) and the social setting (alone or with others). In evaluating all of these dimensions simultaneously, a more comprehensive picture of the person and their needs will evolve and assist in care planning.

In psychosis, prominent symptoms, particularly in onset, are the presence of hallucinations and delusions. An individual's clinical presentation will vary depending on factors such as their psychological health status before the use of drugs. It is important to recognize that psychosis may be a result of an existing mental health disorder or due to another cause altogether. Therefore a clinical assessment by a trained mental health professional is required, and the criteria recommended by the *Diagnostic and Statistical Manual of Mental Disorders, DSM-5* (American Psychiatric Association, 2013) may be used to assist diagnosis. The DSM-5, used by clinicians in order to classify mental disorders, including those associated with drug or alcohol use, identifies eleven separate categories of substances related to mental disorders: alcohol, caffeine, cannabis, hallucinogens, inhalants, opioids, sedatives, hypnotics, anxiolytics, stimulants, tobacco, and other or unknown substances. Table 11.1 presents a simple classification of common psychoactive drugs.

A person experiencing alcohol-related psychosis may present clinically similarly to someone who has taken a drug other than alcohol or who has another medical, neurological or psychological

Table 11.1 Classification of common psychoactive drugs

Drug	Drug class
Alcohol	Depressant
Amphetamine (sulphate, dexamphetamine, methamphetamine)	Stimulant
Anabolic-androgenic steroids	Synthetic variants of the male sex hormone testosterone
Benzodiazepines	Depressant
Cannabis	Alters perception
Cocaine, crack cocaine, Ecstasy (MDMA)	Stimulant
Gamma-hydroxybutyrate (GHB)	Depressant
Heroin, methadone	Depressant
LSD, magic mushrooms	Hallucinogen
Nitrites (amyl nitrite, butyl nitrite, isobutyl nitrite)	Depressant
Volatile substances (e.g., aerosols)	Depressant

11

condition. A formal assessment by a trained nurse or doctor will assist in formulating a diagnosis to inform the treatment and care plan. Identifying the kind and amount of drug being used is vital in terms of determining what kind of acute detoxification medical treatment may be required and what the likely effect on the person's emotional health is likely to be.

3.3 Caring for clients with drug- or alcohol-induced psychosis

Clinical interventions should be initiated based on the person's clinical presentation, mental and physical health needs, and identified associated risks. Mental healthcare interventions for alcohol or drug issues may be delivered by a multidisciplinary team in a range of healthcare environments, and this tends to depend both on the nature and severity of the problem and on the services available. The more serious the mental health problem, the more likely the person is to require hospitalization.

Drug- and/or alcohol-induced psychosis is considered to be a serious mental health issue. The appropriate approach to responding to a client presenting with a significant co-morbid mental health disorder such as psychosis, and those at high risk of suicide, would be to refer them to a psychiatrist. This would enable an assessment to be undertaken and the formulation of a treatment and risk-management plan (Norman and Ryrie, 2013). Treatment for psychosis tends to involve the prescription of anti-psychotic medication, cognitive behavioural therapy and psychosocial interventions such as family therapy. A person experiencing alcohol-induced psychosis is likely to be alcohol dependent and therefore would require medically assisted alcohol detoxification in a hospital (NICE, 2010)

A range of evidence-based interventions designed to address the needs of clients with drug-related issues are highlighted by the Department of Health (2007a). These include health promotion, care planned counselling, needle exchange, a controlled substance use plan, maintenance, a planned reduction regime, gradual withdrawal, detoxification, structured day programmes, community prescribing, inpatient substance misuse treatment, residential rehabilitation, psychosocial interventions and brief advice. An important first step when encountering a person suspected of misusing alcohol or drugs is to identify the relevant substance and the severity and nature of the abuse. There is a range of standard treatment options available depending on the issues the person is experiencing, ranging from brief interventions to alcohol detoxification (NICE, 2010; National Treatment Agency, 2006). With severe alcohol misuse, abrupt withdrawal can increase the risk of potentially life-threatening seizures. It is therefore best not to recommend the complete cessation of drinking but instead refer the person to alcohol services for rapid assessment and treatment. Identifying behaviours associated with substance misuse is of vital importance. It can help identify potential risks – e.g., serious misuse when alone could increase the risk of suicide because of a lack of protective factors; conversely, depending on the circumstances, it might identify that the individual is at increased risk of vulnerability to others. A comprehensive risk assessment and understanding of both the circumstances and the motivations is thus essential in order to safeguard the individual with a referral of appropriate urgency.

The government's *Drug Strategy* (Home Office, 2010) reinforces the importance of a recovery-oriented treatment approach in supporting clients with alcohol or drug misuse issues. The driver for this approach is the increased impetus placed on prevention, enhanced enforcement through criminal justice interventions, and recovery-oriented treatment services. Wellbeing, citizenship, and recovery from dependence are the overarching principles in this strategy.

While the range of evidence-based interventions available to treat clients who misuse drugs or alcohol is increasing, Van Wormer and Thyer (2010) underline important cross-cutting issues. They suggest that, rather than there being one single type of intervention, each individual requires a unique approach; addressing alcohol and drug use in isolation is insufficient, and, in order for treatment to be effective, the person's global needs ought to be taken into account, in a timely manner, and with a realistic time frame in mind.

Case Study 11.4: Jim starts drinking

Jim enjoys alcohol and would previously have described himself as a 'social drinker'. More recently, in response to his experiences of hearing derogatory voices and having ideas that others are acting against him, he has started to drink heavily and alone. This consists of several litres of strong cider a day, usually starting at lunchtime. Jim cannot afford to drink this amount every day and he has noticed that, on the days when he drinks less, he feels unwell. He experiences shaking, sweating and nausea and feels anxious. Jim tells student nurse Beth about his drinking, and she refers him to the local alcohol service for an assessment. Because his increased intake of alcohol is a relatively recent development and he is able to cut down independently, the recommendation is a controlled reducing regime. This involves a gradual reduction, recorded by Jim in a drinking diary, and monitoring and support from an alcohol nurse.

11

Activity 11.1

What aspects of Jim's alcohol use should Beth pay attention to in particular in terms of screening him for risk and the urgency of referral and intervention? What basic techniques of CBT might she use to talk about his experience of psychosis that could be contributing to his alcohol use? (refer to case study 11.3 to help you with this).

Summary

▶ This chapter has critically examined the nature and complexity of psychosis and the role of substance and alcohol misuse in relation to this.

▶ The application of relevant psychological theories of psychosis has been introduced.

▶ Theories of causation, definitions, implications, research and evidence-based interventions have been discussed and examples have been offered through a series of client case studies.

▶ The role of the nurse in the application of evidence and theory to practice has been explored with the aid of the case studies.

Questions for discussion

1 What new pieces of information have you learnt about the causes of altered states of psychosis and drug and alcohol use?

2 How can an understanding of the psychological models of psychosis inform how you work with people with these kinds of difficulties?

Further reading

Marshall, E. J., Humphreys, K., and Ball, D. M. (2010) *The Treatment of Drinking Problems. A guide for the helping professions.* 5th edn, Cambridge: Cambridge University Press.

Sacks, O. (2012) *Hallucinations.* London: Picador.
An eloquently written book, providing an overview of different conditions and where hallucinations may arise.

Grant, A., Biley, F. C., and Walker, H. (eds) (2011) *Our Encounters with Madness.* Ross-on-Wye: PCCS Books.
This edited collection of first-hand accounts of psychosis or 'madness' from those with lived experience of the condition makes for enlightening reading.

Part IV
Communication and Therapeutic Talk

CONTENTS

Leading on from the previous chapters on mental health, Part IV looks specifically at core interactional skills that underpin good communication and therapeutic relationships. As outlined by the Nursing and Midwifery Council in their essential skills cluster, these skills should not be the sole province of mental health nurses; they should be basic skills required by all nurses in order to enhance the nurse–patient relationship. This section begins with an overview of the development of cognitive behavioural therapy (CBT) and the theories underpinning this broad therapeutic approach. It demonstrates how CBT has become the most widely used form of therapy within the NHS and healthcare generally. The 'application' of CBT is explored to demonstrate how it is used in practice, how it is defined and distinct from other approaches, and the skills and techniques it involves. The importance of a therapeutic relationship is also explored, as this is often something which is wrongly assumed to be lacking in CBT. The chapter includes some examples of the experiences of panic and health anxiety as well as more complex mental health difficulties such as trauma and psychosis. Relating the topic to previous chapters, it also discusses some of the wider applications of CBT for the management of other conditions, such as chronic pain and long-term health conditions.

Chapter 13 explores the role of personal relationships in the process of counselling. The psychoanalytic approaches of Freud, the humanistic and client-centred therapeutic approach of Carl Rogers, and Kelly's personal construct theory are all introduced, together with how such approaches can be practically applied by nurses in healthcare settings. Of particular importance are the types of relationship that appear best able to empower patients and increase their wellbeing.

Chapter 14 introduces motivational dialogue as a form of intervention that is increasingly being used in a variety of healthcare settings. It provides a practical guide to this intervention, exploring what motivates people and why some individuals continue with destructive and harmful behaviours despite being told of the consequences. The chapter looks at the model of change, exploring how one conversation can start the process of change, before going on to discuss the role nurses can play in motivating patients. Brief one-off conversations can form the basis of motivational dialogue and can be used effectively in pressured services such as A&E departments, GP practices and community settings.

Jane Toner

CHAPTER CONTENTS

KEY ISSUES IN THIS CHAPTER:

▶ The background and development of therapy and cognitive behavioural therapy (CBT)
▶ The recent growth of CBT within current government policy and the NHS
▶ Using CBT principles and skills in nursing practice

BY THE END OF THIS CHAPTER YOU SHOULD BE ABLE TO:

▶ understand what CBT is and how to describe it to patients
▶ understand how CBT can be useful for nurses in a range of clinical areas of mental health and physical healthcare
▶ understand the principles of CBT and how these can relate to 'normal' difficulties as well as more complex needs
▶ understand how CBT works to help people break patterns of thinking and behaviour.

1 Introduction

CBT is a therapy that focuses upon the *cognitive* aspects (thoughts, beliefs, attitudes) and *behavioural* aspects (what we do, how we do this) of someone who is experiencing difficulties.

The aim of this chapter is to explore the development and principles of CBT and their relevance for staff working in a range of healthcare settings. Firstly we will look at what CBT is, how the therapy has developed and how and why it has become the therapy of 'choice' in many areas of mental health. We will then move on to look at its application, referring to a case example throughout. Finally, we will look briefly at how 'CBT' can be applied to physical health difficulties and how the same principles and techniques we use with mental health problems can be adapted to work with chronic health problems.

2 Cognitive behavioural therapy: what is it?

Consider how people react to a diagnosis of cancer. There is a range of differing responses to such news. Some individuals think: 'This is the end, this is a death sentence.' They may then become very low in mood, stop going out and reduce their activity levels, and become isolated and distressed. Somebody else may think: 'I've got to fight this; I won't let it beat me.' They may feel frustrated that this has happened, but they then change to a healthier lifestyle and research ways to beat cancer. They may feel more positive and use their friends and colleagues for support.

It is this difference in beliefs that CBT therapists are interested in. CBT is based on the premise that our behaviours and our emotions/ feelings about an event or a situation are very personal, are different from the ways in which other people react and are dependent upon how we internally *interpret* a situation. Our 'internal world' of thoughts (what we call 'cognitions') is important to a CBT therapist, who aims to understand what is going on in someone's internal world, why it is happening, and how they can help and guide someone to reduce the distress and problematic behaviours that occur.

The 'cognitions' in CBT are the thoughts, beliefs, words and images that go through our minds. For someone with social anxiety problems, the things going through their mind in a social situation might be: 'I must look stupid, people must see I'm blushing, people are thinking I'm quiet and boring.' For some people these social anxiety cognitions may be in the form of an image (seeing themselves bright red, and mumbling their words); cognitions may also be in the form of a memory of a time they remember being in a bad situation and feeling anxious. Some people are very aware of these cognitions, but others need help to access such thoughts, images and beliefs.

CBT is a structured and often time-limited therapeutic approach, based upon an open, honest and collaborative relationship between the therapist and the client. It has been shown to be an effective therapy with a range of mental health and emotional difficulties, such as low mood, various anxiety problems, psychosis and some long-term physical problems. CBT has been shown to be as effective as medication for many types of depression and anxiety disorders and, unlike drugs, with few side effects; yet there are long-lasting benefits (Hollon et al., 2005).

3 Background and history of CBT

CBT developed through an integration of behavioural theory and cognitive psychology and a response to Freudian dominance in the nineteenth century. In Freud's 'psychodynamic' perspective, emphasis was placed on unconscious processes and the dynamic interactions and conflicts between the id, the ego and the superego, which were theoretical forces Freud believed were within us all (Freud, 1958). Freud's psychodynamic approach is also discussed in chapters 1 and 13.

3.1 Behavioural theory

In response to Freud's theoretical approach, behavioural theorists, in particular John B. Watson (1878–1958), placed an emphasis on the observable relationship between a stimulus and a response and the learning and 'association' that occurs between these two events; we learn by linking things together and by having things reinforced. Bandura (1977) further developed this by describing 'social learning theory', showing that learning also takes place by observing and imitating others. We therefore learn developmentally by observing and copying those around us, and we can influence behaviour socially and vicariously. Within CBT approaches today, behavioural theory and social learning are considered as important aspects in maintaining distress and problematic behaviours; the principles are also used to help patients relearn more functional ways of behaving. The behaviourist approach is also discussed in chapter 1.

12

3.2 Cognitive psychology

Fundamentally, cognitive theory hinges around the idea that a person's emotions/feelings and behaviour are dependent upon (or strongly linked to) their cognitions (see also chapter 1). Ellis (1962) described an ABC model, where A is an event, B is the belief about the event, and C refers to the emotional and behavioural consequences of B given A – see figure 12.1.

As you can see from figure 12.1, there are a range of beliefs that can occur in response to an event, and they have differing emotional and

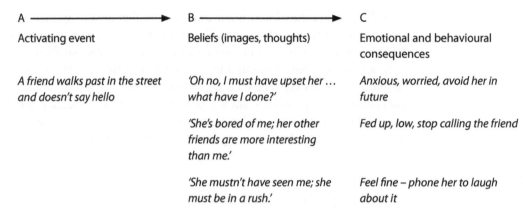

A ⟶	B ⟶	C
Activating event	Beliefs (images, thoughts)	Emotional and behavioural consequences
A friend walks past in the street and doesn't say hello	*'Oh no, I must have upset her … what have I done?'*	*Anxious, worried, avoid her in future*
	'She's bored of me; her other friends are more interesting than me.'	*Fed up, low, stop calling the friend*
	'She mustn't have seen me; she must be in a rush.'	*Feel fine – phone her to laugh about it*

Figure 12.1 The cognitive ABC model

behavioural consequences. Certain kinds of beliefs and cognitions are associated with different emotions and certain behaviours. Negative beliefs and negative self-evaluation is often associated with low mood and depression. Beliefs about being unable to cope and being at risk are often linked to some form of anxiety. Aaron T. Beck, one of the key individuals involved in developing cognitive therapy, recognized that the thoughts that clients are experiencing and the way they 'interpret events' can maintain different emotional states such as depression (Beck et al., 1979). His initial cognitive therapy for depression also drew upon the work of Albert Ellis (1962) and George Kelly's (1955) personal construct theory. Cognitive therapy and behavioural theory grew together to become CBT.

4 CBT and the role of the nurse

As caring professionals, we all want to use approaches and techniques that work. Recently we have seen the development of evidence-based practice, which is an interdisciplinary approach to clinical practice formally introduced into the UK health service widely in 1992. The principle is that all clinical decisions should be made based upon research that has been carried out according to appropriate and recognized standards.

CBT has repeatedly been shown to be an effective approach. As a result, the UK National Institute for Health and Care Excellence (NICE) has incorporated CBT interventions within their guidance for many mental health and emotional difficulties. This includes the use of CBT for depression (NICE 2009), Post traumatic stress disorder (PTSD) (NICE 2005), anxiety and panic (NICE 2004a), and schizophrenia and psychosis. Psychological therapies are therefore an important part of NHS mental healthcare, and the need for specialist nurse therapists who can help to provide this input is significant (Davies-Smith (2006). Additionally, an important role for the nurse is knowing when and where to seek psychological help for patients.

More recently, the government has funded and implemented the Improving Access to Psychological Therapies initiative (see www.iapt.nhs.uk). This initiative was driven by a need to help individuals experiencing mental health problems in the community to get back into the workforce (Layard et al., 2006, 2007). Professor Lord Layard, who has been referred to as the government's 'happiness tsar', recognized that therapies such as CBT could help people return to work but that the approaches weren't being offered routinely in the NHS on account of a lack of skills. Significant numbers of nurses and other professionals within the NHS are now being trained in CBT as part of this initiative.

5 Mental health problems: what are they?

Traditional medical approaches often view a mental health disorder as something which is very different from 'normal', and this is seen as 'pathologizing' mental health problems. In CBT, such problems are seen as being linked to a bias or an exaggeration of a normal process. This psychosocial ethos helps us to understand that mental health problems are not weird or odd but can happen to anyone. When emotions are heightened we can all experience exaggerated or biased thoughts – taking things personally, for example, or assuming everything is going to go wrong on the basis of one thing failing. This is quite normal and something we can all relate to at some point in our lives. It can become a problem, though, if we do this too much or too often. CBT tries to help individuals recognize that they have 'got into' these patterns of thinking, which can maintain the problems they are experiencing. Unfortunately, for some, such patterns are very well established; they have become entrenched, and people get 'stuck'. Table 12.1 outlines some of these cognitive biases with examples.

Table 12.1 Cognitive biases		
Thinking patterns (or biased thinking)	**Description**	**Examples of biased thinking**
Jumping to conclusions	Making an interpretation in the absence of facts	'Everyone will just think I'm boring, so there's no point going out.'
Mind-reading	Assuming what others are thinking and making this fact without evidence	'He's wondering why I even came out tonight and would rather be with his friends.'
Personalizing	Assuming responsibility when bad things happen	'This evening didn't go well; if I'd have been chattier it would have been fine; it's my fault again!'
Catastrophizing	Predicting the worst outcome based upon something minor going wrong	'I don't feel well. I'm going to be off sick again, and my boss will go mad and sack me.'

12

Table 12.1 (continued)		
Thinking patterns (or biased thinking)	**Description**	**Examples of biased thinking**
All or nothing	Events/things are at one extreme or another rather than on a spectrum of possibilities	'I can't get this task right. I'm absolutely rubbish at this job, so I may as well leave.'
Emotional reasoning	Assuming what you are feeling is fact	'I feel ugly tonight. I must look ugly to others.'
Unrealistic and high standards	Using an overly high criterion for judgement of self or others; using 'should', 'ought', 'must'	'I should be able to get this right the first time. I ought to be able to do better.'

Activity 12.1

We all slip into the cognitive biases listed in table 12.1 from time to time. Think about occasions when you might have thought in these ways and about which biases you use the most.

---

6 The maintenance of difficulties

CBT recognizes that individuals can get themselves stuck and lost in cycles of problem thoughts, behaviours and emotions and need help to see a way out. It focuses on five clear areas or 'systems' that are seen to interact with each other:

1 cognitions (thoughts, images, beliefs)
2 emotions/feelings
3 behaviour
4 physiology (bodily sensations/states)
5 environment and triggers.

Figure 12.2 demonstrates how these five 'systems' can be laid out in a cyclical way. The arrows represent potential points of interaction and maintenance occurring between the differing systems.

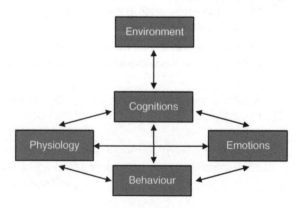

Figure 12.2 Five systems model (Greenberger and Padesky, 1995)

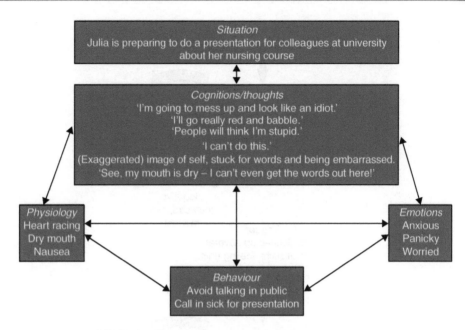

Figure 12.3 The five systems model using public speaking as an example

All of these five 'systems' interact with each other in a cyclical way and, in this respect, can both reinforce each other and maintain the problems that are occurring. This is demonstrated in figure 12.3, where Julia's thoughts and images while preparing for the presentation are making her feel anxious and 'panicky'; physiological symptoms of stress are then triggered. The idea that she won't be able to get the words out is reinforced by her mouth being dry, which perpetuates her anxiety. Her behavioural strategy is then to avoid going to the presentation, which will reduce these symptoms – in the short term. In the long term, though, continual avoidance is resulting in Julia missing key activities, falling behind with her course and spending reduced time with her peers; ultimately, it is also having a negative impact on her mood. A cognitive behavioural therapist would spend time with Julia talking through these longer-term implications, being careful not to blame her for this pattern of events but collaboratively helping her to change her current behaviour. This would involve exploring and challenging some of the thoughts and thinking biases that she is experiencing. Ultimately the aim would be to break the patterns and cycles she has been falling into.

The important concept to establish here is that the interaction of these five systems *maintains* the difficulties: people get 'stuck' in patterns of behaviour and thinking and cannot get out of them; that is why help is needed. Such patterns and how the CBT therapist can help to break them are the subject of the next section.

Researchers and CBT clinicians have also developed 'disorder-specific' formulations – diagrams which show the key relationships and key cognitions involved in certain difficulties. Figure 12.4 demonstrates the typical pattern that occurs during a panic attack, and each arrow

12

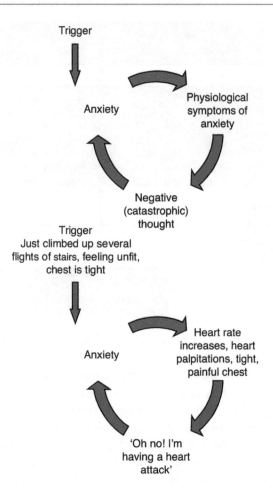

Figure 12.4 Panic cycle

represents a maintenance pathway that can be targeted within CBT. The 'trigger' is a tightness in the chest following exertion. This causes some anxiety, which results in the person experiencing the normal physiological symptoms of anxiety – increased heart rate, increased awareness of heart rate and a tight chest. This individual genuinely misinterprets these symptoms as evidence of a heart attack, which inevitably causes more anxiety, and the vicious cycle goes on and on.

7 The application of CBT

In this section we will explore how CBT is actually carried out with clients. Importantly, therapy is not about telling someone how to think and feel, or giving advice, or telling someone to feel better; it is about providing them with the tools and guidance to change what they are doing. CBT isn't concerned with 'changing someone's mind' about the way they are thinking, feeling and behaving but with enabling them to see the problematic cycles in which they are involved and so how to move forward.

Case Study 12.1 (Part 1):

John is fifty-eight and married. He has worked all his life as a builder, doing shift work, lives with his wife of twenty-four years, and has three children and three grandchildren who live within 10 miles. John had an accident in his car eight months ago which resulted in problems with his mobility, and he had to give up work. He had no pension and was now worried about his finances. Following the accident he had a bad back and knees, and he continues to have problems with his legs so now walks with a stick. John's mood is low: he is unhappy about being unable to work and about losing his mobility. He has reduced his activity levels significantly and feels anxious going out to new places. He regularly attends his local doctor's surgery for his physical problems, but the doctor and nursing staff are also worried about his low mood.

8 The relationship in CBT

As professionals who perform a caring role, we need to be able to engage with others and to try and view the world from the patient's perspective. This is even more significant in cognitive behavioural therapy, where the core skills such as listening, honesty, being open, and being able to develop rapport are essential. A client needs to feel comfortable with the therapist to be able to express distress and to speak about concerns and fears; indeed, in CBT the therapist will often ask the client to face these fears and try new things, and this is more difficult if rapport and trust have not been established. The therapeutic relationship is also seen as a 'model' for working on and through difficulties and then transferring this into everyday life.

Case Study 12.1 (Part 2):

On placement with the practice nurse, student nurse Beth spoke to John about a referral to the therapy service attached to the doctor's surgery. John was sceptical but said he would try this. Upon meeting with the CBT practitioner, John spoke about how he wasn't sure about CBT and he wasn't used to talking about things. Developing a relationship here was key; the therapist had to work hard to ensure that they defined 'CBT' and how it could be helpful for John. The spirit of 'give it a go' was presented to him. It was also important in the early sessions to allow John to express how he had been feeling and to tell his 'story' of how he had reached the position he is in. He had to feel respected and listened to, so the therapist needed to give sensitive non-verbal and verbal cues to encourage him to speak and to validate his feelings, frustrations and experiences. The two also discussed some reasonable short-term goals that John would like to achieve to give the therapy some direction and to find out what was important for him. His initial goals were to get out of the house a bit more and to sleep better at night. Choosing and exploring such goals was done carefully to try and encourage John to think ahead (which can be difficult for those with low mood and depression), but it is very important to ensure the goals are achievable.

12

Activity 12.2

Based on what you have learnt in this chapter so far, how would you 'sell' the rationale of therapy to somebody like John? Think about how you would explain what CBT is and how it could help.

CBT is carried out using specific techniques called guided discovery and 'Socratic' questions – questions that guide discovery and understanding. The therapist asks lots of questions, carried out in a curious, inquisitive and supportive way, to find out what is going on from the client's perspective and to help find a way forward. Christine Padesky (1993) provides a classic summary of the four stages of questions that are used throughout sessions.

1   *Ask information questions*: Questions should be relevant, something the client knows but may not be accessing or paying attention to at this time. The aim is to help the difficulties become concrete and understandable – for example:

   - When did the problems start?
   - How do you feel when …?
   - Which bit of this bothers you the most?
   - Why do you think this is happening?
   - How did you used to react?

2   *Listen*: Truly listening to someone and understanding where they are coming from is a hard task and takes a lot of skill and focus, but this is essential and needs to be genuinely carried out. Listening is honed for key words, key emotions and things that may be incongruent or inconsistent. An example of this might be someone talking about a traumatic incident but presenting as being very emotionally cut-off, minimizing what happened or even laughing about it.

3   *Summarize*: Therapists are taught to summarize what they are hearing; this is done to check understanding but also to slow the process down, to reinforce key ideas and to pull key information together – for example:

   - So it sounds like, when this happened, you talked about feeling frustrated but also very sad and upset. Have I heard that correctly?

4   *Synthesizing questions*: These questions are used to draw links and pull together ideas using the cognitive and behavioural theory. The questions, which are quite sophisticated, should enable new explanations and understandings.

Case Study 12.1 (Part 3):

Information questions were used initially with John to discover his perception of what was happening at that time. It was important to convey that the therapist was genuinely interested in his experiences and wanted to

Case Study 12.1 (continued)

know more. Questions in the first session included: 'Tell me how you spent your time yesterday' and 'How was this different from last year?' With regard to future goals, questions might include: 'How would you like things to be different in three months time?' or 'If we can't improve your mobility, how else could things be different?'

The therapist listened intently to what John was saying, asking more about things that felt particularly significant, focusing upon how he described his mood problems, the words used, and particularly when he spoke with a higher degree of distress and emotion.

Summarizing and reflecting back what he had said ensured that the therapist had clearly understood what John meant and demonstrated that he was being listened to – for example: 'You've said a few times now, John, that you feel "useless", and you used the words "finished" and "on the scrapheap". That must be a terrible way to feel and shows what a big impact all this has had on you.'

9 Formulation

Formulation is the process of developing a joint understanding of what is going on for the client/patient; it is a map of what is happening informed by CBT theory. It highlights the relationships between different thoughts and emotions; a formulation also describes patterns for that individual, noting how problems and difficulties are maintained (i.e., how the problem keeps going and how someone becomes 'stuck' in these patterns). It is important that the formulation guides the clinical interventions to help the client move forward. During a session, while asking relevant questions, listening, summarizing and synthesizing information, the therapist will be drawing out links and patterns with the patient and 'formulating' what they think is going on.

Basic CBT formulations (also known as five systems formulations; see figures 12.2 and 12.3) are often used early on in the therapy process to show the relationships between thoughts, feelings, emotions and triggers. They help to share understanding, to introduce the key CBT concepts to clients, and to show relationships between the systems. Figure 12.5 provides a 'five systems' formulation for our case study, John. After the therapist had drawn several of these maintenance formulations, John began to recognize that he was avoiding activities and that often, by avoiding things, he was feeling worse and doing even less. He described feeling stuck in this pattern and hated feeling the way he does, but he believes he's so 'useless' that he thinks others will believe the same.

Through the course of therapy, we may move onto more complex formulations than the one described in figure 12.5, incorporating how early experiences may contribute to current difficulties – any traumatic events and key relationships and attachment experiences that may

12

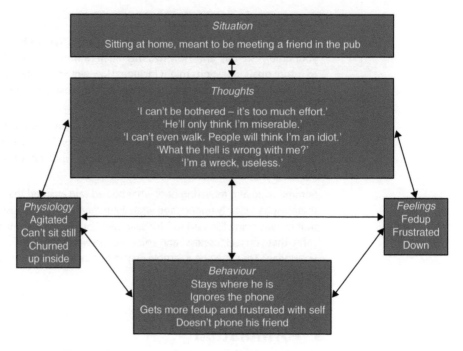

Figure 12.5 Five systems formulation for John

be important to understand what is going on. In these formulations, the therapist would gauge the deeper beliefs and values that individuals hold about themselves, others around them and the world. These would be defined as *core beliefs* in CBT. For John in our case study, we recognized that he had long-held beliefs that 'men needed to work' and that to be out of work was unacceptable and something to be looked down upon and judged by. The formulation used to map out John's difficulties could be either this generic five systems model or one of the 'disorder-specific' models that have been developed and were discussed earlier in this chapter.

10 Cognitive and behavioural interventions and strategies

The formulation should guide the therapist as to which of the range of strategies and techniques may help their patient. Patients are encouraged to practise strategies between sessions to reinforce them and to make them part of day-to-day life. Behavioural strategies are frequently used earlier on in the therapy, often for those experiencing low mood and poor motivation. Learning new skills is also part of CBT, and the patient is encouraged to use these skills in everyday life, both during the course of therapy and in the future. Cognitive strategies are those involved with identifying, exploring and challenging the way individuals are thinking and the way they are interpreting events.

Table 12.2 summarizes some of the key cognitive and behavioural techniques, some of which are also presented in the continuing case study below.

Table 12.2 Behavioural and cognitive strategies		
	Cognitive strategies	**Behavioural strategies**
Purpose	Strategies used to identify the problematic way of thinking, to explore these unhelpful cognitions and introduce new ones	To encourage or to reinforce behavioural change which should facilitate and reinforce cognitive change
Example techniques	*Thought monitoring* Recording frequently occurring beliefs and spotting cognitive biases: people may need a lot of practice and assistance to do this within sessions to help them to identify key thoughts. When regularly occurring negative automatic thoughts/beliefs have been identified, the therapist can help the person explore these thoughts and their impact on a day-to-day basis and establish whether they are valid or led by thinking/cognitive biases. *Thought evaluation* Exploring and questioning the evidence that the patient holds for their beliefs and also developing 'counter-evidence' for alternative and healthier beliefs. These more valid and reasonable thoughts can be put in place and, with practice, the client can begin to implement and adopt these thoughts in real life. *Finding alternative strategies* Other 'cognitive strategies' can include • techniques to develop mindfulness • techniques to develop new cognitive skills such as distraction or controlled worry periods.	*Activity monitoring* Used to find out how patients are doing on an everyday basis and to explore what effect their activity type and activity levels are having upon their experiences and their mood. It is used to highlight the link between key situations, feelings, thoughts and behaviours and to identify triggers for problems and patterns of behaviours. It can be helpful to 'scale' or rate the level of emotions in particular situations. *Activity scheduling* This involves detailing how a person is spending their time and adapting their schedule to include more pleasurable and meaningful activities that will promote and enhance their mood and levels of enjoyment and fulfilment. *Exposure work* A strategy aimed at gradually mastering a problem; the primary method is to develop a hierarchy of difficult situations and then conquer them, with support, one step at a time. *Behavioural activation* Scheduling activities to encourage people to approach the activities that they are avoiding and focusing on the 'cognitions' that they are using to avoid activities. *Role play* Practising new behaviours and developing cognitive changes. *Relaxation* A way to help clients manage anxiety responses and promote self-awareness and self-monitoring.

Source: Adapted from Toner (2012).

12

Case Study 12.1 (Part 4):

Activity monitoring was used to find out how John was spending his time and how he felt during each activity. This proved to John that he was avoiding activities, thinking this was the easier option, whereas actually it was having a detrimental effect on his mood and was getting worse week by week. Several sessions were spent discussing activities and pastimes that John used to enjoy and devising plans and steps to encourage him to re-engage in a couple of activities. With guidance and support, John began a few extra activities in *activity scheduling* – e.g., to go daily to the shop to buy a paper, which he did early to ensure there were fewer people to see him. He reported back at the following session that, although he hadn't managed this every day, on the days he had done so he felt marginally better. Rather than feeling 3/10 (on a scale from bad to good), he felt 4/10, which was an improvement! He was avoiding family because of the loudness of grandchildren, which tired him out; he was also avoiding friends, as he was ashamed of his lack of mobility. As a hometask he began to re-engage with these activities. Firstly, he examined why he had been doing this and found that he was thinking: 'They'll just tire me out too much. I can't face them.' This was adapted to: 'It'll be tiring, but I might enjoy it', and John was able to face the activity and get some benefit from it.

John had lots of negative thoughts that he and the therapist discussed, and they began the *thought evaluation* process with these. One key thought was that John was 'finished' now that he wasn't working. The evidence both for and against this thought was examined. On balance, John concluded that he wasn't 'finished' but that he was a different man with a different future. Sessions were spent talking about his re-evaluation of who he was and what the future would be without his job and his mobility. John's original thoughts about 'retirement' were considered and adapted to allow for his mobility problems, but some activities that, once retired, he had hoped to do more of remained accessible to him.

Within this chapter, we have introduced the theory underpinning CBT and demonstrated the skills and techniques used with a client in mind. The final section will briefly demonstrate how CBT can be used for physical difficulties.

11 Application of CBT to chronic health conditions

Cognitive behaviour therapy has been shown to be useful in a range of physical health difficulties, and in this section we are going to explore its use and application for chronic fatigue syndrome/ME and chronic pain.

It is important to stress that, in using CBT to help physical health conditions, we are not stating that it can cure the symptoms. The aim is to help people cope better with those symptoms, which in turn can help with their experience of a chronic health condition and improve their general level of functioning. When people are experiencing physical health problems they may get trapped into a negative spiral of negative thoughts, negative emotions, physical sensations and behaviours. CBT helps individuals to break these negative patterns and cycles and improve their quality of life. Additionally, depression and anxiety is more common in patients who are experiencing long-term physical health conditions (Hunter et al., 2013). Such health problems can either exacerbate an existing problem or cause depression, which can have huge implications for the treatment of these patients and how they are able to manage their conditions.

Chronic fatigue syndrome, or ME (myalgic encephalomyelitis/encephalopathy), is a condition with a range of symptoms, such as fatigue, headaches, concentration difficulties and muscular pain. Sufferers are unable to work or to attend to many activities of daily living. The causes and progress of ME are not fully understood, but research has shown that involvement in a course of CBT can help individuals to manage the condition better and improve functioning and quality of life (NICE, 2007). The literature shows that, once other physical causes have been excluded, CBT may be helpful as long as individuals are fully involved and fully engaged in the process. This therefore means that those professionals who are introducing the concept of CBT to an individual with CFS/ME need to be able to inspire and encourage the sufferer to engage fully in the therapy.

Activity 12.3

What do you think about the use of psychological therapy for individuals with health problems? Imagine how someone with CFS/ME might feel if you tell them they are going to have therapy to help with their condition. How would you word this so that a patient would be likely to engage with and benefit from CBT?

CBT has also been shown to help chronic pain. The rationale for its use is that the experience of pain is a complex experience that is influenced by the underlying physical problem but also by the way the person is thinking, feeling and behaving in relation to the pain. Many models for managing chronic pain are available. One classic article which has clear guidance is by Keefe (1996), who discusses a three-stage plan.

12

1 Help the patient to understand that cognitions and behaviour can influence their experience of pain and can influence how they can have some control over the experience of pain.
2 Introduce coping skills training, such as progressive muscular relaxation, brief relaxation or mindfulness. Activity scheduling and distraction techniques can also be used. Cognitive restructuring can help sufferers identify and challenge pain-related cognitions

and replace these with more constructive and balanced thoughts and beliefs.

3   Patients are encouraged to implement and maintain these coping strategies in day-to-day life. Support and guidance is given with regard to how to implement these strategies in the long term.

Summary

▶ The key issue in CBT is how individuals interpret events and situations; this is very personalized and determines how we think, feel and behave.

▶ CBT is an active, collaborative and time-limited therapy and involves a range of approaches.

▶ CBT is based on cognitive psychology principles and behavioural theory.

▶ CBT has a broad evidence base and, because of this, is recommended for use within the NHS for a range of mental health difficulties and to help those who experience some chronic health problems.

▶ The relationship is key; therapy will be more successful if good rapport and trust is able to develop.

▶ Many cognitive and behavioural techniques are based upon a 'map' of difficulties that are drawn up between the patient and therapist in the early sessions and reviewed throughout.

Questions for discussion

1   What are your thoughts about mental health problems and where they come from?

2   Do you feel that an awareness of mental health issues and knowing about psychological treatments such as CBT is relevant to your nursing role?

3   How do you feel about working with individuals with mental health difficulties?

4   Would you feel able to recognize someone with mental health difficulties and would you feel able to recommend CBT or other psychological therapy?

Further reading

Espie, C. A. (2010) *Overcoming Insomnia and Sleep Problems: A Self-Help Guide Using Cognitive Behavioural Techniques.* London: Constable & Robinson.

An easy to read guide to applying CBT to physical health problems and common problems such as sleep difficulties. It can be given to patients as a self-help guide.

Hays, A., and Iwamasa, G. Y. (eds) (2006) *Culturally Responsive Cognitive-Behavioral Therapy: Assessment, Practice, and Supervision*. Washington, DC: American Psychological Association.
This book provides the reader with thought-provoking chapters that need to be considered when applying CBT to a range of individuals and their specific cultural needs.

Westbrook, D., Kennerley, H., and Kirk, J. (2011) *An Introduction to Cognitive Behaviour Therapy: Skills and Applications*. 2nd edn, London: Sage.
This book presents a good explanation of CBT with key mental health disorders and key models used in the NHS today. It also has a good explanation of the political and economic benefits of CBT.

Chris Williams's 'Five Areas approach', www.fiveareas.com.
This includes downloadable resources for use in sessions and while learning about the application and theory of CBT.

12

Peter Spencer

KEY ISSUES IN THIS CHAPTER:

▶ The background to counselling, psychotherapy and coaching
▶ Role relationships in counselling
▶ Psychoanalysis
▶ Client-centred counselling
▶ Personal construct theory and therapy
▶ A critique of therapy culture

BY THE END OF THIS CHAPTER YOU SHOULD BE ABLE TO:

▶ define the basic concepts involved in counselling
▶ identify different approaches to counselling
▶ demonstrate how you might apply this practically
▶ propose what you consider to be the best approach to counselling for a given situation
▶ evaluate the effectiveness of counselling approaches.

1 Introduction

In recent years there has been an increasing interest in the field of counselling, apparent in a significant rise in the number both of counsellors and clients/patients and of areas in which counselling is used (such as careers and family counselling). Counselling also has a greater profile in the media and research literature. For example, in 1993 there were fewer than 500 citations of the word 'counselling' in British newspapers, whereas in 2000 there were more than 7,000 (Furedi, 2004).

Burnard (1989: 11) states that, rather than just those with professional certification, 'We are all counsellors, anyone who works in one of the health professions and comes into contact with people who are distressed in any way.' Thus a nurse can expect to find themselves in the role of an informal counsellor during the course of their work. The British Association for Counselling (BAC, now the British Association for Counselling and Psychotherapy, BACP) offered this definition of counselling:

> The overall aim of counselling is to provide an opportunity for the client to work towards living in a more satisfying and resourceful way. The term counselling includes work with individuals, pairs or groups of people, often but not always referred to as clients. The objectives of particular counselling relationships will vary according to the client's needs but may well be concerned with developmental issues, addressing and resolving specific problems, making decisions, coping with crisis, developing personal insight and knowledge, working through feelings of inner conflict or improving relationships with others. The counsellor's role is to facilitate the client's work but in ways which respect the client's values, personal resource and capacity for self-determination. (BAC, 1993: 6)

Dexter and Russell (1997) suggest that counselling is a return to the old roots of the practice of psychotherapy. However, it might be suggested that, in the broadest terms, psychotherapy is pre-dated by pastoral counselling such as is provided by the clergy and nurses, whose implicit or explicit role description has always included some aspect of what might be termed informal counselling. Frank (1982) suggests that the defining characteristic of psychotherapy is that it is a planned relationship between a socially sanctioned person and a person in the role of sufferer, patient or client which is often emotionally charged. The term 'coaching' represents a new approach to counselling, which can be described as a time-limited intervention useful for people wanting change, either in their personal or in their professional life, involving goal-setting and action planning with the aim of the client achieving their full potential by improving behaviour and/or performance (Berriman, 2007).

13

While there are subtle differences between counselling, psychotherapy and coaching in terms of clients and length of engagement, there is also much overlap, with eclectic therapists using a variety of methods simultaneously (Myers, 1998). It has even been suggested that exercise could be seen as a form of psychotherapy (Spencer, 1990a, 1990b), in that it leads us to feel better, increases our self-esteem and confidence, can help to break the cycle of depressed and anxious thoughts and, hence, can reduce unhelpful and pessimistic thinking (Wood, 1983).

Whatever else counselling, coaching and psychotherapy might be (or how they are defined), they all clearly involve a relationship between therapist/healer/nurse and client/patient. Perhaps the key point is to explore these relationships and to evaluate their effectiveness.

Activity 13.1

It might be interesting to think of the roles the nurse might adopt in a counselling situation. For example, one could play the role of a friend or a parent. Although most approaches to counselling would not regard this as best practice, the role of a friend could be likened to that of a listener and supporter, whereas the role of a parent is more akin to that of an advisor.

List some other roles that might be suitable, along with the typical traits of those roles. For each role, make a list of advantages and disadvantages that make or don't make that role suitable for counselling. Which, out of these, seem most appropriate for a counsellor and why?

Does the type of question being presented determine the most useful role relationship? Reassess the roles you have identified for the case of (a) relationship problems; (b) work-related problems; (c) traumatic events.

Think back to times when patients or colleagues have come to you with a personal problem. What kind of role relationship do you often find yourself adopting? Looking back on the advantages and disadvantages of different roles, do you think adopting this role is the most effective in the long run?

Particularly in the context of a hospital setting, where patients come with the expectation of being given a prescription or direct advice concerning their condition, people will often ask a counsellor for a precise prescription of how to live their lives. 'Do I finish or continue that relationship?' is a typical question (Spencer, 1983; Spencer and Bannister, 1983), and the kind of role adopted will influence the counsellor's approach.

Before we look at specific approaches to counselling, a clear statement should be made regarding the importance of its ethical basis. Different professional bodies will have their own variants of ethical procedures, but perhaps it is worth stating the vision and values of the Samaritans. While the Samaritans are not a typical counselling organization, in that their approach is highly non-directive, their ethical stance is worth considering. Their vision is that:

- fewer people die by suicide
- people are able to explore their feelings
- people are able to acknowledge and respect the feelings of others.

Their values are:

- the importance of having the opportunity to explore difficult feelings
- that being listened to in confidence, and accepted without prejudice, can alleviate despair and suicidal feelings
- that everyone has the right to make fundamental decisions about their own life.

Whatever role relationship and type of counselling is adopted, at the core is the fact that it is an ethical relationship reflected in the above.

There are three main approaches to counselling, one of which (CBT) has been discussed in the previous chapter. This present chapter will examine the remaining two – psychoanalysis (psychodynamic), the original invention of Sigmund Freud, and client-centred counselling, which will include the work of both Carl Rogers and George Kelly. Both psychodynamic and humanistic approaches contain many subtle differences within those two broad labels, but all share basic similarities in common. For example, while Sigmund Freud was the father of psychoanalysis, his work was criticized and developed by proponents of other psychodynamic approaches, such as Adler (1870–1937), Jung (1875–1961), Anna Freud (1895–1982), Erikson (1902–1994), Melanie Klein (1882–1960), Donald Winnicott (1896–1971) and John Bowlby (1907–1990).

Similarly, Rogers's ideas were developed by a range of people. George Kelly will be one considered in this chapter. Another approach is that of Fritz Perls (1893–1970), who was trained as a psychoanalyst but then moved towards humanistic ideas. In his gestalt therapy Perls highlighted the idea that our experiences of reality depend on how we view the world. This core idea, as we shall see, is central to the approaches of Rogers and Kelly.

2 Psychoanalysis

Psychoanalysis is both a theory of personality and a technique of therapy originally put forward by Sigmund Freud (1856–1939), though, as we have seen above, developed and criticized by many practitioners both during his lifetime and after his death. The approach is often referred to as psychodynamic. Freud was trained in medicine and later specialized in neurology, and it was during his clinical work that he came across the phenomenon of hysteria. Essentially what Freud observed was that patients could present with conditions such as paralysis of a limb without there being identifiable physical causation.

13

> **Case Study 13.1:**
>
> The experience of physical symptoms without there being an obvious physical cause is still a puzzle for medicine. While psychodynamic approaches would now not be considered effective vis-à-vis such symptoms, the more usual being cognitive behaviour therapy, the problem remains the same as that which Freud observed in Vienna.
>
> Student nurse Beth was spending time observing work in a pain clinic. One patient, Sharon, was a middle-aged woman who had suffered from disabling back pain for three years. Various medications had been tried, but with little success. It emerged that, in discussion with the psychologist, she had been through a difficult divorce a few months before the pain began and was bringing up three children on her own. She said she felt she was 'carrying a heavy load on her back', and she began to explore, with the psychologist, any possible links between events in her life and her back pain and how she might change her thinking and behaviour to manage the pain more effectively.

Freud developed this 'talking cure' as an attempt to provide the patient with an insight into their distressing symptoms. Once this insight had been attained, the cure, theoretically, was accomplished. As we shall see, the evidence of effectiveness, in the long term, is debatable. Further, it was sometimes difficult to understand at exactly which point this had been achieved.

At first Freud tried hypnosis but did not find this successful. Later he tried a 'pressure' technique, where he placed his hand on the patient's brow, but finally he came to use the process of 'free association', in which the patient lay on a couch and was encouraged to speak of the first thing that appeared in consciousness, without any censure. Freud listened especially for any slips of the tongue (nowadays referred to as 'Freudian slips') and was interested in the dreams that his patients had, as this was thought to indicate the unconscious processes underlying the hysteria. These dreams or slips of the tongue were often interpreted by the analyst. The role relationship has been compared to that of a priest listening to a penitent during confession.

Freud developed a complex theory of personality and personality development. Students who wish to focus on the theory of Freud are referred to the further reading section and especially the books by Hough (2012), who goes into some detail of the theory, and Sutherland (2010), who relates a critique of Freudian approaches from the viewpoint of his own experiences as a patient.

In this chapter we shall focus on two clinical aspects of psychodynamic work most relevant to the experience of the nurse: defence mechanisms and transference.

Very early on, Freud observed the important process of transference. In positive transference the patient transferred warm feelings from a previous relationship onto the analyst. In negative transference the patient projected more hostile feelings. In counter-transference the analyst transferred their own feelings onto the patient, such as sexual emotions or anger. Freud felt that transference was important, not just as an indicator of the patient's emotional life and a clue to earlier relationships but also as a means of changing these unconscious feelings towards significant others. You may already have experienced a patient becoming warmly attached to you, or perhaps aggressive for no apparent reason. In Freudian terms this demonstrates the process of transference. You may also yourself have felt feelings of warmth or irritation towards patients, and this counter-transference can be a real and difficult challenge for the nurse, both ethically and therapeutically.

Freud also observed in his clinical work the phenomenon of defence mechanisms, which appeared to be a person's way of protecting themselves from the anxiety-producing effects of frustration. Listed below are some of the more commonly used defence mechanisms.

- *Repression* is where a person pushes uncomfortable feelings into the unconscious. It could be a memory, a goal, a conflict, or anything that leads to frustration.
- *Sublimation* is the use of a substitute activity to satisfy a drive, such as the sex drive, in a more socially acceptable way. This could be, for example, through science, writing or art.
- *Projection* is where we attribute our own motives to someone else. A person who has strong aggressive or sexual feelings may attribute them to someone else. Scapegoating, where we attribute negative connotations to an external person or group, is another example.
- *Rationalization* refers to the situation where a person explains actions in such a way that more acceptable motives are ascribed to them. Beating a child might be 'explained' as an act 'for the child's own good' rather than an act of aggression.
- *Displacement* describes the process where an unacceptable act is displaced onto another object. A man angry at his boss but afraid to challenge him may come home and be aggressive towards his wife. A child who feels he has been replaced in his parents' affections by a new baby may destroy a toy.
- *Fantasy* – if they are unable actually to carry out an act they desire, a person may fantasize or daydream about it.
- *Reaction formation* describes the process whereby a person believes that the motive they have is the opposite of their real motive. A person who harbours aggressive feelings towards another may show overly caring behaviour.

13

Activity 13.2

Read again the list of defence mechanisms. Can you think how these are demonstrated in everyday life or in the practice of nursing? Could these mechanisms explain some cases of aggression or blame towards nurses?

Freud's theories have attracted criticism because of their unscientific nature. For example, how can one test the notion of repression and the unconscious? If we do not observe phenomena, can we really test their existence? Certainly there may be simpler explanations for these phenomena. Nevertheless, even accepting that Freudian theory may be unscientific, it does not negate the possibility that the therapy of psychoanalysis may be successful in some cases, and that the phenomena of free association, dreams and slips of the tongue, defence mechanisms and transference may be relevant to many approaches in counselling and therapy. At the very least, Freud highlighted the importance of careful listening to the patient, even to details that may seem unimportant, and that the relationship between therapist and patient is complex and vital to the success of therapy.

3 Client-centred psychotherapy

In contrast to psychodynamic approaches, Carl Rogers (1902–1987) developed client-centred psychotherapy (CCP), sometimes described as non-directive counselling (Rogers, 1951). Rogers focused on the development of the self and the 'me' part of the self-concept, which was considered the most important part of personality development (Rogers, 1961). This self-concept was influenced by the person's experience with others and their evaluations. At the core of the theory is the idea that, if the correct conditions are provided, the person will grow towards independence and be self-directing. Rogers's theory is therefore important not just for counselling and therapy but also for education (Spencer and Tordoff, 1983).

In comparison to psychoanalysis, CCP is a much more optimistic theory, focusing on the present and future rather than the past, believing that the clients have the necessary ability to grow and solve problems within themselves. The role relationship in CCP is thus something akin to a listening friend rather than a brooding priest listening to confession, or perhaps that of a 'psychological midwife' who is assisting, but not controlling, the emergence of new ways of behaving and feeling.

One of the key techniques the counsellor uses is that of active listening and reflection. The counsellor feeds back what they are hearing to the client in order to enable them to consider different ways of experiencing and acting. Just the word 'client' rather than 'patient' emphasizes this activity on the part of the person concerned: rather than passively receiving information about how to live their lives, the person moves forward in their own way.

Listening is the most important tool that the counsellor possesses, and in many ways the most difficult. It is very easy to bring our own judgements to bear on what the person is trying to tell us. It is very difficult to have any kind of therapeutic relationship with someone without that person feeling that they are being listened to. As well as finding a quiet place to listen to someone, it is important to clear out our own 'noise'. This 'noise' includes our own prejudices and biases. Furthermore, it is not just the words that need to be attended to but the body language and silences, which can often tell us more of a person's deeper feelings than the spoken word. For example, a furrowed brow, tight fists and tense shoulders might contradict the fact that the patient has told us that they are not anxious. Tics, the speed of speech, facial expressions and the posture of a person can often indicate more of their psychological state than a verbatim record of their speech. The nurse should be willing to pause, wait and be comfortable with silences in order to enable the patient to find the right words to express their feelings and also to attend closely to the non-verbal cues during these silences.

> **Case Study 13.2:**
>
> Student nurse Beth met David while he was waiting for his first appointment in a psychiatric outpatient clinic. He was looking sad and was staring at the floor. Beth asked him what he was hoping to receive from the counselling. David hesitated for a while, but then said that neither his family nor his school ever listened to his own thoughts and feelings, and he was hoping that today he would be listened to seriously and have his own viewpoint appreciated. When Beth asked what he wanted, David said that he wasn't sure, but he hoped that, by being listened to, potential new ways forward would become clear.

One way in which the therapist can transmit the idea that the patient is being listened to is to summarize and reflect back to them what they have said. The counsellor can then begin tentatively to explore, with the client, a range of possible options for future directions. A number of thought experiments may be discussed, such as, 'What might happen if you …' or 'How would you feel if that happened?' These open questions enable the patient to focus on and develop their own feelings and thoughts. Through this process, a plan of action can be put together, which might involve a simple change, such as visiting a local leisure centre. It is not the size of the step that is important but the direction of movement.

At the end of a session it is important that things are not left 'dangling'. One technique is to inform the person that there are only a few minutes left until the end of the interaction, and to try to reflect on what has been said and to summarize what has been discussed. In this way, while the problem might not be solved, there is a logical starting point at the next session, when the counsellor might say, 'Remember last time we discussed the idea of visiting a leisure centre?'

In the final stage of goal-setting and action planning it is important to bring a focus to the future. For example, a goal such as 'I will try to be a happier person' is far too vague and difficult to quantify. Some key points of goal-setting are listed below. Goals should be:

13

- clear and specific
- realistic
- cost effective
- adequate
- in keeping with the client's values
- achievable within a realistic time frame
- the client's own (this is perhaps the most important).

For example, rather than the vague 'I want to be happier', the goal could be 'This next week I shall try to arrange three occasions to engage in activities I enjoy.' Goals should not be about other people. When a client says, 'I have discussed this with my partner and they think I should ...,' the counsellor might ask, 'And what do you think about that?'

Box 13.1 Summary of client-centred psychotherapy strategies

1 Actively listen.
2 Summarize and reflect back.
3 Ask open questions.
4 Set goals and plan actions.
5 End the session effectively.

Egan (1994) incorporated many of Rogers's ideas into a model described in box 13.2.

Box 13.2 Model for client-centred psychotherapy

Stage 1 Review of the present situation
Stage 2 Development of a new or preferred scenario
Stage 3 Action planning

Through the use of these skills and strategies, Rogers believed that the 'actualizing' tendency (the natural urge to grow) that we all have could be developed. However, it is the attitude of the therapist and the relationship that develops between the counsellor and the client that, for Rogers, was the most important determinant of therapeutic effectiveness. Rogers put forward core conditions that he felt were crucial to the development of the person in therapy – acceptance, genuineness and empathy.

- *Acceptance* The therapist should show unconditional positive regard for the client. It is a kind of non-possessive care. It is not that the client is viewed as a perfect human being or that they have not made 'mistakes' in the past, but rather that the therapist communicates confidence and hope in the client's capacity to undergo the sometimes necessary pain of change successfully, and that they have value in their own right.
- *Genuineness* The therapist should aim to present themselves without a mask or persona. The therapist is a human being, in the

same way that the client is, and should not hide behind a mask. This can be difficult. For example, in a hospital, all the cues indicate that the person is a 'patient' waiting to have therapy *done* to them rather than seeking to find the resources to heal from within. One solution can be for the therapist to give a little of themselves away, perhaps some disclosure about life that is relevant to the process, with honesty and humility. This need not be something shocking or even terribly important – just something to show that the therapist is a 'real' human being, not hiding behind a façade.

- *Empathy* This is not to be confused with sympathy. Empathy is the ability to stand inside the client's shoes and understand what the situation feels like from their perspective. This may also be difficult, and will be heavily dependent on the situation. Again, a little disclosure from the therapist might enable the client to feel that their words and feelings are truly being understood. One way might be for the counsellor to recall a time when they felt isolated and abandoned by other people, such as being bullied at school because of their hair colour. This might at least indicate to the client that the counsellor has some appreciation of the types of feelings being experienced. In certain situations, empathizing will seem incredibly hard, such as the case of someone who has committed a crime. In this case, the therapist could show some empathy for the *feelings* exhibited by the client, such as regret or anger which may have fuelled the actions, without endorsing the client's actions.

Through this approach, centred on the relationship between the client and therapist and the attitude of the therapist to the client, Rogers very much simplified approaches to counselling. When compared to the many technicalities of psychoanalysis, Rogers offered a far simpler approach to counselling, moving away from the medical framework: 'To me it appears that only as the therapist is completely willing that any outcome, any direction, may be chosen – only then does he realize the vital strength of the capacity and potentiality of the individual for constructive action' (1951: 49).

4 Personal construct therapy

In this section we shall consider the work of George Kelly, who, as well as demonstrating another type of humanistic approach, links together some of the ideas of the previous chapter and the chapter following. He places emphasis on the way we view the world and the ways in which we can explore the world to bring about change in ourselves and our circumstances.

George A. Kelly (1905–1967) developed a theory of personality and therapy, called personal construct theory (PCT), which was based explicitly on the model that people were *scientists*. The model is essentially that, as scientists, we all develop a 'theory' about the world and see the world through this theory. This is our personal construct system, which can be considered to be a set of goggles through which we see and make sense of the world. Kelly says that people never react simply to a stimulus but, rather, to what they interpret that stimulus to be.

These constructs enable us to make predictions about the world, and our behaviour is considered to be an experiment to test out our view of reality. If our anticipations of events are confirmed ('validated' in Kelly's terms), then our construct system is strengthened, but if our expectations do not match the outcomes, then we are left in a slightly anxious situation and we have to modify, or at least develop, our construct system (Kelly, 1955).

If people are acting as scientists, however, why do they sometimes find themselves in different types of predicaments and dilemmas? People may sometimes be not effective scientists but, rather, 'bad scientists'. For example, we might spend all our time searching for findings that reinforce our theories of the world (the *inductive* method) rather than really trying to test our theories effectively. This would involve trying to falsify our best-loved notions in what is termed the *deductive* method (Popper, 1959). A person who is racially prejudiced may all the time look for examples to confirm their prejudices but ignore any evidence that may contradict their assumptions.

The role relationship in PCT is one of a research supervisor to a research student, thus maintaining the model of the person as scientist. Translated to the position of the nurse, this means that the nurse acts as someone who allows the patient to develop their own approach to choices and decisions. Kelly suggests, as reinforced by later workers (Bannister and Fransella, 1989), that PCT is a reflexive theory. What this means is that the individual 'giving' the therapy is not seen as a completely different kind of person from the individual 'receiving' the therapy. Thus the patient has more connection and involvement with their own predicament but may need a listening and reflective nurse to enable them to move forward.

Activity 13.3

Take these three 'elements', as Kelly would describe them, and say why any two are different from the third:

tea	coffee	cider

You might say tea and coffee are refreshing and cider is not, or that tea and coffee are warm and cider is cold, or that coffee and cider are fun and tea is not. Thus the constructs we have elicited are bipolar constructs of the elements tea, coffee and cider:

refreshing – not refreshing	warm – cold	fun – not fun

Kelly termed this a 'triadic' method. Now complete this method, but this time with people as the 'elements'. For example, the elements could be:

patient	teacher	friend

Activity 13.3 (continued)

What constructs do you discover? What do you think it says about your way of viewing the world, especially your views of your relationships with patients? You may even like to use the elements of:

who I was   who I am now   who I would like to be

What do these constructs tell you about the direction in which your life is going? You might like to do the exercise with a friend or colleague and discuss and compare your findings.

To utilize PCT, the therapist might elicit constructs from the patient, put together what their construct system looks like, and then feed this back to the patient. The patient can then stand back and, perhaps for the first time, realize how they are viewing the world and how such views might be creating difficulties. The two may devise 'experiments' together for the patient to try out and bring back to the therapist at the next session. Note the similarity with the approach of Rogers in terms of goal-setting. For example, for the socially anxious patient, an experiment could be to visit a community centre and to try to mix with people, or to join a club so as to test whether their anxieties are based in reality. The idea is that these experiments can enable the person to change their views on the world. The act of visiting a community centre is an experiment that will help the person to find out that it is not devastating and/or frightening to talk with other people. Experiments could also be developed to show the person that, if people do ignore them, it is not the end of the world.

PCT can be very effective, and often an individual can go on to change their aspirations significantly depending on the results of their experiments. Lowering our aspirations, or modifying our aspirations to become more achievable, is one way in which we can easily boost our self-esteem. To summarize Kelly's work:

> Kelly stresses that a person is in business to understand their own nature and the nature of the world and to test that understanding in terms of how it guides them and enables them to see into the immediate and long-term future. Thus the model person of construct theory is 'The Scientist'. He is saying that we have our own view of the world (our theory), our own expectations of what will happen in given situations (our hypotheses) and that our behaviour is our continual experiment with life. (Bannister and Fransella, 1989: 8)

13

---

5 Evaluation of therapies

Given there are different approaches and many different styles and techniques of counselling, which is the most effective? The question is more easily asked than answered, partly because it depends on how we measure it. For example, one could measure:

- the client's perception
- the clinician's perception
- outcome research, where one measures according to specified criteria.

As can be appreciated, different therapists in different traditions may have very different perceptions of 'success'.

Although psychoanalysis had been around for more than forty years, possibly the first systematic evaluation was that by H. J. Eysenck (1952), who found that, while 66 per cent of the patients experiencing eclectic (using a mixture of approaches) therapy improved, only 44 per cent of those undergoing psychoanalysis improved, and 71 per cent showed spontaneous remission. It seemed as if patients got better left to their own devices or when enjoying eclectic therapy. However, Bergin (1971), using the same data as Eysenck but with different criteria, found 66 per cent of the eclectic groups and 91 per cent of the psychoanalysis group got better, but only 30 per cent of the untreated group recovered. In a study looking at patients' views, Kotkin et al. (1996) found that 42 per cent of patients said that therapy helped a lot, 44 per cent said it helped somewhat, and only 1 per cent said it made things worse.

Michael Eysenck, the son of H. J. Eysenck, states: 'It is now clear that therapy works, in the sense that therapy is better than no therapy, although there is no clear evidence that one type of therapy is generally superior to another' (1998: 585). Luborsky et al. (1975), looking at these kinds of findings, quoted the Dodo bird in *Alice in Wonderland* at the end of a rather strange race: 'Everyone has won and all must have prizes.' Davey defines the Dodo bird verdict:

> Adherents of a wide variety of psychotherapeutic approaches ... claim success in treating psychological disorders ... early meta-analyses of outcome data indicated that all main therapeutic approaches are equally effective, known as the 'Dodo bird' verdict. It is clear from the evidence that patient improvement is heavily influenced by common factors shared by all psychotherapies. (Davey, 2006: 375)

Put together, these findings suggest that the various therapies might not be as different as they seem and that, rather than approaches to counselling being very different, they may share common features responsible for their effectiveness.

5.1 Common factors of therapies

What are these common factors? Jackson (1992) suggests that what all successful therapies do is:

- give hope
- enable a person to gain a new perspective on themselves and the world
- provide an empathic, trusting and caring relationship.

Blatt et al. (1996) also stated that the most effective therapists were perceived as most empathic and caring. Myers (1998) summarizes the findings of research into the efficacy of counselling as follows.

- Untreated people often improve anyway.
- Regardless of the type of approach, those who receive psychotherapy are more likely to improve.
- Mature, articulate people with specific problems benefit the best.
- Placebo, sympathy and friendly counsel of healthcare professionals often produces improvement. This effect is clearly important for the nurse. The placebo effect may be seen not as an artefact to be eliminated from research but as a valuable therapeutic tool.

Torrey (1986) points out that, if they were to be effective, witch doctors, shamans, psychiatrists – in fact, healers everywhere – all needed to possess warmth and empathy. Bandura (1977) proposed that self-efficacy is the variable that all successful therapies produce in people – that is, the idea that a person can effectively produce positive changes in their life. There is also evidence that those who feel they have effective supportive relationships are less likely to seek therapy than those without such relationships (O'Connor and Brown, 1984), which reinforces the idea of the importance of such a relationship in therapy.

Some further evidence of the importance of common factors, irrespective of approach, comes from a study by Spencer (1998) of thirty-nine people who had recovered from chronic fatigue syndrome (CFS). The stated reasons for their recovery were acupuncture, amytryptaline, Chinese medicine, cognitive behaviour therapy, colonic irrigation, counselling, diet, early diagnosis, graded activity, homeopathy, hypnotherapy, immunoglobulin injections, kinesiology, nystatin, oestrogen patches, polarity therapy, positive thinking, propolis, Prozac, reflexology, running, spiritual healing, total rest in the early stages, transcendental meditation, vitamin supplements and yoga. So, for the thirty-nine persons studied, there were twenty-six methods of recovery cited, some of which seem, at first sight, contradictory. What these findings suggest is that the support of the therapist and the hope engendered may have been the key common factors aiding recovery, irrespective of the type of therapy.

All of the counselling approaches we have looked at in this chapter seem, to a greater or lesser extent, to share these common factors. They give hope, a new way at looking at things, and a safe, secure and supportive relationship. In the future, research needs to focus more precisely on these common factors and also to discover the finer details of which particular approaches benefit specific persons and specific difficulties.

13

5.2 Critique of counselling

It has already been noted that there has recently been a rapid expansion in counselling. For some, this very expansion may lead to an over-reliance on professionals for what was once regarded as everyday problems and difficulties with living that people used to tackle effectively on their own. Furedi argues that the traditional support structures, such as the local community, are being superseded by professional counsellors: 'By recognising the authority of the therapist the individual accepts a relationship of dependence and acquiescence so this subordinate status becomes a way of life' (2004: 96). If one of the important processes in counselling is to promote independence, then it may be that the over-extension of counselling to situations previously considered to be normal actually does the opposite. Possibly even more worrying is the idea that this focus on the individual, who becomes 'pathologized' by the attention, might take our attention away from factors in *society* that need to be changed.

The philosopher Friedrich Nietzsche took a very different view of life's difficulties, believing that they were a source of growth, and that through facing these challenges head on we become more fulfilled people. Alain de Botton, a populist philosopher, suggests that everyone's life is difficult, but it is the *manner* in which we tackle these 'slings and arrows' that can make us better people: 'Not everything that makes us feel better is good for us. Not everything which hurts may be bad' (de Botton, 2000: 244). Perhaps the role of the nurse can be very effective here. Without putting themselves forward as a professional counsellor, they may nevertheless use counselling approaches to enable the patient to become self-sufficient and independent, thus avoiding the possibly negative labelling arising from the patient needing to visit a professional counsellor.

Case Study 13.3:

In psychiatric outpatients, student nurse Beth had been observing the work of a psychologist with David, a young man who had suffered from depression after failing, on the third attempt, to get into medical school. His parents and friends had suggested that he move into an allied profession such as social work, but David had been reluctant to follow these paths, had become withdrawn, and had stopped trying either to look at courses in these allied areas or to do voluntary work connected to these professions.

The psychologist used a technique in which David had been presented with cards on which were written names of professions. Three of these cards were picked at random for each trial, and David was asked to say in what way two of them were different from the third. In one trial, the cards 'bricklayer', 'social worker' and 'accountant' were considered.

Beth was quite surprised when David said that bricklayer and social worker were different from accountant because they were, in his view of the world,

Case Study 13.3 (continued)

poorly paid and of low status, whereas accountants were highly paid and of high status. Personal constructs were identified:

high status – low status   high pay – low pay

When David was presented with the cards 'doctor', 'social worker' and 'accountant', he said that a doctor and an accountant are highly paid and had high status and a social worker was relatively lower paid with lower status. Thus the problem seemed to be that he was viewing the world in a very different way from his parents, who had always wished him to become a doctor, because, in their view, that was a worthwhile, ethical and helping profession. David secretly had not shared these views, but was a little ashamed and worried that to admit to being interested in high status and high pay would diminish him in the eyes of his parents. His parents were invited to the sessions and, when they heard of these findings, reluctantly accepted them. The remainder of the work with David was aimed at reinforcing his self-esteem and image.

To test out these constructs, a volunteering opportunity was arranged via the local Jobcentre for David in an accountancy office. He immediately found this to his liking, and his appearance improved, as did his self-confidence, when he found himself in an environment with like-minded people. When his parents saw the change, his confidence and his more positive attitude, they too began to see that this was indeed the direction in which David needed to move and became very positive about the idea and proud of their son. His father admitted that he himself had always wished to be a doctor, and that he had assumed (projected) that his son would feel the same way about things. When David realized this, he saw that his parents' motives for him were guided (if a little misguided) by love.

Beth had been impressed by the way that being able to see, accept and be empathic about the view of the world of another person could produce such positive change. She decided that, the next time she became angry about someone's behaviour or thinking, she would try to stand in their shoes for a while and attempt to understand the direction from which they were approaching the situation.

Summary

There are many varieties of counselling, psychotherapy and coaching.

▶ All depend on the relationship between the therapist and the patient/client.

▶ Most approaches, though based on different theories (the Dodo hypothesis), appear equally effective.

▶ This has led to the idea of there being common factors among approaches.

▶ These common factors include hope for the client, a new perspective on themselves and the world, and a supportive relationship based on acceptance, genuineness and empathy.

13

▶ Further research on effectiveness may focus more precisely on the best fit between approaches and particular difficulties.

▶ Recently some concerns have been raised about the over-extension of counselling to situations that were previously considered to be a normal part of living.

Questions for discussion

1 What do you consider are the skills, qualities and behaviours that the nurse should exhibit to be effective in a counselling context?

2 What are the best practical arrangements for a situation to be conducive for the nurse to listen to the patient? What skills can the nurse develop to enable listening to be effective?

3 What emotions, positive or negative, might occur between the nurse and the patient? In what ways could the nurse handle these emotions ethically and professionally?

Further reading

Furedi, F. (2004) *Therapy Culture*. London: Routledge.
Practical, critical analysis of some of the possible negative effects of the growth of counselling.

Hough, M. (2012) *Counselling Skills and Theory*. London: Hodder Education.
A book covering a wide range of counselling techniques, supported by practical examples.

Joseph, S. (2011) *What Doesn't Kill Us: A Guide to Overcoming Adversity and Moving Forward*. London: Piatkus.
This text looks at post-traumatic growth, continuing the ideas touched upon at the end of the counselling chapter. Relevant case histories support the findings. The title is taken from Nietzsche and illustrates that there is much that is positive that can develop from negative experiences.

Lopez, S. J., and Snyder, C. R. (eds) (2009) *Oxford Handbook of Positive Psychology*. 2nd edn, Oxford: Oxford University Press.
An overview of the developing field of positive psychology, illustrating how psychology can be used to enable people to develop.

Sutherland, S. (2010) *Breakdown: A Personal Crisis and a Medical Dilemma*. London: Pinter & Martin.
A personal account of his breakdown by a professor of experimental psychology and his experiences of therapy on his way to recovery.

CHAPTER 1

Motivational Dialogue

Gillian Tober

KEY ISSUES IN THIS CHAPTER:

▶ Motivation, behaviour and change
▶ Patient motivation in maintaining and changing health behaviours
▶ The role of the nurse in eliciting motivation to change
▶ The application of core motivational change skills to improvement in patient health-related behaviours

BY THE END OF THIS CHAPTER YOU SHOULD BE ABLE TO:

▶ understand motivation, behaviour and motivational change
▶ understand the role of the nurse in motivational change
▶ practise skills for encouraging motivational change in patients
▶ practise skills for encouraging readiness to plan behaviour change in patients
▶ develop opportunities to learn, apply and maintain these skills.

1 Introduction

In the hospital and other healthcare settings you will come across people whose health status is impaired by choices they themselves are making. Sometimes, indeed often, these choices are hard to understand. People persist in drinking a lot of alcohol when they are told that the painful conditions they experience are caused by this drinking; people continue to smoke cigarettes in the face of increasing breathing difficulties or repeated chest problems. Overeating and lack of exercise are also associated with commonly occurring physical conditions in impaired health. Understanding what maintains the seemingly irrational continuation of these behaviours is the first step in deciding and implementing the kind of responses that are likely to stimulate change.

Data on the prevalence of drinking alcohol, smoking cigarettes, obesity rates and other lifestyle-related behaviours are frequently publicized and can be found in the UK on the Department of Health website or via the Health and Social Care Information Centre (2011), which also describe the harms resulting from these behaviours. The informed nurse would expect to keep abreast of population health and its various sources of influence (commercial pressure to purchase, peer pressure to consume, the addiction-forming potential of behaviours and substances). By way of introduction, it is useful to stake the claim that it is the role of the nurse in any setting to take a holistic view of the patient, their health behaviours and needs; having addressed this question, the theory and practice that enables the nurse to address behaviours that contribute to the health status of the patient are explored.

The challenge of a patient's acceptance of diagnoses and the consequent requirement to change lifestyle behaviours, with the attendant changes in self-image, are discussed elsewhere in this book (see in particular chapter 2, which deals with psychological models of health beliefs and behaviour). It is worth considering that material when addressing the need to bring about volitional behaviour change to promote improved health or prevent further deterioration. Medication adherence, changes in diet, daily routine, drinking alcohol, smoking and physical mobility all present a challenge to population and individual health, and consequently there is a challenge to apply pressure to change these behaviours at the individual as well as the societal level.

2 The role of the nurse in behaviour change

What do you consider to be the role of the nurse in the care of patients? Is it to focus on specific conditions regardless of the circumstances that might cause or contribute to the maintenance of that condition? Or is the role broader than that, requiring the nurse as health professional to take the view that a patient's lifestyle choices, whether with reference to consumption, exercise or sexual activity, are within their legitimate sphere of activity and intervention? The official view is the latter, and government policy and practice guidelines make this clear. The Department of Health identified concerns related to excessive drinking and, in developing its national alcohol strategy (DoH, 2007), and subsequently (DoH, 2008b), published guidance on implementing routine screening, identification and brief interventions. The implementation of this guidance has improved (Patton and O'Hara, 2013) but remains variable in ways that appear to depend upon multiple factors, including the perception of role legitimacy, knowledge of how to apply the guidance, perceived support and follow-on resources.

In a complex healthcare system, with its multiple components, disciplines and practices, there is a role to play at each stage of patient contact. At the first contact stage, in primary care and in accident and emergency departments, there are guidelines to inquire about drinking, smoking, diet and exercise as primary prevention measures as well as screening for the detection of disease. Some of these occur as regular requirements, while others are part of regular campaigns or research programmes. There are then condition-specific requirements to inquire about these behaviours for the purpose of preventing further deterioration. The primary care nurse has a role in both types of prevention, as drinking, smoking and other health-related behaviours can be identified as soon as a patient registers at a practice, as well as at identifiable developmental points in the lives of young people. In a hospital the role is more likely to be one of secondary prevention. Wherever the subject is addressed, there is recognition that most health-related behaviours are connected to attitudes that are entrenched in personal choices or family, social and cultural values. A change in behaviour, where it is required in order to avoid or manage disease, is not straightforward and, moreover, is likely to be contingent on a change in attitude. Attitude change in health behaviours has always been perceived as a challenge – a task that requires time and specialist knowledge – and this may be the root of the perception that this is not the role of the nurse, who does not have time to address patients' attitudes or to facilitate 'lifestyle' behaviour change (Raistrick et al., 2007, 2014).

Activity 14.1

Think of three reasons to inquire about a patient's drinking.

Think of three things that might inhibit you from inquiring.

List three things that would change your reluctance to inquire.

Think of three ways to overcome your reluctance.

14

What contribution can and does the nurse provide? If your responses to the first point in activity 14.1 are clear and you feel confident to overcome any reluctance you might have, the way forward may be straightforward. The responses you have given will depend upon your own attitude to drinking alcohol, your previous experience of dealing with people who drink excessively, and your confidence in your reasons and ability to address the behaviour.

Thus there is the task to address our own attitudes and behaviours before we can address attitudes to health behaviours in patients. To say 'This is not my job' when faced with a difficult task is a method of maintaining professional self-esteem in light of perceived professional failure (Cartwright, 1980). The case for early intervention, or intervention as early as possible, is to prevent increasing problems and poorer prognosis down the line. The same principles, which we revisit below, are relevant here: learning the skills of motivational dialogue gives confidence to practice and belief in one's ability to perform the required tasks; knowledge of the benefits of intervention gives optimism of outcome expectations – in other words, persuades us that there is a point in taking action.

Case Study 14.1:

Paul is a new patient registering at the GP practice. As part of her placement assessment, student nurse Beth is being supervised conducting basic health checks on new patients. Among her tasks, Beth administers the AUDIT (Alcohol Use Disorders Identification Test) (Babor et al., 2001), which, in measuring quantity and frequency of alcohol consumption and some commonly occurring consequences, is capable of detecting dependence; she also measures the patient's blood pressure. Paul's blood pressure is high, and when she measures this Beth detects a faint smell of alcohol on his breath. The time is 11 a.m.

Paul has reported that he drinks on more than four days of the week and that on one occasion per week his drinking exceeds 6 units of alcohol. He has answered positively to questions from Beth about other people expressing concern, very occasionally not doing what was expected of him following drinking, and not remembering everything that happened after a drinking session. According to the instructions for interpreting the AUDIT responses, Beth notices that the patient obtains a score that falls in a category of risky drinking, attracting the guidance to give advice, including a recommendation to monitor drinking.

What are the possible scenarios from the patient's perspective? Paul may say: 'I didn't realize that I was drinking this much and I must cut down forthwith.' The best thing Beth can do is to probe a little as to how he will set about cutting down, demonstrating interest and concern and reinforcing the idea, and to offer a follow-up appointment, saying: 'That sounds like a good plan. Come back and see me in a fortnight so you can tell me how you are getting on.' We are more likely to pursue a course of action if we express a commitment to another person, and even more likely to pursue it if the other person expresses that they care whether we do or not.

An alternative scenario is that the patient says any or all of the following: 'These government guidelines, they are all rubbish, not scientific.' 'What are they based on?' 'Everyone I know drinks the same amount as me.' 'This was highly unusual.' 'I have been having a difficult time.' 'It's my only form of relaxation, enjoyment.' 'I wouldn't go out if I didn't drink' – and so on. These many statements denote a different attitude on the part of the patient. In situations like this it is probable that the response of the nurse may have an even greater effect on the patient's behaviour.

We will work with the second scenario – the first, as suggested, being straightforward. The patient in the second scenario can be said to be ambivalent at best about their drinking and is more likely to be actively resistant to change. This is a good point to examine some theories of motivation and behaviour change.

3 Theories of behaviour and behaviour change

There are several theories of behaviour change, some emphasizing the role of cognitions over the role of experience and some placing greater weight on the primary role of experience, where attitudes change in the light of new experiences (see chapter 2, which discusses psychological models of health beliefs and behaviour). Some theories place greater emphasis on the role of reasoning and rational thinking and decision-making, while others emphasize pressures such as social desirability and modelling in learning new behaviours. It might be worth starting with an understanding of the more or less universally accepted principles of behaviour modification that have been demonstrated in classical (Pavlov, 1927) and operant conditioning (Skinner, 1969) and build on these foundations to understand thinking and change with reference to the more complex behaviours (see also chapter 2).

Behavioural learning theory tells us that people are more likely to repeat a behaviour that has rewarding consequences and less likely to repeat one that has punishing consequences or no consequences at all. This is essentially an operant conditioning theory of behaviour. Rewarding consequences can be the experience of pleasure, called positive reinforcement, or the removal or avoidance of pain, called negative reinforcement. They can also be the expectation of reward or of the removal of pain. Observations of these phenomena have been made in the laboratory, but they also reflect our everyday experience. Behaviours are learnt and extinguished on the basis of these principles of reinforcement.

Skinner and subsequent behavioural researchers have demonstrated in the laboratory, and replicated *in vivo*, the principles of

14

reinforcement that consequences occurring immediately following the behaviour are the most rewarding compared with consequences that are delayed. This makes sense, in that consequences occurring immediately after the behaviour are more likely than consequences that are delayed to be associated with that behaviour – i.e., they will be attributed to the behaviour rather than to some other cause and are therefore more likely to be perceived as a reward for the behaviour. Bandura (1977) added to operant conditioning theory the dimensions of cognitions and social value that draw our attention to the value placed by the individual on consequences, including their social as well as their physical value. In human behaviour the social rewards can be more highly valued in some instances. Learning to smoke cigarettes would be an example. The first ever cigarette is commonly described as physically punishing (characterized by feelings of nausea and dizziness) but socially rewarding (characterized by acceptance by a desired social group, excitement or feelings of rebelliousness). For smoking to continue, it is likely that a higher value is placed on the social reward (Russell, 1971). The pursuit of the reward then becomes a driver, otherwise known as a cue or a trigger, for the behaviour. Such drivers, as expectations of reward, form a component of motivation. Experience of the reward strengthens this motivation, though, if the reward has been strong enough and desirable enough in the past, the behaviour does not need to be rewarded on every occasion. An equally powerful, and some would say even more powerful, reinforcement schedule is known as intermittent reinforcement, which helps to explain many drug-taking behaviours and gambling. Such behaviours that are not rewarded on each occasion – indeed, may be very infrequently rewarded – demonstrate the strength of the role of expectations in shaping behaviour.

Once behaviour is learnt through these sorts of processes, how might it be changed? Learnt behaviour will be 'unlearnt' through a number of reverse processes. Reinforcement may fail to occur at all, in which case the expectation of it eventually diminishes. This can be either the expectation of a pleasurable consequence or the avoidance of a painful one – the alcohol, for example, no longer has the desired effect – or the consequence of the behaviour changes to being immediately punishing (the principle of immediacy is critical here), such that a painful response is elicited. Another route to extinction of a behaviour occurs when circumstances change and the reinforcing consequences are no longer valued by the individual. Alternative consequences take their place. Lifestyle changes, such as finding new friends, moving on to a new occupation, starting a new family, and so on, tend to rearrange the value people place on particular consequences. And then there are times where this is not the case, where the consequences of the behaviour, no matter how seemingly unpleasant, outweigh the consequences of alternative behaviours or remain more highly valued than their absence.

Case Study 14.2:

Paul looks at his AUDIT score and sees that it places him in the category of risky drinking. Student nurse Beth tells him his blood pressure is high. Paul's circumstances are that he has recently retired and has moved, with his wife, to live closer to their grandchildren, so they can help with their care. Paul has arthritis, so he finds the activities required with small children more difficult than his wife does, and he was unsure that this was what he wanted to do. He was concerned that he would be leaving some lifelong friends and neighbours, his much loved garden and his familiar routines. In order to meet new people he had taken to frequenting the local pub, and this was becoming part of his daily routine. His wife thought this was no bad thing, though she wished that he would develop some more physically active interests. The benefits to Paul of his drinking are the socializing, making some local contacts, getting out of the house, and avoiding some of the more boisterous childcare activities – longer-term gains, but important short-term gains as well – coupled with the relaxing effect of the alcohol itself. He had made sure that his drinking did not interfere with mealtimes and family routines and responsibilities. Now here was Beth telling him it was not alright. Paul's first reaction is to feel defensive. Why should he not have a bit more to drink? He is retired, he is mainly in good health, his arthritis restricts what he can do, and he enjoys drinking.

4 Motivational balance and change

Paul's motivation to drink in the way he does is easy to understand. He experiences short-term benefits as the relaxing effect of the alcohol, the greater ease in situations with new social contacts, having a reason or purpose in getting out of the house, and feeling that there is some structure to his day outside of the domestic routine. If this drinking pattern puts this patient's health at risk, what if anything is going to change it? If Paul experiences no negative (or punishing) consequences from his drinking, how might he be persuaded to cut down in order to reduce the risk of future health problems and/or the development of dependence? Theorists of motivational change have suggested that the first step is the introduction of ambivalence about the behaviour. Prochaska and DiClemente (1992) describe the circumstances of developing ambivalence in line with behavioural learning theory: some negative consequences occur, either gradually or suddenly; drinking no longer fits with changed circumstances so is perceived to 'get in the way' – for example, in the case of adopting new responsibilities or interests, or new friends whose activities are different. Other people express concern. All sorts of things can happen to shift the balance of consequences of the behaviour. Ambivalence denotes the experience of feeling two ways about something: on the one hand, there are the rewarding consequences, the comfort derived from the effects and

14

from the habit but, on the other hand, some negative consequences or implications have been introduced.

Ambivalence is uncomfortable and needs to be resolved. We do not tolerate ambivalence – the feeling of conflict resulting from holding inconsistent thoughts simultaneously – or having thoughts and behaviours that are inconsistent – for example, 'I like smoking but I know it damages my health.' Festinger (1957) referred to this as cognitive dissonance and developed our understanding of how such dissonance can motivate behaviour change or cognitive (pertaining to thinking) change. To regain consistency, it follows logically that something needs to change, and this can be either the thoughts or the behaviour. Which of these two courses of action is pursued depends on many things.

Activity 14.2

Think of a behaviour you have changed, preferably something you have given up.

Think back to the time when the behaviour was routine and valued.

Think about why you decided to give it up.

Think about what the process of deciding to give it up entailed.

Looking at the questions in activity 14.2, what did you find your decision to change your behaviour was based upon? What were the thought processes or the experiences involved? Research points to two almost equally important components of motivation to change a behaviour: the first is the belief that life/health/wellbeing will be enhanced specifically by cessation of the behaviour, that things will be better as a result of the change – a perception that health, for example, or a specific health condition will deteriorate seems insufficient, albeit that it might be useful in initiating thoughts about change. There needs also to be an expectation of benefit, called positive outcome expectancy. Think of the very different rates of smoking cessation in people diagnosed with lung cancer compared with those diagnosed with coronary heart disease or having suffered a heart attack. Believing things will improve seems to be the source of the variation in these rates of change. In the first instance, few people quit smoking, because they do not believe it will make any difference to their life expectancy; in the second instance, far more people quit smoking precisely because they believe it will. But even in the second instance not everyone quits. There remains the problem of self-efficacy, the belief in one's ability to do it, the second essential component of a good-quality decision to change (i.e., one that is likely to be put into practice). Bandura (1997) developed our understanding of the role of self-efficacy in motivation for behaviour change.

4.1 Addressing motivation to change

If these are the naturally occurring processes, what, if anything, can the nurse or other healthcare professional do to instigate such motivational change? The question is how best to address this state of ambivalence without driving the patient into an entrenchment of their commitment to the current behaviour. When providing answers to activity 14.2, some people might have said that they were persuaded to change by an argument that convinced them it was a good idea. The essence of such persuasion is that someone else is not arguing with you that it would be good for you to change or telling you what to do, but drawing to your attention something that is of value to you rather than to them. In other words, for us to be persuaded that we want to try to change, we need to value the reason for acting; it needs to be our reason, not someone else's. This suggests that great caution is required in broaching behaviours that evoke feelings of ambivalence.

Case Study 14.3:

Student nurse Beth asks Paul if they might have a brief discussion about his drinking in order to help her to understand how it fits into his life. She expresses interest in his perspective on this. She suggests that he describe a typical day so she can begin to identify his thoughts about his drinking by the tone of his voice and the way he describes it. She might then ask what he thinks about his AUDIT score and elicit his understanding of how risky drinking is defined. Paul expresses his defensive position about his drinking and thinks the limits as prescribed by the Department of Health are excessively low. Beth might then pick up on Paul's positive response to the question of whether anyone else has criticized or expressed concern about his drinking and ask him to describe their point of view. This enables her further to make a judgement about whether Paul has any ambivalence about his drinking and, if so, what that might be based on. He describes a couple of arguments with his wife when he has stayed at the pub longer than he said he would, and Beth inquires whether this was his intention and how he would have preferred things to have been. Paul then expresses concern about the way that sometimes he does drink more than he intends and that he thinks, once he has had a couple of drinks, his resolve to go home weakens and he becomes more amenable to people offering him further drinks and encouraging him by saying 'Just one more for the road'.

In case study 14.3, by making inquiries, Beth has enabled Paul to expand his thoughts about his drinking. She has managed, by listening and asking open questions, and inviting the patient to elaborate, to elicit some concerns. Once these have been described, it is then more likely to be possible to move to the question of how he would prefer things to be with reference to his drinking.

14

Activity 14.3

This is something you can try at home. Ask a friend about a highly valued behaviour about which they feel somewhat ambivalent, then try to persuade them to give it up; use any means you think will work. Tell them what you think about it and what you think they should do. It would be a good idea to record what happens and what the thoughts and feelings of the other person are. Then say you want to start again and ask them to describe the behaviour and use your best listening skills, exploring what they say, encouraging them to expand, really getting their view about the advantages of the behaviour. If there is any expression of a downside or reservation, ask them to expand on this. Explore this in the same way and then ask how they would prefer things to be.

The second time, use open questions – for example, 'What is the best thing about it?' and 'What do you like least about it?' – and follow these with selective reflective listening. This means that you may repeat certain phrases and statements, but not all. For instance, you might say: 'You love the way it makes you feel a bit rebellious, and at the same time this makes you wonder, is this a good idea? Why do I want to feel like this?' You can start to shape the direction of the dialogue by selecting out those expressions of concern about the behaviour – the basis of the ambivalent feelings – and by avoiding reinforcing the idea that everything is alright.

In activity 14.3 you explored two ways of proceeding when someone expresses ambivalence about a behaviour. In the first condition it is likely that you elicited a defensive response, an entrenchment of thinking and a rationalization for the continuation of the behaviour. In the second you probably elicited a more considered position with possible room for considering change. That is because in the first condition you are judging the other person and suggesting they are not doing the right thing, and moreover that you understand this and they do not. This elicits a defensive reaction because it is experienced as an attack. Defensiveness is a normal response. In the second condition you are communicating respect for the other person's point of view and will therefore be able better to explore what that point of view is.

The challenge of dealing with a subject which the patient is ambivalent about discussing introduces the rationale for using a motivational interviewing approach. Motivational interviewing is the method of choice to deal with situations like this because it minimizes the likelihood of provoking further resistance in the patient. The core skills in this approach are the art of eliciting the patient's point of view and avoiding telling them what to do. Evoking the patient's perspective will help to identify their own thoughts and then their own reasons for change, not those of someone else. In our current example, health-based drinking limits may or may not be meaningful to the patient; what is likely is that people who are drinking to excess will experience some adverse effects that they would wish to avoid. The same goes for other health-related behaviours. Unless they are able to identify these for themselves, they are unlikely to concur with exhortations to change their behaviour.

Two core skills described in activity 14.3 merit close examination and are the foundation of motivational interviewing practice: open questions and selective reflections.

What are open questions? Who?, What?, Where?, When?, and How? are useful opening words and less likely to result in a closed question, unlike 'Do you? Can you? Have you? Is it?', which precede a closed question. An open question does not and cannot predetermine the reply, cannot be answered by 'yes' or 'no'. Thus an open question more genuinely communicates an interest in what the respondent has to say.

Another thing about open questions is that, if the question itself contains no options from which to choose (is it this or is it that?) and therefore no hint of what the inquirer thinks, it is easier to express a non-judgemental position. The reason for using open questions is simply that they enable you to find out more, to withhold your own position (usually implicit in the closed question) and to express interest in what the respondent has to say. This is a valuable skill to practise, because open questions are useful in any situation where you want to get the view of the respondent rather than their reaction to a suggestion made by you.

A reflection may be a repetition of what the recipient has said, but applied excessively this can be irritating and not much use. A more useful reflection might be more complex, bringing together two or more strands of what the recipient has said. The art of reflection is the method of demonstrating interest, attention and concern. The selective nature of reflection suggested here is the method of reinforcing components of the recipient's speech, enabling the inquirer to steer the dialogue in the desired direction. Drinking to excess and other potentially damaging health-related behaviours may be difficult to talk about; there may be a lot invested in their continuation despite the experience of some adverse consequences. Encouragement to talk about these problematical things by expressing interest and concern and a positive attitude to what the recipient has to say has the potential to reduce resistance and any attempt to change the subject.

If you think of speech as a behaviour, then reflecting back speech is a way of reinforcing it. Reflections can be reinforcing if they accurately amplify what the speaker has said because they make the speaker feel listened to and therefore interesting and valued. This in itself is encouragement to keep talking. For example, if Paul were to say, 'I have been enjoying the company and chance to make new friends at the pub, but it seems to bother my wife and that doesn't feel great', the reflection might be: 'You are troubled by your wife's reaction and perhaps you want to get to the bottom of what you might do about that.'

Activity 14.4

Practise the discipline of asking open questions; sometimes this is not as easy as it sounds. Health service practitioners are taught to ask closed questions in order to establish concrete facts, and that habit generalizes rather easily. So be vigilant and, when you find you have asked a closed question, stop and modify it into an open question. You will then see there is no circumstance in which you cannot do this.

For example, ask someone else to tell you about something they enjoy doing but feel two ways about. Use only open questions. Reflect selectively the ambivalent components of their speech, reflect both sides of their own position, as expressed, for example: 'On the one hand you think that ... and on the other hand you say that ...' Then ask: 'Where does this leave you?' 'What might you want to do next?'

See whether you can reach a positive conclusion about the way forward and try to restate this in a summary.

If you have been successful, you may have felt that the dialogue flowed well, that the recipient thought it was worth having even if some of it was difficult. You may even have elicited a positive intention to act differently, to change something. Let's examine how we might use this approach in our example case.

Case Study 14.4:

Paul is worried about the revelation that his drinking pattern includes a higher quantity and frequency of drinking than is recommended to be safe. Occasionally he has not felt great in the morning, and once or twice he has taken a mouthful of wine remaining in a bottle from the night before to 'steady his nerves' and has noticed that it does precisely that; it reduces the tremor in his hands. He thinks it is not a great idea, in spite of the short-term relief, and that it was particularly not a good idea before his visit to the doctor. He has resolved to cut down his drinking on each occasion when this happened but somehow has not put his plan into practice.

Student nurse Beth is not going to be likely to persuade Paul to reduce his drinking by telling him he should because it would be good for his future health. This is not a current concern for him. If Beth tells Paul he needs to cut down his drinking, she is not telling him something he does not know. The fact of her telling him sounds like a criticism and may make him feel 'told off'. This would be quite punishing for Paul and may result in his attempting to avoid seeing Beth in the future. It would certainly close down rather than open up the discussion. He may therefore respond by defending himself, and the interaction will not be conducive to having a helpful conversation. The job for Beth is to find out what, related to drinking, might be a current concern for him. She wants Paul to feel able to tell her that his drinking is a concern and that for some reason he has not been able to reduce it.

This will more likely present a basis from which they can have a discussion of what might help.

Asking open questions obtains Paul's perspective and enables Beth to communicate interest in his situation, as well as empathy, reflecting understanding of how things are for him. Such reflection will help to reinforce, to encourage him to question his drinking and increase the likelihood that he will see her as an ally, a source of help and support.

Beth can ask, 'What have you tried?', 'What would you like your day to look like?' or 'What other things would you like to be doing?' If Paul is able to express how he would prefer things to be, then the scene is set for making a plan of action involving specific behaviour changes and identification of support to put them into practice. If, on the other hand, Paul expresses resistance to talking about change, then further exploration of his current circumstances or a self-help leaflet and the offer of a follow-up appointment would be the way forward. The follow-up appointment is important because it demonstrates the nurse's concern for the patient.

This sounds as though it could take a lot of time, but in fact it takes a few minutes, and the evidence says it is a few minutes well spent if you get agreement from the patient just to think about it. The same scenario can be played out in the hospital ward, at the outpatient clinic, or at an ante-natal clinic, for example (Raistrick et al., 2006). The principle is one of avoiding offering criticism that elicits a defensive response. Remember the evidence that simply raising the question of drinking as a routine will result in a proportion of people reducing their consumption (Wallace et al., 1988).

4.2 Estimating motivation to change

Throughout this chapter the nature and importance of motivation has been emphasized because it plays an important role in the question of whether or not people will change a problem behaviour. The components of motivation have been described: motivation for a specific behaviour is defined by the reinforcement potential or actual reinforcement of that behaviour. If the behaviour is reinforced either by having pleasurable consequences or by resulting in avoidance of unpleasant consequences, it is likely to be repeated. If the consequences are non-existent, not valued or punishing, the behaviour is likely to recur; value, strength and immediacy are all considerations in understanding the reinforcement potential of consequences. There may be several consequences, some immediate, some intermediate and some delayed; there may be stronger and weaker, more and less highly valued consequences. All these factors make up the balance that characterizes motivation. There are differences between motivation to continue a behaviour and motivation to give it up. Motivation to stop doing something is different again from motivation to do something different in its place. We may not like something we are doing (reinforcement for

14

the behaviour is weak or non-existent), but there is a fear of stopping because of the consequences. For example, will Paul feel isolated and lonely if he stops drinking? Does he think that the habit is now too strong to break and, if he tries, he will fail? He might prefer not to try so that he will not know whether this is the case.

> ### Case Study 14.5:
>
> As student nurse Beth gets him to describe it, Paul begins to think that there are drawbacks to his drinking. He turns over in his mind that he might be, or be becoming, 'an alcoholic', and he finds this thought to be alien and unacceptable; he wonders whether this is what his wife thinks and does not like the idea. He wonders whether anyone has thought he is not fit to look after his grandchildren. At this point his thoughts become clearer, and he thinks that he wants to do something about this now. He asks Beth what she suggests he should do.

Different types of speech can be understood as either supporting the continuing behaviour, known as sustain talk (Miller and Rollnick, 2013), or talking about change and finally making a commitment to change (Amrhein et al., 2003). Paul is moving in this direction. Although his drinking often causes him to relax and experience pleasure, he increasingly feels 'rough' the next day, and this feeling is becoming more important to him than the feeling of relaxation derived more immediately from drinking. He values his time with his family above all else. That is irreplaceable, whereas his drinking friends are replaceable with people who are doing other, non-drinking things. He is ready to take some serious action to change this developing lifestyle involving regular visits to the pub and almost daily drinking, and to replace it with an entirely different routine.

Beth perseveres with the open questions and selective reflections: What do you want your day to look like? When do you want to start this new regime? Who are you going to tell? In what way can they support you? Although there is no resistance to change, there is a risk of making suggestions that are quite wide of the mark; only Paul knows what the right, realistic and desirable things are for him to do. It is a good idea to avoid missing out on eliciting these. Thus, even if the patient asks for the nurse's advice, it may be useful to refrain from making suggestions but, rather, to encourage the patient to make some and then explore which offer the best chance of success. Equally, if the patient really does seem devoid of ideas, making suggestions based upon the formula 'Other people have found that ...' may be the way forward.

The goal of the motivational dialogue is to elicit this kind of change talk, denoting the patient's reasons for wanting to change and his ambitions about what he will achieve when he does change, culminating in his making a commitment to commence reduction or plan a quit date.

There have been numerous methods devised and described for measuring motivation to change, but the preferred method for everyday purposes would be the development of our clinical skills to detect motivational state, rather than using a more time-consuming validated measure. In the context of our dialogue about the behaviour – whether it is drinking, smoking, diet or exercise – impressions of motivation can be derived from tone of voice, volume of speech, language chosen (indicating warmth or distaste for the behaviour) and frank statements. Once statements about desire to change have been elicited, the strength of this desire can be gauged using a ten-point analogue scale: 'On a scale of 0 to 10, how important is it for you to stop smoking (or drinking, or whichever specific behaviour and behavioural goal is the focus)?', and 'On a scale of 0 to 10, how confident do you feel that you can change your …?'

Why is it necessary to assess motivational balance? Because it determines the content and direction of the dialogue in the following way: some people lack the expectation that change will be beneficial and others lack belief in their ability to change. Knowing whether either (or both) is the case enables the nurse to focus the motivational dialogue: there is no need to waste time trying to enhance self-efficacy when it is strong, and likewise with positive outcome expectancy. If the patient is convinced that life will be better if they drink less, but is ambivalent about whether they can achieve the change, this is the question upon which to focus. Addressing the weaker component of motivation to change is the better use of limited time.

4.3 Making the most of opportunities

The body of research on motivational interviewing is wide ranging, as it has been applied, in many contexts, to many health behaviours and attempts to change them (Hettema et al., 2005; Apodaca and Longabaugh, 2009; Miller and Rollnick, 2013). Some studies refer to its application in specialist settings, while others look at its use as a style of consultation to be used in generalist settings or in an opportunistic way. Some of these opportunities are more apparent than others, and in this chapter we have focused primarily on the general practice setting, where the scene is set for the discussion of drinking, smoking, diet and exercise, at least in new patients, by virtue of the health screening required at this point. Other settings are less obvious but might present an unmissable moment, an opportunity that presents itself and can be utilized for a possibly useful conversation. The rationale is the evidence that just having the conversation does more good than not having it at all. An example of an opportunistic intervention is described in a study of interventions delivered by the suture nurse when she raises the subject of drinking while suturing injuries sustained as a result of drinking (see box 14.1). The recipient is quite literally a captive audience, and therefore the communication of concern and respect implicit in the motivational interviewing style is all the more important, since at least for a few moments the patient cannot get up and walk away (Smith et al., 2000).

14

Box 14.1 A motivational interview

The dialogue might go like this:

Nurse: How did you get this injury?

Patient: We were in a taxi queue and these men tried to get in front of us; we objected. I wish we had kept our mouths shut.

Nurse: What happened?

Patient: They went for us. It was obvious looking back on it. They were drunk and we were drunk.

Nurse: What would you do differently next time?

Patient: All of it. Not get in a taxi queue. Keep our mouths shut. Not drink so much.

Nurse: You think you might drink less. How much do you reckon you had had?

These are examples of open questions. The nurse stays with what the patient is saying and then selectively chooses the drinking subject when the patient offers a list of behaviour change suggestions. She reflects what he says about drinking too much and then asks him to elaborate. This is how to get a conversation going about drinking. It is a brief exchange to be followed by inquiring about what sort of plan of action might work. This, like many other situations the nurse will encounter, may or may not lend itself to follow-up. If the patient is required to return for follow-up, then a brief mention in their case notes might prompt the same or another healthcare practitioner to inquire. If there is no scope for follow-up in this clinic, then the nurse would do well to ask the patient who he might tell about his plan and emphasize that doing this will increase the likelihood of his putting it into action. This principle was discussed earlier in this chapter: the benefit of sharing a plan increases the likelihood of being asked to report progress on it, and being accountable for our actions increases the likelihood of carrying them out.

Activity 14.5

Review the situations with which you are familiar in the various departments you have observed, and think of four or five opportunities like this where you could have initiated a conversation. Ask your colleagues to do the same exercise and share your thoughts.

Get groups of three together to rehearse motivational interviewing skills in each of the scenarios you describe:

Step 1 Inquire about the behaviour using open questions.

Step 2 Ask the respondent to elaborate and reflect back thoughts and expressed feelings.

Step 3 Pick up on any ambivalence and ask for elaboration, reflecting concerns and expressions of desire to change.

Step 4 Ask how the recipient would prefer things to be.

Step 5 Ask what would help to achieve this aspiration.

Step 6 Make a behaviour change plan and arrange a time to report back.

You can elaborate on the above task in many ways; each member can have a turn to take the role of the nurse, the patient and the invigilator who stops the dialogue when the nurse asks a closed question, sounds judgemental or confrontational, misses the point, or goes off on a tangent. The invigilator needs to be strict to be useful.

A variation on this is to practise *in vivo* and make a recording. Then play it back and use the above criteria for self-assessment and critical reflection. Getting other people's feedback is useful when it is accurate. New skills are not acquired without repeated practice, and they are not maintained unless they are subject to observation and feedback from knowledgeable colleagues.

Summary

▶ Motivational interviewing is a style of consultation that communicates respect and concern.
▶ It is a style of consultation that is usable in any situation.
▶ It provides the skills to adhere to guidance on addressing difficult subjects and challenges of behaviour change.
▶ It increases the likelihood of future attendance and adherence with plans and behaviour change goals.
▶ Developing and sustaining motivational interviewing requires practice.

Questions for discussion

1 Explore the range of health behaviours that can be explained by conditioning theory.
2 In what ways might conditioning theory assist the nurse in making treatment plans?
3 Reflect on your experience in using motivational dialogue with patients who are resistant to change or ambivalent about embarking on changes to their health behaviour. What were the challenges? How did you attempt to overcome them? How successful were your interventions? What other interventions might you use next time?

Further reading

Tober, G., and Raistrick, D. (2007) *Motivational Dialogue*. London: Routledge.

14

Conclusion

Psychology and Working as a Nurse

Sally Sargeant, Patricia Johnson and Patricia Green

KEY ISSUES IN THIS CHAPTER:

▶ The transition from being a student nurse to establishing a career as a qualified nurse
▶ Power and interprofessional relationships
▶ Stress and burnout
▶ Continuing professional development

BY THE END OF THIS CHAPTER YOU SHOULD BE ABLE TO:

▶ place social psychological theories alongside issues relevant to working in nursing
▶ appreciate the issues faced by both newly qualified and experienced nurses that relate to behavioural science
▶ understand characteristics of group dynamics that contribute to interactions between professionals.

1 Introduction

It goes without saying that working as a nurse has its inherent challenges and difficulties. There are few health service jobs without them. However, with a basic understanding of the dynamics of intra- and interprofessional communication, you will be equipped to anticipate and appreciate the complexities of working in what is considered to be a demanding but ultimately rewarding and positively recognized profession. Additionally, an appreciation of some of the theoretical principles behind occupational aspects of nursing – for example, teamwork, intergroup conflict and decision-making – will strengthen your capacity to deliver and maintain quality healthcare. This chapter provides an opportunity to review some of the preceding content of the book in the context of what it means to be a professional nurse.

Reflection in healthcare practice is now integral to healthcare training in many disciplines, with written reflections often forming part of the coursework and continuing professional development portfolios required of students and qualified nurses. Reflection has also been studied in context as an intervention that improves professional development. This chapter continues with the case study format of previous chapters but includes more examples to represent reflections that Beth has had in various areas of practice. These range from observations when newly qualified as a nurse to five years' post-qualification experience.

2 Reality shock

Case Study 15.1:

Beth completes her first day as a qualified nurse in an unfamiliar hospital on the women's surgical ward and feels quite lost. In her reflection she describes feeling very new and junior, not knowing where she was meant to be or how work was allocated. She questions if she has anything to contribute as a nurse given the established sets of rules, practices and actions that she does not yet quite understand in this new environment. She even finds herself repulsed by strange smells. Many unfamiliar things disconcert her, despite the fact that she felt prepared when she finished her formal studies in nursing.

The transition from a university to a work environment can be challenging and is a particularly relevant issue to consider within healthcare. 'Reality shock' is a term that is often used to describe this transition and the mismatch of expectations and outcomes that accompany it. Put simply, reality shock is a 'jarring feeling or experience that results from a wide difference in what was anticipated or expected and what the situation actually is' (http://thelawdictionary.org/reality-shock/). This definition alludes to what is essentially a bicultural conflict between the training situation and a workplace situation. It is a phenomenon that has been well documented among nurses and is not uncommon in other healthcare specialties. According to Saewert (2011), reality shock is characterized by four main phases.

1 *Technical mastery*: This involves not simply the acquisition of new skills but finding the opportunity to practise them within a new workplace setting. At the start of a new job it is likely that beginners' enthusiasm will manifest in a positive and optimistic disposition. However, this can also be accompanied by a sense of how much one does not know in comparison to older, more experienced colleagues.
2 *Social integration*: Working towards being accepted by colleagues.
3 *Moral outrage*: The most complex of the stages, in which a new graduate may feel disconcerted by the variation in quality of practice between professionals.
4 *Outcome*: This can take different directions, many of which can be negative. However, it is possible to adjust and maintain positive strategies to manage the discomfort encountered in the previous stage.

Despite the negative outcomes, such as loss of self-confidence, that can sometimes occur as a result of reality shock, there are strategies that newly qualified nurses can deploy to manage the uncomfortable feelings that arise from the transition from academic study to professional practice – these are addressed later in this chapter within the section on burnout. Additionally there are recommendations from the profession to place responsibility with employers to provide transitional support and resources for newly qualified nursing graduates as they move from being a beginner to an experienced practitioner (Boychuk Duchscher, 2009).

3 Interprofessional relationships

Case Study 15.2:

Beth's next entry in her reflective diary focuses on the doctor–nurse relationship. Earlier in the day she called a registrar and conveyed a symptom presentation for a post-operative patient, a pyrexial woman with a reddened leg experiencing difficulty bearing weight. Beth thinks she knows what the problem is, but nevertheless still presented the signs and symptoms to the doctor. She feels uncertain whether or not she should convey her opinions to the doctor, while knowing that they are the ones who are supposed to make a diagnosis.

The issues of power have been addressed elsewhere in this book (chapter 4) in relation to nurses' relationships with patients. However, there are issues of power and conformity that exist in relationships between other health professionals. Case study 15.2 focuses on the

15

much discussed relationship between nurses and doctors and exemplifies the changing status of nursing as a profession over the years; however, it alludes to the hierarchies in healthcare that are omnipresent and sometimes challenging. While relationships with doctors are mostly positive and many professionals report good working rapport, there is also an acknowledged asymmetry. Historically, the relationship between doctors and nurses has been vexed, due, in part, to evolving professional roles. This led to negative stereotyping of nurses not trained under the traditional hospital apprenticeship system and poor interprofessional collaboration, as doctors sought to maintain their power and control over patients and healthcare provision (Mckay and Narasimhan, 2012). This was articulated in earlier research, where nurses were challenged by doctors' behaviour and themselves behaved in ways that contradicted their own professional standards and instincts. Chapter 1 addresses issues of power and conformity in some detail, but the topic is worth revisiting here as there are surprising influences that other colleagues and perceived powerful others can exert over individual decision-making processes. For example, as outlined in chapter 1, Hofling et al. (1966) tested nurses' readiness to comply with doctors' instructions by setting up a scenario in which a fictitious drug was presented to them and a researcher posing as a doctor instructed them to administer the drug to a patient. Despite several rules being in place that gave ample reasons not to administer the drug, all but one of the twenty-two nurses in the study complied with the instruction. Fortunately, they were intercepted at an appropriate juncture.

While this experiment was admittedly conducted at a time when professional hierarchies were markedly different, it remains worth noting, given the extensive research into conformity and obedience that is discussed in other chapters. Effective leadership skills and placing of authority are crucial to manage such potential extremities of conformity which could, at worst, place patients at risk. Nurses now occupy roles which capitalize on extensive leadership and clinical skills and are key players in the multidisciplinary management of patients and health service delivery. Whether you are in a managerial position or newly qualified, it is important to identify leadership styles and consider what your own style is. With more nurses choosing to specialize in research or designated clinical areas, positions of management and leadership have increased, and a knowledge of leadership styles is advantageous not only in managing others but also in enabling an individual to prioritize and maintain awareness of their own strengths and limitations. Autocratic leaders display undesirable characteristics, such as assuming absolute responsibility for decision-making and being intolerant of others' views, in contrast to democratic leaders, who adopt a more consultative approach and involve others in decision-making and planning. Whether you are a leader or a team member, it is important to understand the importance of working within what can be quite large healthcare teams who may be responsible for the care of individual patients.

4 Teamwork

> **Case Study 15.3:**
>
> Beth has been working for several months now. Her latest reflective diary entry for her professional development portfolio requires her to comment on her experiences of teamwork. She documents that working as part of a team is one of the things she enjoys most about nursing. Although the main focus is on patient care, Beth thrives on being part of that team and appreciates the support that her colleagues provide when the workload is tough or if there is a difficult patient. Sometimes her colleagues are off sick and not replaced. Another time a doctor might have a bad day and make things difficult for those working with her. Yet the collective positivity that Beth feels from working together for the patients, despite the circumstances, confirms to her the plusses of entering the profession.

The reflection in case study 15.3 touches on the importance of group solidarity and cohesion. It directly addresses the benefits of belonging to an established occupational group and having shared responsibilities. It could arguably be an account that relates a busy day of any type of worker. However, the psychology of belonging to a group here is fundamental to the success of working within the complex systems of healthcare – systems that are spoken and unspoken.

Humans are by nature social beings, and a strong sense of personal and professional identity is central to our daily functioning. We belong to all kinds of groups, some of which are determined by our occupations, hobbies and interests. Others might be determined by our support for a sports team or other social roles. A group to which we belong is known as an 'in-group', and those to which we do not belong are 'out-groups'. Generally, in-group members hold their group in positive regard and look less favourably on out-groups (Taylor and Doria, 1981). This is known as in-group favouritism and can partially account for the cohesion and support that is generated in pressured situations.

A key theory within psychology that accounts for many inter-group processes and behaviours is social identity theory (SIT) (Tajfel and Turner, 1979). Before the exposition of SIT, Tajfel and his colleagues (1971) conducted experiments that identified how conflict and hostility can occur in group situations, and how the 'mere existence of social categories or groups can be sufficient to provide the framework for this behaviour' (Martin et al., 2010: 702). One such experiment was the minimal group paradigm, which involved the random allocation of children to two groups (the children thought they were allocated according to a preference for a painting by Paul Klee or Wassily Kandinsky). When the children were asked to distribute 'money' (not real currency) among all the group members, they showed a tendency to allocate it to the group in which they belonged, thereby discriminating against the other group (they did not know the identity of group members). While such categorization does not always produce discriminatory behaviour, this particular experiment has been replicated many times in psychological research and generally shows a tendency towards in-group favouritism.

However, we cannot attribute in-group favouritism solely to inter-group conflicts and discrimination. It is too naïve to assert that the nurses harbour negative feelings towards anaesthetists and surgeons because they belong to different professional groups. Elements of blame are also aligned to a further development in the psychological studies of in-group and out-group behaviour, which is that of the inter-group sensitivity effect (ISE). Hornsey, Oppes and Svensson (2002) conducted a series of experiments that investigated the perceived sensitivity to criticism from out-group members. Across all studies that were conducted, the authors concluded that criticism is perceived more negatively if delivered from an out-group member rather than an in-group member. Some aspects of the ISE are directly linked to the perceived power inequalities between professionals, and it is often the negative criticism that emerges from a professional out-group rather than actual membership of a group that is the cause of conflict. The important message from this is that it is perfectly normal to resent criticism from those who are not part of your professional group and to respond more positively to someone within your group. However, always remember that successful patient care relies on multidisciplinary teams working together. If someone challenges your actions, it is unwise automatically to assume that they are wrong based upon their group membership.

Given that we are sensitive to out-group criticism, problems also arise in the expectations of how a team is meant to perform. While healthcare staff in various occupational capacities work together to contribute to a team effort in practical outcomes, such as surgical procedures, it is also necessary to maintain and express one's own concerns, opinions and doubts, particularly where patient safety is concerned. There are many psychological theories pertaining to group dynamics, but there are some key terms that are useful to bear in mind when faced with a situation that is common to healthcare. One such area would be decision-making processes of groups. It might seem easy to make a decision as a group rather than as an individual, but there are other processes that can impede the process or even skew an outcome. There are many ways in which decisions can be reached, as identified by the following typology (Davis, 1973).

- *Unanimity*: Everyone agrees with a decision, or dissenters are persuaded to agree.
- *Majority wins*: A majority decision is accepted as the group decision.
- *Truth wins*: A position which is clearly accurate is the basis of the decision.

- *Two-thirds majority*: No decision is made unless this threshold is reached.
- *First shift*: A group aligns itself with the first opinion that is volunteered by any member.

Such processes are hard to negotiate when a group consists of members of similar backgrounds. In healthcare this is even more complex when multidisciplinary teams are required to make decisions in a clinical setting, and also within team meetings, often about the care of an individual patient. Often group decision-making processes do not pose problems, but the last point above – 'first shift' – is something to be aware of. Such a shift can lead to a phenomenon known as groupthink. Groupthink was a term coined by Janis (1972) and is defined as a tendency to reach group consensus with minimal dissent – at the expense of other reasonable decision-making processes. Groupthink tends to occur within a pressured situation, and a group that is susceptible to this phenomenon is likely to consist of a tightly cohesive group of people with a charismatic leader. In the decision-making process there is minimal or no assessment of strengths and weaknesses contributing to a desired outcome, and, in spite of what could be an erroneous decision, group members share the illusion that it is right and actively discourage opposition. This is of relevance to nurses who are part of multidisciplinary decision-making teams. They may encounter persuasive colleagues who do not necessarily have as their priority the best outcome for the patients, but may instead be driven by other factors.

Similarly, another phenomenon that should be considered in group decision-making processes is that of polarization. Usually groups will make unremarkable decisions, but, if a group has a tendency to make more extreme decisions, the resulting decision will naturally be more risky. This has enormous implications in healthcare and therefore endorses the rationale for multidisciplinarity within teams, ensuring that there are different appraisals of risk and minimizing the possibilities of groupthink and polarization.

5 Relationships with patients and oneself as a nurse

> **Case Study 15.4:**
>
> Beth is five years into her career and, despite the positivity she felt when she last wrote in her reflective diary, she now feels slightly disillusioned and anxious. When she started working in the hospital environment she acknowledged how privileged she was as a nurse – the limitless permission to gain entry into the most intimate lives of patients she has never met before and seeing them at their worst and their best. She has cared for

15

> **Case Study 15.4 (continued)**
>
> people who aren't bothered about their health and aggressive and angry people whom she doesn't like – while managing to maintain a non-judgemental disposition. She has seen the joy experienced by new parents and patients who have been given the all-clear, through to those who are at the end of their lives. She feels emotionally exhausted and wonders how her colleagues seem to handle it all.

The scenario of case study 15.4 is the one that best exemplifies the great variety of contexts in which nurses work, together with the joyful highs and significant lows that accompany them. The degree of access to lives described here is often on a level that other health professions do not see and contributes to the robust establishment of professional identity.

The desire to promote and deliver optimal care and gain maximum trust from patients and families can easily manifest as unhelpful traits such as perfectionism and increased self-criticism – which are at best unhelpful and perpetuate the belief that no one makes errors of practice and/or judgement. But human nature is human nature, and no one in any profession, health-related or otherwise, can claim immunity from this. Additionally, healthcare is seen as a high-risk profession, and the complexity of healthcare systems and practice heighten the quest for positive outcomes.

A major component of decision-making and action-taking is communication. This is not necessarily based always on verbal expressions but also on sets of practices, assumptions and protocols that exist within occupational settings. Implicit knowledge is absorbed and is not always easily verbally expressed. The complexity of healthcare systems can seem initially daunting. Several decades ago, healthcare personnel consisted primarily of doctors and nurses with distinct role divisions and expectations. Today's healthcare systems are much more complex, with nurses working within different specialities alongside technicians and other healthcare personnel contributing to the care of individual patients. Such complexity is also accompanied by the need for good communication and interprofessional learning. Communication in practice is not simply a matter of what we say to one another. It is also in written forms such as patient notes, memos and policy documents. Other communication is non-verbal, and there are sets of practices within healthcare that may not be explicitly verbalized but packaged into a set of assumptions that are hidden. Within such complexity it is understandable and inevitable that things do not always go to plan. Negative clinical outcomes may or may not be the result of errors, but they certainly contribute towards the feelings of stress and self-recrimination as articulated in case study 15.4.

6 Burnout

It is possible for a health professional, when exposed to periods of prolonged stress, to become 'burnt out'. Sometimes this term is used synonymously with stress, but there are subtle differences that distinctively characterize burnout. Burnout occurs as a state of physical, mental and emotional exhaustion. In contrast to stress, which heightens our engagement with a situation, burnout renders an individual disengaged and personally detached from their occupational circumstances. It is also accompanied by a reduced sense of personal accomplishment, high levels of job dissatisfaction, and absenteeism. Typically, burnout may occur after years in practice, but it is not unheard of for recently qualified nurses and other health professionals to experience it. However, the most important factor to consider here – whether as a newly qualified or an experienced nurse – is how to develop and maintain strategies to minimize stress and ultimately prevent burnout.

Maslach (2007) identified six factors that relate directly to occupational burnout: lack of control, high workload, the absence of fairness, value conflicts, insufficient rewards and lack of community. Many of these factors can be applied to health professions, given the number of different specialty groups that now contribute towards patient care and the complexity of healthcare systems operating at administrative levels. Therefore it is crucial to ask how healthcare professionals, and specifically nurses, can take active steps to mitigate these factors and ultimately try to prevent burnout.

There are of course informal social routes to debriefing – for example, a glass of wine after work with colleagues – but there are other ways to address stress and prevent burnout within the workplace setting. It is important actively to comprehend and practise some of these strategies early on in one's career to avoid prolonged stress leading to burnout.

In nursing training, and sometimes medical training more generally, there are moves to encourage reflective practice, a phrase that is often used but not always sufficiently placed to equip future health professionals how to use it well. Becoming a reflective practitioner is more than just becoming aware of your thoughts and feelings about adverse or difficult events. It is a process of metacognition – of learning to think about thinking – and thereby enables an individual to ask themselves relevant questions about their personal and professional reactions to a challenging situation. This can be done retrospectively, but it is ideally practised while executing tasks too. If something does not feel quite right, having the confidence to take a step back and think about these uncomfortable responses, and share them with someone else, is critical to the process of reflection.

Another key strategy to minimize burnout and ensure adequate support for staff is having a mentor. Ideally this would be a more

15

experienced member of staff who is able to advise on everyday practice, policy and future career developments. Even if you are not formally assigned a mentor in your occupational setting, you can always personally identify a more experienced member of staff and ask them to mentor you, and therefore ensure that you have a point of reference for career progression.

7 Continuing professional development and specialist training

Case Study 5.5:

Beth is now five years into her career and reflects on how much she has learned. She is thinking about specializing as a mental health nurse, despite feeling after qualifying that she would never do another course or put herself under the stress of exams again. She thinks the new nurses and doctors who are recent graduates look so young and inexperienced and finds it hard to believe that she was once like that.

Thinking about career progression naturally leads us to consider further training or study. After a long period of time working as a nurse, it is likely that one will gradually build the confidence and implicit knowledge that comes with experience. The acquisition of such knowledge naturally leads to a judgement about new colleagues and the ideals that they may bring to the profession. Effectively, this is another illustration of the formation of in-groups and out-groups, with the latter being the more inexperienced cohorts that emerge in the workplace. It is perhaps easy to be dismissive of newer colleagues' enthusiasm and tempting to fall into the 'in my day we did it like this' camp. Continuing professional development is a critical pathway that ensures that best practice is continually observed and updated, and it is also a way in which nurses can liaise and network with other nurses in different environments and clinical specialties.

Given the range of continuing professional development options that are available, from one-off workshops through to higher degree courses that can be completed while still working, it is unsurprising that nurses find it difficult to meet the challenges of balancing work and study. With this in mind, it is useful to consider how we respond to teaching and the differences in learning styles that we exhibit. Psychologists and education professionals have developed numerous measures of learning styles; indeed, psychology has an established pedigree of theoretical evidence, from the constructivist arguments of Piaget (1950) and Bruner (1960), through to specific measurement scales such as the Student Process Questionnaire (SPQ) (Biggs, 1987). The SPQ contains a series of statements that reflect whether someone is a deep learner (e.g., using a range of modalities to absorb knowledge) or a surface learner (e.g., a preference for rote learning), or whether they maintain an achieving approach (e.g., a constant drive to gain high grades). By reflecting on and identifying what type of learner you are, it is possible to devise strategies to manage effective learning alongside paid work.

Retention of information is also dependent on memory – something that could easily form another chapter, if not a book. While this is not an appropriate juncture to introduce a lengthy discussion on memory, it is important to recognize some of the cognitive biases we hold that inevitably affect our learning and subsequent decision-making. In the context of medicine, Crosskerry (2003) documents a comprehensive list of biases that influence diagnostic and treatment procedures. These biases are equally appropriate to nursing practice and healthcare in general. One example of such a bias is ascertainment bias, in which current thinking is shaped by prior expectation. Stereotyping, which is representative of ascertainment, can mean that readily available information that might contribute to a clinical decision may be lost based on prior expectation. Similarly, availability bias can affect learning and decision-making; if an event happens frequently, it is more likely to come to mind, therefore maximizing the chance of a diagnosis. Conversely, if something has not been witnessed for a long time, it may be missed, as it does not readily spring to mind. To try and ameliorate such biases, Crosskey advocates strategies already recommended here, such as mentorship, reflection and continued professional development.

8 Conclusion

Beth's reflections have covered a range of issues within the context of professional nursing that are relevant to occupational, social, educational and cognitive psychology. While her observations may instigate questions about emotional attachment, retention of information and teamwork, among other things, they also convey the richness of experience of working as a nurse. Nursing is a profession that has grown immensely over the years and from which many rewards can be gained. Research opportunities, continued professional development and conferences all provide networks in which the profession continues to strengthen and progress. Psychology assists this strengthening process by enabling nurses to understand their patients in ways that were not considered several decades ago. Additionally, psychology assists nurses in recognizing the social occupational processes in which they work and, most importantly, enables them to consider their own position as a practitioner – both as an individual and as a team member.

We wish you a long and fulfilling career.

15

Summary

▶ The transition between being a student nurse and establishing a career as a qualified nurse can be challenging and should not be underestimated.

▶ The power inherent in interprofessional relationships, including managing leadership roles, requires careful attention and management.

▶ Nurses need to be alert to signs of stress to try and manage their professional lives effectively and prevent burnout. Reflective diaries and clinical supervision can aid with this.

Questions for discussion

1 How does being identified as a member of a specific occupational group influence your thinking and actions within the workplace?

2 What influence do you think social identity theory has on workplace relations?

3 What strategies can you develop to assist in your adjustment to a professional role and successful career progression?

Further reading

Hargreaves, J., and Page, L. (2013) *Reflective Practice*. Cambridge: Polity.

Hochschild, A. (1983) *The Managed Heart: Commercialization of Human Feeling*. Berkeley: University of California Press.
This classic text looks at how nurses and other professionals manage the emotional component of their work.

Benner, E. (1984) *From Novice to Expert: Excellence and Power in Clinical Nursing Practice*. Menlo Park, CA: Addison-Wesley.
Benner's book builds on theories from cognitive psyhcology, arguing that, as they become more experienced, nurses rely more on intutitive judgements than rational, cognitive judgements. Through worked examples, Benner leads the reader from how the novice nurse goes through a series of stages in order to become the expert nurse.

Schon, D. A. (1983) *The Reflective Practitioner: How Professionals Think in Action*. London: Temple Smith.
A classic text on how professional learning is a continual process of reflection on experience and expertise.

References

Aghotor, J., Pfueller, U., Moritz, S., Weisbrod M., and Roesch-Ely D. (2010) Metacognitive training for patients with schizophrenia (MCT): feasibility and preliminary evidence for its efficacy, *Journal of Behaviour Therapy and Experimental Psychiatry* 41: 207–11.

Ainsworth, M. D. S. (1978) *Patterns of Attachment: A Psychological Study of the Strange Situation*. Hillsdale, NJ: Lawrence Erlbaum Associates.

Ajzen, I. (1985) From intentions to actions: a theory of planned behaviour, in J. Kuhl and J. Beckman (eds), *Action-Control: From Cognition to Behaviour*. Berlin: Springer, pp. 11–29.

Almeida, D. (2005) Resilience and vulnerability to daily stressors assessed via diary methods, *Current Directions in Psychological Science* 14: 64–8.

Alzheimer's Society (2009) *Counting the Cost: Caring for People with Dementia on Hospital Wards*. London: Alzheimer's Society.

Alzheimer's Society (2013) *Low Expectations: Attitudes on Choice, Care and Community for People with Dementia in Care Homes*. London: Alzheimer's Society.

American Psychiatric Association (2013) *Diagnostic and Statistical Manual of Mental Disorders, DSM-5*. 5th edn, Washington, DC: American Psychiatric Association.

Amrhein, P. C., Miller, W. R., Yahne, C. E., Palmer, M., and Fulcher, L. (2003) Client commitment language during motivational interviewing predicts drug use outcomes, *Journal of Consulting and Clinical Psychology* 71: 862–78.

Andersen, B., Anderson, B., and deProsse, C. (1989a) Controlled prospective longitudinal study of women with cancer, I: Sexual functioning outcomes, *Journal of Consulting and Clinical Psychology* 57(6), 683–91.

Andersen, B., Anderson, B., and deProsse, C. (1989b) Controlled prospective longitudinal study of women with cancer, II: Psychological outcomes, *Journal of Consulting and Clinical Psychology* 57(6), 692–7.

Andershed, B. (2006) Relatives in end-of-life care, part 1: A systematic review of the literature the last five years, January 1999 – February 2004, *Journal of Clinical Nursing* 15: 1158–69.

Andershed, B., and Ternestedt, B. (2001) Development of a theoretical framework describing relatives' involvement in palliative care, *Journal of Advanced Nursing* 34: 554–62.

Apodaca, T. R., and Longabaugh, R. (2009) Mechanisms of change in motivational interviewing: a review and preliminary evaluation of the evidence, *Addiction* 104(5): 705–15.

APPGD (All-Party Parliamentary Group on Dementia) (2008) *Always a Last Resort: Inquiry into the Prescription of Antipsychotic Drugs to People with Dementia Living in Care Homes.* London: The Stationery Office.

Asch, S. E. (1951) Effects of group pressure upon the modification and distortion of judgment, in H. S. Guetzkow (ed.), *Groups, Leadership and Men.* Pittsburgh: Carnegie Press.

Asch, S. E. (1955) Opinions and social pressure, *Scientific American* 193: 31–5.

Asch, S. E. (1956) Studies of indepencence and conformity: a minority of one against a unanimous majority, *Psychological Monographs: General and Applied* 70(9): 1–70.

Aziz, C., and Ahmad, A. (2006) The role of the thalamus in modulating pain, *Malaysian Journal of Medical Sciences* 13(2): 11–18.

Babor, T. F., Higgins-Biddle, J. C., Saunders, J. B., and Monteiro, M. G. (2001) *AUDIT, the Alcohol Use Disorders Identification Test: Guidelines for Use in Primary Health Care.* 2nd edn, Geneva: World Health Organization.

BAC (1993) *Code of Ethics and Practice for Trainers in Counselling and Counselling Skills.* Rugby: British Association for Counselling.

Bakish, D. (1999) The patient with comorbid depression and anxiety: the unmet need, *Journal of Clinical Psychiatry* 60(6): 20–4.

Ball, J. E., Murrells, T., Rafferty, A. M., Morrow, E., and Griffiths, P. (2012) 'Care left undone' during nursing shifts: associations with workload and perceived quality of care, *BMJ Quality & Safety*: doi:10.1136/bmjqs-2012-001767.

Ballatt, J., and Campling, P. (2011) *Intelligent Kindness: Reforming the Culture of Healthcare.* London: RCPsych Publications.

Bandura, A. (1965) Influence of models' reinforcement contingencies on the acquisition of imitative responses, *Journal of Personality and Social Psychology* 1(6): 589–95.

Bandura, A. (1977) *Social Learning Theory.* Englewood Cliffs, NJ: Prentice Hall.

Bandura, A. (1986) *Social Foundations of Thought and Action.* Englewood Cliffs, NJ: Prentice Hall.

Bandura, A. (1997) *Self-Efficacy: The Exercise of Control.* New York: W. H. Freeman.

Bandura, A., O'Leary, A., Taylor, C., Gauthier, J., and Gossard, D. (1987) Perceived self-efficacy and pain control: opioid and non-opioid mechanisms, *Journal of Personality and Social Psychology* 53: 563–71.

Banerjee, S. (2009) *The Use of Antipsychotic Medication for People with Dementia: Time for Action.* London: Department of Health.

Bannister, D., and Fransella, F. (1989) *Inquiring Man: The Psychology of Personal Constraints.* London: Croom Helm.

Bartlett, R. (2000) Dementia as a disability: can we learn from disability studies and theory? *Journal of Dementia Care* 8(5): 33–6.

Baze, C., Monk, B., and Herzog, T. (2008) The impact of cervical cancer on quality of life: a personal account, *Gynecologic Oncology* 109: S12–S14.

Beail, N. (1998) Psychoanalytic psychotherapy with men with intellectual disabilities: a preliminary outcome study, *British Journal of Medical Psychology* 71: 1–11.

Beail, N., and Warden, S. (1996) Evaluation of a psychodynamic psychotherapy for adults with intellectual disabilities: rationale, design and preliminary outcome data, *Journal of Applied Research in Intellectual Disabilities* 9(3): 223–8.

Beck, A. T. (1967a) *Depression: Causes and Treatment*. Philadelphia: University of Pennsylvania Press.

Beck, A. T. (1967b) *Depression: Clinical, Experimental and Theoretical Aspects*. New York: Harper & Row.

Beck, A. T. (2008) *Depression: Causes and Treatment*. 2nd edn, Philadelphia: University of Pennsylvania Press.

Beck, A. T., Rush, A. J., Shaw, B. F., and Emery, G. (1979) *Cognitive Therapy of Depression*. New York: Guilford Press.

Beecher, H. K. (1956) Relationship of significance of wound to pain experienced, *Journal of the American Medical Association*, 161: 1609–13.

Benkel, I., Wijk, H., and Molander, U. (2009) Family and friends provide most social support for the bereaved, *Palliative Medicine* 23: 141–9.

Benson, B. A. (1986) Anger management training, *Psychiatric Aspects of Mental Retardation Reviews* 5(10): 51–5.

Benson, B. A., and Havercamp, S. M. (1999) Behavioural approaches to treatment: principles and practices, in N. Bouras (ed.), *Psychiatric and Behavioural Disorders in Developmental Disabilities and Mental Retardation*. Cambridge: Cambridge University Press.

Bentall, R. P., Kaney, S., and Dewey, M. E. (1991) Paranoia and social reasoning: an attribution theory analysis, *British Journal of Clinical Psychology* 30(1): 13–23.

Bentall, R. P., Kinderman, P., and Kaney, S. (1994) The self, attributional processes and abnormal beliefs: toward a model of persecutory delusions, *Behaviour Research and Therapy* 32: 331–41.

Bergin, A. E. (1971) The evaluation of therapeutic outcomes, in A. E. Bergin and S. L. Garfield (eds), *Handbook of Psychotherapy and Behavior Change: An Empirical Analysis*. New York: Wiley, pp. 217–70.

Bergvik, S., Sorlie, T., Wynn, R., and Sexton, H. (2010) Psychometric properties of the Type D scale (DS14) in Norwegian cardiac patients, *Scandinavian Journal of Psychology* 51(4): 334–40.

Bernstein, D. A., and Borkovec, T. D. (1973) *Progressive Relaxation Training: A Manual for the Helping Professions*. Champaign, IL: Research Press.

Berriman, J. (2007) Can coaching combat stress at work? *Occupational Health* 59(1): 27–30.

Biggs, J. B. (1987) *Student Approaches to Learning and Studying.* Melbourne: Australian Council for Educational Research.

Birks, J. (2006) Cholinesterase inhibitors for Alzheimer's disease, *Cochrane Database of Systematic Reviews,* www.ncbi.nlm.nih.gov/pubmed/16437532

Black, L., Cullen, C., and Novaco, R. (1997) Anger assessment for people with mild learning disabilities in secure settings, in B. Stenfert Kroese, D. Dagnan and K. Loumidis (eds), *Cognitive-Behaviour Therapy for People with Learning Disabilities.* London: Routledge.

Blatt, S. J., Sanislow, C. A. III, Zuroff, D. C., and Pilkonis, P. A. (1996) Characteristics of effective therapists: further analyses of data from the National Institute of Mental Health Treatment of Depression Collaborative Research Program, *Journal of Consulting and Clinical Psychology* 64(6): 1276–84.

Boduszek, D., Adamson, G., Shevlin, M., and Hyland, P. (2012) The role of personality in the relationship between criminal social identity and criminal thinking style within a sample of prisoners with learning difficulties, *Journal of Learning Disabilities and Offending Behaviour* 3(1): 12–24.

Boecker, H., Sprenger, T., Spilker, M., Henriksen, G., Koppenhoefer, M., Wagner, K., Valet, M., Berthele, A., and Tolle, T. (2008) The runner's high: opioidergic mechanisms in the human brain, *Cerebral Cortex* 18(11): 2523–31.

Bonaz, B., Baciu, M., Papillon, E., Bost, R., Gueddah, N., Le Bas, J., Fournet, J., and Segebarth, C. (2002) Central processing of rectal pain in patients with irritable bowel syndrome: an fMRI study, *American Journal of Gastroenterology* 97(3): 654–61.

Bond, G. R., Resnick, S. G., Drake, R. E., Xie, H., McHugo, G. J., and Bebout, R. R. (2001) Does competitive employment improve non-vocational outcomes for people with severe mental illness? *Journal of Consulting and Clinical Psychology* 69(3): 489–501.

Bond, R., and Smith, P. (1996) Culture and conformity, *Psychological Bulletin* 119: 111–37.

Bonica, J. (1979) Editorial: the need of a taxonomy, *Pain* 6(3): 247–52.

Borkovec, T. D., Newman, M. G., and Castonguay, L. G. (2003) Psychotherapy for generalized anxiety disorder, *CNS Spectrum* 8: 382–9.

Bowlby, J. (1953) Child Care and the Growth of Love. London: Penguin.

Bowlby, J. (1980) *Attachment and Loss,* Vol. 3: *Loss, Sadness and Depression.* London: Hogarth Press.

Boychuck Duchscher, J. (2009) Transition shock: the initial stage of role adaptation for newly graduated registered nurses, *Journal of Advanced Nursing* 65(5): 1103–13.

Bradford Dementia Group (2005) *DCM 8 User's Manual.* Bradford: University of Bradford.

Breedlove, S., Watson, N., and Rosenzweig, M. (2010) *Biological Psychology: An Introduction to Behavioral, Cognitive, and Clinical Neuroscience*. 6th edn, Sunderland, MA: Sinauer Associates.

Brehm, J. W. (1966) *A Theory of Psychological Reactance*. New York: Academic Press.

Bronfenbrenner (1979) *The Ecology of Human Development*. Cambridge, MA: Harvard University Press.

Brooker, D. (2004) What is person-centred care in dementia? *Reviews in Clinical Gerontology* 13(3): 215–22.

Brooker, D., and Surr, C. (2005) *Dementia Care Mapping: Principles and Practice*. Bradford: University of Bradford.

Brown, A. S., Cohen, P., Harkavy-Friedman, J., Babulas, V., Malaspina, D., Gorman, J. M., and Susser, E. S. (2001) Prenatal rubella, premorbid abnormalities, and adult schizophrenia, *Biological Psychiatry*, 49(6): 473–86.

Brown, J., and Addington-Hall, J. (2008) How people with motor neurone disease talk about living with their illness: a narrative study, *Journal of Advanced Nursing* 62: 200–8.

Brown, J., Chatterjee, N., Younger, J., and Mackey, S. (2011) Towards a physiology-based measure of pain: patterns of human brain activity distinguish painful from non-painful thermal stimulation, *PLoS ONE* 6(9): 1–8.

Brown, J., Sheffield, D., Leary, M., and Robinson, M. (2003) Social support and experimental pain, *Psychosomatic Medicine* 65(2): 276–83.

Browne, C. J., and Shlosberg, E. (2005) Attachment behaviours and parent fixation in people with dementia: the role of cognitive functioning and pre-morbid attachment style, *Aging and Mental Health* 9(2): 153–61.

Bruner, J. (1960) *The Process of Education*. Cambridge, MA: Harvard University Press.

Buhagiar, L., Cassar, O., Brincat, M., Buttigieg, G., Inglott, A., Adami, M., and Azzopardi, L. (2013) Pre-operative pain sensitivity: a prediction of post-operative outcome in the obstetric population, *Journal of Anaesthesiology Clinical Pharmacology* 29(4): 465–71.

Burman, E. (2008) *Deconstructing Developmental Psychology*. 2nd edn, London: Routledge.

Burnard, P. (1989) *Counselling Skills for Health Professionals*. London: Chapman & Hall.

Bury, M. (1982) Chronic illness as biographical disruption, *Sociology of Health and Illness* 4: 167–82.

Bury, M. (2004) Researching patient–professional interactions, *Journal of Health Service Research Policy* 9: 48–54.

Butcher, S., Killampalli, V., Lascelles, D., Wang, K., Alpar, E., and Lor, J. (2005) Raised cortisol: DHEA ratios in the elderly after injury: potential impact upon neutrophil function and immunity, *Aging Cell* 4: 319–24.

Caplan, G. (1964) *Principles of Preventative Psychiatry*. New York: Basic Books.

Carr, D. C., and Comp, K. (2011) *Gerontology in the Era of the Third Age: Implications and Next Steps*. New York: Springer.

Cartwright, A. (1980) The attitudes of helping agents toward the alcoholic client: the influence of experience, support training and self-esteem, *British Journal of Addiction* 75: 413–31.

Carver, C. S., Scheier, M. F., and Segerstrom, S. C. (2010) Optimism, *Clinical Psychology Review* 30(7): 879–89.

Caspi, A., Moffitt, T. E.,Cannon, M., McClay, J., Murray, R., Harrington, H., Taylor, A., Arseneault, L., Williams, B., Braithwaite, A., Poulton, R., and Craig, I. W. (2005) Moderation of the effect of adolescent-onset cannabis use on adult psychosis by a functional polymorphism in the catechol-O-methyltransferase gene: longitudinal evidence of a gene x environment interaction, Biological Psychiatry 57: 1117–27.

Cavallini, M. C., and Bellodi, L. (2005) Epidemiology of anxiety disorders, in E. J. L. Griez, C. Faravelli, D. Nutt and J. Zohar (eds), *Anxiety Disorders: An Introduction to Clinical Management and Research*. Chichester: John Wiley.

Caycedo, N., and Griez, E. J. L. (2001) Generalised anxiety disorder, in E. J. L. Griez, C. Faravelli, D. Nutt and J. Zohar (eds), *Anxiety Disorders: An Introduction to Clinical Management and Research*. Chichester: John Wiley.

CDCP (Centers for Disease Control and Prevention) (1996) *Prevention of Plague: Recommendations of the Advisory Committee on Immunization Practices (ACIP)*. Morbidity and Mortality Weekly Report 45(RR-14).

Cervero, F. (2012) *Understanding Pain: Exploring the Perception of Pain*. Cambridge, MA: MIT Press.

Charmaz, K. (1991) *Good Days, Bad Days: The Self in Chronic Illness and Time*. New Brunswick, NJ: Rutgers University Press.

Charmaz, K. (1999) Stories of suffering: subjective tales and research narratives, *Qualitative Health Research* 9(3): 362–82.

Clemerson, G., Walsh, S., and Isaac, C. (2014) Towards living well with young onset dementia: an exploration of coping from the perspective of those diagnosed, *Dementia: The International Journal of Social Research and Practice* 13(4): 451–66.

Cloitre, M., Cohen, L. R., and Koenon, K.C. (2006) *Treating Survivors of Childhood Abuse: Psychotherapy for the Interrupted Life*. New York: Guilford Press.

Clow, A. (2004) Cortisol as a biomarker of stress, *Journal of Holistic Healthcare* 1: 10–14.

Coffin, P., and Sullivan, S. (2013) Cost-effectiveness of distributing naloxone to heroin users for lay heroin overdose reversal, *Annals of Internal Medicine* 158(1): 1–9.

Cohen, L., Cole, S. W., Sood, A. K., Prinsloo, S., Kirschbaum, C., Arevelo, J. M. G., Jennings, N. B., Scott, S., Vence, L., Qi, W., Kentor,

D., Radvanyi, L., Tannir, N., Jonasch, E., Tamboli, P., and Pisters, L. (2012) Depressive symptoms and cortisol rhythmicity predict survival in patients with renal cell carcinoma: role of inflammatory signaling, *PLoS ONE* 7(8): e42324; doi: 10.1371/journal.pone.0042324.

Cohen, S., and Wills, T. A. (1985) Stress, social support and the buffering hypothesis, *Psychological Bulletin* 98(2): 310–57.

Cohen, S., Frank, E., Doyle, W., Skoner, D., Rabin, B., and Gwaltney, J. (1998) Types of stressors that increase susceptibility to the common cold, *Health Psychology* 17: 214–23.

Coltheart, M., Langdon R., and McKay, R. (2011) Delusional belief, *Annual Review of Psychology* 62: 271–98.

Conner, M. (2014) Extending not retiring the theory of planned behaviour: a commentary on Sniehotta, Presseau and Araújo-Soares, *Health Psychology Review*, http://dx.doi.org/10.1080/17437199.201 4.899060.

Corcoran, R., and Frith, C. D. (2005) Thematic reasoning and theory of mind: accounting for social inference difficulties in schizophrenia, *Evolutionary Psychology* 3: 1–19.

Corner, L., and Bond, J. (2004) Being at risk of dementia: fears and anxieties of older adults, *Journal of Aging Studies* 18(2): 143–55.

Costa, P. T., and McCrae, R. R. (1992) The five-factor model of personality and its relevance to personality disorders, *Journal of Personality Disorders* 6(4): 343–59.

Cox, J. J., et al. (2006) An SCN9A channelopathy causes congenital inability to experience pain, *Nature* 444: 894–8.

Coyne, J., Stefanek, M., and Palmer, S. (2007) Psychotherapy and survival in cancer: the conflict between hope and evidence, *Psychological Bulletin* 133: 367–94.

Cracknell, R. (2010) The ageing population, www.parliament.uk/documents/commons/lib/research/key_issues/Key-Issues-The-ageing-population2007.pdf.

Craig, R., and Mindell, J. (eds) (2014) *Health Survey for England*. London: Health and Social Care Information Centre.

Craske, M. G., and Waters, A. M. (2005). Panic disorder, phobias, and generalized anxiety disorder, *Annual Review of Clinical Psychology* 1: 197–226.

Crittenden, P. M., and Ainsworth, M. D. S. (1989) Child maltreatment and attachment theory, in D. Cicchetti and V. Carlson (eds), Handbook of Child Maltreatment. Cambridge: Cambridge University Press, pp. 432–63. www.patcrittenden.com/include/docs/Crittenden_Ainsworth_1989.pdf.

Croiset, G., Heijnen, C., Veldius, H., de Weid, D., and Ballieux, R. E. (1987) Modulation of the immune response by emotional stress, *Life Sciences* 40(8): 775–82.

Crosskerry, P. (2003) The importance of cognitive errors in diagnosis and strategies to minimize them, *Academic Medicine* 78: 775–80.

Cummings, J. L., Mega, M., Gray, K., Rosenberg-Thompson, S., Carusi, D. A., and Gombein, J. (1994) The neuropsychiatric inventory: comprehensive assessment of psychopathology in dementia, Neurology 44(12): 2308.

Cunningham, C., McClean, W., and Kelly, F. (2010) The assessment and management of pain in people with dementia in care homes, Nursing Older People 22(7): 29–35.

Cupps, T., and Fauci, A. (1982) Corticosteroid-mediated immunoregulation in man, Immunological Review 65: 133–55.

Dabo, F., Nyberg, F., Zhou, Q., Sundström-Poromaa, I., and Akerud, H. (2010) Plasma levels of β-endorphin during pregnancy and use of labor analgesia, Reproductive Sciences 17(8): 742–7.

Daemmrich, A. (2013) The political economy of healthcare reform in China: negotiating public and private. Springer Link, doi: 10.1186/2193-1801-2-448.

Dagnan D. (2012) Cognitive therapy, in R. Raghavan (ed.), Anxiety and Depression in People with Intellectual Disabilities: Advances in Interventions. Brighton: Pavilion.

Damasio, A. R. (1999) The Feeling of What Happens. New York: Harcourt, Brace.

Darke, S., Kaye, S., McKetin, R., and Duflou, J. (2008) Major physical and psychological harms of methamphetamine use, Drug and Alcohol Review 27(3): 253–62.

Davey, G. (ed.) (2006) The Encyclopaedic Dictionary of Psychology. London: Hodder Arnold.

Davies-Smith, L. (2006) An introduction to providing cognitive behavioural therapy, Nursing Times 102: 26, 28–30.

Davis, J. H. (1973) Group decision and social interaction: a theory of social decision schemes, Psychological Review 80: 97–125.

Day, A., Therrien, D., and Carroll, S. (2005) Predicting psychological health: assessing the incremental validity of emotional intelligence beyond personality, Type A behaviour, and daily hassles, European Journal of Personality 19(6): 519–36.

De Botton, A. (2000) The Consolations of Philosophy. London: Penguin.

De Felipe, C., et al. (2006) Altered nociception, analgesia and aggression in mice lacking the receptor for substance P, Nature 392: 394–7.

De Jong, G., van Sonderen, E., and Emmelkamp, P. (1999) A comprehensive model of stress: the roles of experienced stress and neuroticism in explaining the stress–distress relationship, Psychotherapy and Psychosomatics 68(6): 290–8.

De Loos, W. S. (2001) Post-traumatic syndromes: comparative biology and psychology, in E. J. L. Griez, C. Faravelli, D. Nutt and J. Zohar (eds), Anxiety Disorders: An Introduction to Clinical Management and Research. Chichester: John Wiley.

De Visser, R. (2009) Psychology in medical curricula: 'need to know' or 'nice to know'? European Health Psychologist 11: 20–3.

DeBellis, R., Smith, B. S., Choi, S., and Malloy, M. (2005) Management of delirium tremens, *Journal of Intensive Care Medicine* 20(3): 164–73.

Deegan, P. E. (1988) Recovery: the lived experience of rehabilitation, *Psychosocial Rehabilitation Journal* 9: 11–19.

Denollet, J., Sys, S., and Brutsaert, D. L. (1995) Personality and mortality after myocardial infarction, *Psychosomatic Medicine* 57: 582–91.

D'Eon, J., Harris, C., and Ellis, J. (2004) Testing factorial validity and gender invariance of the pain catastrophizing scale, *Journal of Behavioral Medicine* 27(4): 361–72.

DeSalvo, L. (1999) *Writing as a Way of Healing: How Telling Our Stories Transforms Our Lives*. London: Women's Press.

Deutsch, M., and Gerard, H. B. (1955) A study of normative and informational social influence upon individual judgment, *Journal of Abnormal and Social Psychology* 51: 629–36.

Dexter, G., and Russell, J. (1997) *Challenging Blank Minds and Sticky Moments in Counselling*. Preston: Winckley Press.

DHSSPS (Department of Health, Social Services and Public Safety) (2010) *Living Matters Dying Matters: A Palliative and End of Life Care Strategy for Adults in Northern Ireland*. Belfast: Department of Health, Social Services and Public Safety; www.dhsspsni.gov.uk/8555_palliative_final.pdf.

Diener, E., and Chan, M. Y. (2011) Happy people live longer: subjective well-being contributes to health and longevity, *Applied Psychology: Health and Well-Being* 3(1): 1–43, http://internal.psychology.illinois.edu/~ediener/Documents/Diener-Chan_2011.pdf.

Dill, D. L., Chu, J. A., Grob, M. C., and Eisen, S. V. (1991) The reliability of abuse history reports: a comparison of two inquiry formats, *Comprehensive Psychiatry* 32: 166–9.

Dobson, K. S., and Dozois, D. J. (2001) Historical and philosophical bases of the cognitive behavioural therapies, in K. S. Dobson (ed.), *Handbook of Cognitive Behavioural Therapies*. New York: Guilford Press.

DoH (Department of Health) (2001a) *Treatment Choice in Psychological Therapies and Counselling: Evidence Based Clinical Practice Guideline*. London: Department of Health.

DoH (Department of Health) (2001b) *Valuing People: A New Strategy for Learning Disability for the 21st Century*, Cm 5086. London: The Stationery Office.

DoH (Department of Health) (2007a) *Drug Misuse and Dependence: UK Guidelines in Clinical Management*. London: The Stationery Office.

DoH (Department of Health) (2007b) *Safe. Sensible. Social: The Next Steps in the National Alcohol Strategy*. London: The Stationery Office.

DoH (Department of Health) (2008a) *End of Life Care Strategy: Promoting High Quality Care for Adults at the End of their Life*. London: Department of Health.

DoH (Department of Health) (2008b) *Reducing Alcohol Harm: Health Services in England for Alcohol Misuse.* London: National Audit Office.

DoH (Department of Health) (2009) *Living Well with Dementia: A National Dementia Strategy.* London: Department of Health.

DoH (Department of Health) (2011) *A Summary of the Health Harms of Drugs.* London: Department of Health.

DoH (Department of Health) (2012) *Prime Minister's Challenge on Dementia: Delivering Major Improvements in Dementia Care and Research by 2015.* London: Department of Health.

DoH (Department of Health) (2013) *More Care, Less Pathway: A Review of the Liverpool Care Pathway.* London: Department of Health.

Donaldson, M. (1978) *Children's Minds.* London: Fontana.

Dunbar, R. (2012) *The Science of Love and Betrayal.* London: Faber & Faber.

Dunbar, R., Baron, R., Frangou, A., Pearce, E., van Leeuwen, E., Stow, J., Partridge, G., MacDonald, I., Barra, V., and van Vugt, M. (2012) Social laughter is correlated with an elevated pain threshold, *Proceedings of the Royal Society of London B* 279: 1161–7.

Eaton, N. R., Krueger, R. F., Keyes, K. M., Hasin, D. S., Balsis, S., Skodol, A. E., Markon, K. E., and Grant, B. F. (2011) An invariant dimensional liability model of gender differences in mental disorder prevalence: evidence from a national sample, *Journal of Abnormal Psychology* 121(1): 282–8.

Ebrahim, S., Wallis, C., Brittis, S., Harwood, R. H., and Graham, N. (1993) Long-term care for elderly people, *Quality in Health Care* 2: 198–203.

Eccleston, C., Palermo, T. M., Fisher, E., and Law, E. (2015) *Psychological Therapy for Parents of Children with a Longstanding or Life-Threatening Physical Illness,* www.cochrane.org/CD009660/SYMPT_psychological-therapy-for-parents-of-children-with-a-longstanding-or-life-threatening-physical-illness.

Edwards, G., Marshall, J., and Cook, C. H. (2009) *The Treatment of Drinking Problems: A Guide for the Helping Profession.* 4th edn, Cambridge: Cambridge University Press.

Edwards, M., and Titman, P. (2010) *Promoting Psychological Well-Being in Children with Acute and Chronic Illness.* London: Jessica Kingsley.

Egan, G. (1994) *The Skilled Helper.* 5th edn, Pacific Grove, CA: Brooks/Cole.

Ehrenreich, B. (2009) *Smile or Die: How Positive Thinking Fooled America and the World.* London: Granta.

Ellis, A. (1962) Reason and Emotion in Psychotherapy. New York: Lyle Stuart.

Elmer, S. (2010) Overcoming barriers to the use of play therapy and direct work with children in social care practice. PhD thesis, Leeds Metropolitan University.

Elmer, S. (2013) Marginalised children in marginalised communities: the challenges for early years and parenting support services where there is domestic violence, *North East Branch Newsletter* [British Psychological Society], winter.

Emerson, E. (1998) Working with people with challenging behaviour, in E. Emerson, C. Hatton, J. Bromley and A Caine (eds), *Clinical Psychology and People with Intellectual Disabilities*. Chichester: John Wiley.

Emerson, E., Hatton, C., Robertson, J., Roberts, H., Baines, S., and Glover, G. (2010) *People with Learning Disabilities in England 2010: Services & Supports*. University of Lancaster, Learning Disability Observatory.

Engel, G. L. (1977) The need for a new medical model: a challenge for biomedicine, *Science* 196: 129–36.

Essex, H., and Pickett, K. (2008) Mothers without companionship during childbirth: an analysis within the Millennium Cohort Study, *Birth* 35(4): 266–76.

Eysenck, H. J. (1952) The effects of psychotherapy: an evaluation, *Journal of Consulting Psychology* 16: 319–24.

Eysenck, H. J. (1970) *The Structure of Human Personality*. 3rd edn, London: Methuen.

Eysenck, M. W. (ed.) (1998) *Psychology: An Integrated Approach*. London: Longman.

Ezzy, D. (2000) Illness narratives: time, hope and HIV, *Social Science and Medicine* 50, 605–17.

Fashner, J., Ericson, K., and Werner, S. (2012) Treatment of the common cold in children and adults, *American Family Physician* 86(2): 153–9.

Faull, C., and Taplin, S. (2012) Adapting to death, dying, and bereavement, in C. Faull et al. (eds), *Handbook of Palliative Care*. 3rd edn, Hoboken, NJ: Wiley-Blackwell, pp. 81–92.

Festinger, L. (1954) A theory of social comparison, *Human Relations* 7: 117–40.

Festinger, L. (1957) *A Theory of Cognitive Dissonance*. Stanford, CA: Stanford University Press.

Fillingim, R. B., Browning, A. D., Powell, T., and Wright, R. A. (2002) Sex differences in perceptual and cardiovascular responses to pain: the influence of a perceived ability manipulation, *Journal of Pain* 3(6): 439–45.

Fink, S. L. (1967) Crisis and motivation: a theoretical model, *Archives of Physical Medicine and Rehabilitation* 48: 592–7.

Flaten, M., Aslaksen, P., Lyby, P., and Bjørkedal, E. (2011) The relation of emotions to placebo responses, *Philosophical Transactions of the Royal Society B: Biological Sciences* 366: 1818–27.

Fletcher, P. C., and Frith, C. D. (2009) Perceiving is believing: a Bayesian approach to explaining the positive symptoms of schizophrenia, *Nature Reviews: Neuroscience* 10, 48–58.

Francis, R. (2013) *The Independent Inquiry into Care Provided by Mid-Staffordshire NHS Foundation Trust, January 2005 to March 2009*. London: The Stationery Office; www.midstaffspublicinquiry.com/report

Frank, A. W. (1995) *The Wounded Storyteller*. Chicago: University of Chicago Press.

Frank, J. D. (1982) Therapeutic components shared by all psychotherapies, in J. H. Harvey and M. M. Parks (eds), *The Master Lecture Series*, Vol. 1: *Psychotherapy Research and Behaviour Change*. Washington, DC: American Psychological Association.

Frankish, P. (1992) A psychodynamic approach to emotional difficulties with a social framework, *Journal of Intellectual Disability Research* 36: 559–63.

Freud, S. ([1915] 1957) Mourning and melancholia, in *The Standard Edition of the Complete Psychological Works of Sigmund Freud*, Vol. XIV: *1914–1916*, pp. 237–58.

Freud, S. ([1922] 2011) *Group Psychology and the Analysis of the Ego*, www.gutenberg.org/files/35877/35877-h/35877-h.htm.

Freud, S. (1958) *On Creativity and the Unconscious*. New York: Harper & Row.

Friedman M., and Rosenman, R. (1959) Association of specific overt behaviour pattern with blood and cardiovascular findings, *Journal of the American Medical Association* 169: 1286–97.

Friedman, M., and Rosenman, R. (1974) *Type A Behavior and Your Heart*. New York: Random House.

Frith, C. D. (1992) *The Cognitive Neuropsychology of Schizophrenia*. Hove: Lawrence Erlbaum Associates.

Furedi, F. (2004) *Therapy Culture*. London: Routledge.

Futterman, A., Kemeny, M., Shapiro, D., and Fahey, J. (1994) Immunological and physiological changes associated with induced positive and negative mood, *Psychosomatic medicine* 56(6): 499–511.

Gamondi, C., Larkin, P., and Payne, S. (2013a) Core competencies in palliative care: an EAPC White Paper on palliative care education, part 1, *European Journal of Palliative Care* 20(2): 86–91.

Gamondi, C., Larkin, P., and Payne, S. (2013b) Core competencies in palliative care: an EAPC White Paper on palliative care education, part 2, *European Journal of Palliative Care* 20(3): 140–5.

Garety, P. A., Hemsley, D. R., and Wessley, S. (1991) Reasoning in deluded schizophrenic and paranoid patients: biases in performance on a probabilistic inference task, *Journal of Nervous Mental Disease* 179: 194–201.

Garety, P. A., Kuipers, E., Fowler, D., Freeman, D., and Bebbington, P. E. (2001) A cognitive model of the positive symptoms of psychosis, *Psychological Medicine* 31: 189–95.

Garra, G., Singer, A., Taira, B., Chohan, J., Cardoz, E., and Thode, H. (2010) Validation of the Wong–Baken FACES pain rating scale in pediatric emergency department patients, *Clinical Practice* 17(1): 50–4.

Gerhardt, S. (2004) *Why Love Matters: How Affection Shapes a Baby's Brain*. New York: Brunner-Routledge.

Gillies, R., Robey, I., and Gatenby, R. (2008) Causes and consequences of increased glucose metabolism of cancers, *Journal of Nuclear Medicine* 49(suppl. 2): 24S–42S.

Gobrial, E., and Raghavan, R. (2012) Prevalence of anxiety in children and young people with autism and learning disabilities, *Advances in Mental Health and Intellectual Disabilities* 6(3): 130–41.

Goffman, E. (1959) *The Presentation of Self in Everyday Life*. London: Penguin.

Goffman, E. (1961) *Asylums: Essays on the Social Situations of Mental Patients and Other Inmates*. London: Penguin.

Goffman, E. (1963) *Stigma*. London: Penguin.

Gottesman, I. I. (1991) *Psychiatric Genesis: The Origins of Madness*. New York: Freeman.

Gottesman, I. I., and Bertelsen, A. (1989) Confirming unexpressed genotypes for schizophrenia: risks in the offspring of Fischer's Danish identical and fraternal discordant twins, Archives of General Psychiatry 46(10): 867–72.

Grande, G., Romppel, M., and Barth, J. (2012) Association between Type D personality and prognosis in patients with cardiovascular diseases: a systematic review and meta-analysis, *Annals of Behavioural Medicine* 43(3): 299–310.

Grant, A., Townend, M., Mulhern, R., and Short, N. (2010) *Cognitive Behavioural Therapy in Mental Health Care* 2nd edn, London: Sage.

Greasley, P. (2010) Is the evaluation of complementary and alternative medicine equivalent to evaluating the absurd?, *Evaluation & the Health Professions* 33(2): 127–39.

Greasley, P., Chiu, L. F., and Gartland, M. (2001) The concept of spiritual care in mental health nursing, *Journal of Advanced Nursing* 33(5): 629–37.

Green, M. F., and Harvey, P. D. (2014) Cognition in schizophrenia: past, present and future, *Schizophrenia Research: Cognition* 1: 1–9.

Greenberger, D., and Padesky, C. A. (1995) *Mind Over Mood: Change How You Feel by Changing the Way You Think*. London: Guilford Press.

Grossarth-Maticek, R., Bastiaans, J., and Kanazir, D. T. (1985) Psychosocial factors as strong predictors of mortality from cancer, ischaemic heart disease and stroke: the Yugoslav prospective study, *Journal of Psychosomatic Research* 29(2): 167–76.

Grov, E., Fossa, S., Bremnes, R., Dahl, O., Klepp, O., Wist, E., and Dahl, A. (2009) The personality trait of neuroticism is strongly associated with long-term morbidity in testicular cancer survivors, *Acta Oncologica* 48: 842–9.

Gustorff, B., Sycha, T., Lieba-Samal, D., Rolke, R., Treede, R.-D., and Magerl, W. (2013) The pattern and time course of somatosensory changes in the human UVB sunburn model reveal the presence of peripheral and central sensitization, *Pain* 154(4): 586–97.

Guthrie, E., Moorey, J., Barker, H., Margison, F., and McGrath, G. (1998) Psychodynamic-interpersonal psychotherapy in patients with treatment resistant psychiatric symptoms, *British Journal of Psychotherapy* 15: 155–66.

Hahm, B., and Bhunia, A. (2006) Effect of environmental stresses on antibody-based detection of escherichia coli O157:H7, Salmonella enterica serotype Enteritidis and Listeria monocytogenes, *Journal of Applied Microbiology* 100: 1017–27.

Hama, S., Yamashita, H., Kato, T., et al. (2008) 'Insistence on recovery' as a positive prognostic factor in Japanese stroke patients, *Psychiatry and Clinical Neurosciences* 62: 386–95.

Harmer, B. J., and Orrell, M. (2008) What is meaningful activity for people with dementia living in care homes? A comparison of the views of older people with dementia, staff and family carers, *Aging and Mental Health* 12(5): 548–58.

Health and Social Care Information Centre (2011) *Statistics on Alcohol: England 2011*, www.hscic.gov.uk/pubs/alcohol11.

Hekler, E. B., Lambert, J., Leventhal, E., Leventhal, H., Jahn, E., and Contrada, R. J. (2008) Commonsense illness beliefs, adherence behaviors, and hypertension control among African Americans, *Journal of Behavioural Medicine* 31: 391–400.

Heider, F. (1958) *The Psychology of Interpersonal Relations*. New York: Wiley.

Heiser, P., Dickhaus, B., Schreiber, W., Clement, H., Hasse, C., Hennig, J., Remschmidt, H., Kreig, W., Wesemann, W., and Opper, C. (2000) White blood cells and cortisol after sleep deprivation and recovery sleep in humans, *European Archives of Psychiatry and Clinical Neuroscience* 250: 16–23.

Helmes, E., Norton, M. C., and Stybe, T. (2013) Personality change in older adults with dementia: occurrence and association with severity of cognitive impairment, *Advances in Aging Research* 2(1): 27–36.

Hemphill, A. L., and Dearmun, A. K. (2006) Working with children and families, in A. Glasper and R. Richardson (eds), *A Textbook of Children's and Young People's Nursing*. Edinburgh: Churchill Livingstone, ch. 2.

Herbert, M. (2003) *Typical and Atypical Development: From Conception to Adolescence*. Oxford: Blackwell.

Herman, J., and Schatzow, E. (1987) Recovery and verification of childhood sexual trauma, *Psychoanalytical Psychology* 4: 1–14.

Hettema, J., Steele, J., and Miller, W. R. (2005) Motivational interviewing, *Annual Review of Clinical Psychology* 1: 91–111.

Higgins, E. T. (1987) Self-discrepancy: a theory relating self and affect, *Psychological Review* 94: 319–40.

Higgins, E. T., Bond, R. N., Klein, R., and Strauman, T. (1986) Self-discrepancies and emotional vulnerability: how magnitude, accessibility and type of discrepancy influence affect, *Journal of Personality and Social Psychology* 51: 5–15.

Hoffman, S. G., and Smits, J. A. J. (2008) Cognitive behavioural therapy for adult anxiety disorders: a meta-analysis of randomized placebo-controlled trials, *Journal of Clinical Psychiatry* 69: 621–32.

Hofling, C. K., Brotzman, E., Dalrymple, S., Graves, N., and Pierce, C. (1966) An experimental study of nurse–physician relations, *Journal of Nervous and Mental Disease* 143: 171–80.

Hollander, E., and Simeon, D. (2008) Anxiety disorders, in R. E. Hales, S. C. Yudofsky and G. O. Gabbard (eds), *American Psychiatric Publishing Textbook of Psychiatry*. 5th edn, Washington, DC: American Psychiatric Publishing.

Hollins, S. (2001) Psychotherapeutic methods, in A. Dosen and K. Day (eds), *Treating Mental Illness and Behaviour Disorders in Children and Adults with Mental Retardation*. Washington, DC: American Psychiatric Press.

Hollins, S. (2003) Counseling and psychotherapy in seminars in the psychiatry of learning disabilities, in W. Fraser and M. Kerr (eds), *Seminars in the Psychiatry of Learning Disabilities*. London: Gaskell.

Hollon, S. D., et al. (2005) Prevention of relapse following cognitive therapy vs medications in moderate to severe depression, *Archives of General Psychiatry* 62(4): 417–22.

Home Office (2010) *Drug Strategy 2010: Reducing Demand, Restricting Supply, Building Recovery: Supporting People to Live a Drug Free Life*, https://www.gov.uk/government/policies/reducing-drugs-misuse-and-dependence.

Horne, R., and Weinman, J. (2002) Self-regulation and self-management of asthma: exploring the role of illness perceptions and treatment beliefs in explaining non-adherence to preventer medication, *Psychology and Health* 17(1): 17–32.

Hornsey, M. J., Oppes, T., and Svensson, A. (2002). 'It's OK if we say it, but you can't': responses to intergroup and intra-group criticism, *European Journal of Social Psychology* 32(3): 293–307.

Hornstein, G. A. (1992) The return of the repressed: psychology's problematic relations with psychoanalysis, 1909–1960, *American Psychologist* 47(2): 254–63.

Hough, M. (2012) *Counselling Skills and Theory*. London: Hodder Education.

Howe, D. (2011) *Attachment across the Life Course: A Brief Introduction*. Basingstoke: Palgrave Macmillan.

Howes, O. D., and Kapur, S. (2009) The dopamine hypothesis of schizophrenia: version III – the final common pathway, *Schizophrenia Bulletin* 35(3): 549–62.

Hudson, P. (2004) Positive aspects and challenges associated with caring for a dying relative at home, *International Journal of Palliative Nursing* 10: 58–64.

Hudson, W., Roerkasse, R., and Wald, A. (1989) Influence of gender and menopause on gastric emptying and motility, *Gastroenterology* 96: 11–17.

Hughes, E. (2009) Dual diagnosis: an integral approach to care for people with co-occurring mental health and substance use problems, in R. Newell and K. Gournay (eds), *Mental Health Nursing*. 2nd edn, London: Churchill Livingstone.

Hunt, J. (2015) Oral statement to Parliament: the Morecambe Bay investigation, https://www.gov.uk/government/speeches/the-morecambe-bay-investigation.

Hunter, M. S., Craig, E., Advani, J., and Hutton, J. (2013) IAPT for people with chronic physical health problems: an audit and evaluation of training, *Clinical Forum* 251: 37–44.

Hurst, C. E. (2012) *Social Inequality: Forms, Causes, and Consequences*. 8th edn, Boston: Pearson.

Husebo, B. S., Ballard, C., and Aarsland, D. (2011) Pain treatment of agitation in patients with dementia: a systematic review, *International Journal of Geriatric Psychiatry* 26: 1012–18.

Hyland, M. (2011) Motivation and placebos: do different mechanisms occur in different contexts? *Philosophical Transactions of the Royal Society B: Biological Sciences* 366: 1828–37.

Ingram, R. E., and Luxton, D. D. (2005) Vulnerability-stress models, in B. L. Hankin and J. R. Z. Abela (eds), *Development of Psychopathology: A Vulnerability Stress Perspective*. Thousand Oaks, CA: Sage.

Iversen, M., Vora, R., Servi, A., and Solomon, D. (2011) Factors affecting adherence to osteoporosis medications: a focus group approach examining viewpoints of patients and providers, *Journal of Geriatric Physical Therapy* 34(2): 72–81.

Jackson, K., and Nazar, A. (2006) Breastfeeding, the immune response, and long-term health, *Journal of the American Osteopathic Association* 106: 203–7.

Jackson, S. W. (1992) The listening healer in the history of psychological healing, *American Journal of Psychiatry* 149: 1623–32.

Jackson, T., Iezzi, T., Chen, H., Ebnet, S., and Eglitis, K. (2005) Gender, interpersonal transactions and the perception of pain: an experimental analysis, *Journal of Pain* 6: 228–36.

Jacobson, E. ([1929] 1938) *Progressive Relaxation*. 2nd edn, Chicago: University of Chicago Press.

Janis, I. L. (1972) *Victims of Groupthink: A Psychological Study of Foreign Policy Decisions and Fiascos*. Boston: Houghton Mifflin.

Janssen, S., and Arntz, A. (2001) Real-life stress and opioid-mediated analgesia in novice parachute jumpers, *Journal of Psychophysiology* 15(2): 106–13.

Jarvis, P., Newman, S., and Swiniarski, L. (2014) On 'becoming social': the importance of collaborative free play in childhood, *International Journal of Play* 3(1): 53–68, doi: 10.1080/21594937.2013.863440.

Jemal, A., Ward, E., and Thun, M. (2010) Declining death rates reflect progress against cancer, *PLoS ONE* 5(3): 1–10.

Johnsen, A., Sundet, R., and Torsteinsson, V. W. (2004) *Self in Relationships: Perspectives on Family Therapy from Developmental Psychology.* London: Karnac.

Johnston, M. (1997) Hospitalization in adults, in A. Baum, S. Newman, J. Weinman and C. McManus (eds), *The Cambridge Handbook of Psychology, Health and Medicine.* Cambridge: Cambridge University Press, pp. 121–3.

Jones, C., Hacker, D., Cormac, I., Meaden, A., and Irving, C. B. (2012) Cognitive behaviour therapy versus other psychosocial treatments for schizophrenia, *Cochrane Database of Systematic Reviews* 4. http://www.ncbi.nlm.nih.gov/pubmed/22513966

Kalueff, A. V., and Nutt, D. J. (2007) Role of GABA in anxiety and depression, *Depression and Anxiety* 24: 495–517.

Kato, C., Petronis, A., Okazaki, Y., Tochigi, M., Umekage, T., and Sasaki, T. (2002) Molecular genetic studies of schizophrenia: challenges and insights, *Neuroscience Research* 43(4): 295–304.

Keefe, F. J. (1996) Cognitive behavioral therapy for managing pain, *Clinical Psychologist* 49(3): 4–5.

Keiling, C., Baker-Henningham, H., Belfer, M., Conti, G., Ertem, I., Omigbodun, Y., Rohde, L., Srinath, S., Ulkuer, N., and Rahman, A. (2011) Global child and adolescent mental health: evidence for action, *The Lancet* 378: 1515–25.

Kelly, G. A. (1955) *The Psychology of Personal Constructs*, Vol. 1: *A Theory of Personality*; Vol. 2: *Clinical Diagnosis and Psychotherapy.* New York: W. W. Norton.

Kelsey, J., and Abelson-Mitchell, N. (2007) Adolescent communication: perceptions and beliefs, *Journal of Children's and Young People's Nursing* 1(1): 42–9.

Keogh, E., and Herdenfeldt, M. (2002) Gender, coping and the perception of pain, *Pain* 97(3): 195–201.

Kessler, R. C. (2000) Gender differences in the prevalence and correlates of mood disorders in the general population, in M. Steiner, K. A. Yonkers and E. Eriksson (eds), *Mood Disorders in Women.* London: Martin Dunitz.

Kessler, R. C., McGonagle, K. A., Zhao, S., Nelson, C. B., Hughes, M., Eshleman, S., Wittchen, H. U., and Kendler, K. S. (1994) Sex and depression in the national comorbidity survey II: cohort effects, *Journal of Affective Disorders* 30: 15–26.

Kiecolt-Glaser, J., Marucha, P., Malarkey, W., Mercado, A., and Glaser, R. (1995) Slowing of wound healing by psychological stress, *The Lancet* 346: 1194–6.

Kienle, G., and Kiene, H. (1997) The powerful placebo effect: fact or fiction? *Journal of Clinical Epidemiology* 50: 1311–18.

Kitwood, T. (1993) Discover the person, not the disease, *Journal of Dementia Care* 1(1): 16–17.

Kitwood, T. (1997) *Dementia Reconsidered*. Buckingham: Open University Press.

Kitwood, T., and Bredin, K. (1992) Towards a theory of dementia care: personhood and well-being, *Ageing and Society* 12: 269–87.

Klass, D., Silverman, P. R., and Nickman, S. L. (eds) (1996) *Continuing Bonds: New Understandings of Grief*. Washington, DC: Taylor & Francis.

Knapp, M., Prince, M., Albanese, E., Banerjee, S., Dhanasiri, S., Fernandez, J. L., Ferri, C. P., Snell, T., and Stewart, R. (2007) *Dementia UK: Report to the Alzheimer's Society*. London: Alzheimer's Society.

Koch, T., Iliffe, S., and EVIDEM-ED project (2010) Rapid appraisal of barriers to the diagnosis and management of patients with dementia in primary care: a systematic review, *BMC Family Practice* 11(52).

Kolcaba, K. Y. (1994) A theory of holistic comfort for nursing, *Journal of Advanced Nursing* 19: 1178–84.

Koolhaas, J., Korte, S., De Boer, S., Van der Vegt, B., Van Reenen, C., Hopster, H., De Jong, I., Ruis, M., and Blokhuis, H. (1999) Coping styles in animals: current status in behavior and stress-physiology, *Neuroscience and Biobehavioral Reviews* 23: 925–35.

Korczyn, A. D., Vakhapova, V., and Grinberg, L. T. (2012) Vascular dementia, *Journal of the Neurological Sciences* 322(1–2): 2–10.

Korotkov, D., Perunovic, M., Claybourn, M., Fraser, I., Houlihan, M., MacDonald, M., and Korotkov, K. (2011) The type B behavior pattern as a moderating variable of the relationship between stressor chronicity and health behavior, *Journal of Health Psychology* 16(3): 397–409.

Kotkin, M., Davie, T. C., and Gurin, G. (1996) The consumer reports mental health survey, *American Psychologist* 51: 1080–2.

Krackow, A. (1995) When nurses obey or defy inappropriate physician orders: attributional differences, *Journal of Social Behaviour and Personality* 10(3): 585–94.

Kübler-Ross, E. (1969) *On Death and Dying*. New York: Macmillan.

Kupper, N., and Denollet, J. (2007) Type D personality as a prognostic factor in heart disease: assessment and mediating mechanisms, *Journal of Personality Assessment* 89(3): 265–76.

Langford, C. P., Bowsher, J., Maloney, J. P., and Lillis, P. (1997) Social support: a conceptual analysis, *Journal of Advanced Nursing* 25: 95–100.

Latham, S. R. (2002) Medical professionalism: a Parsonian view, *Mount Sinai Journal of Medicine* 69: 363–9.

Lau, R. R., and Hartman, K. A. (1983) Common sense representations of common illnesses, *Health Psychology* 2: 167–86.

Lau-Walker, M. (2006) A conceptual care model for individualized care approach in cardiac rehabilitation – combining both illness representation and self-efficacy, *British Journal of Health Psychology* 11: 103–17.

Layard, R., and Dunn, J. (2009) *A Good Childhood: Searching for Values in a Competitive Age.* London: Penguin.

Layard, R., Bell, S., Clarke, D. M., Knapp, M., Meacher, M., Priebe, S., and Wright, B. (2006) *The Depression Report: A New Deal for Depression and Anxiety Disorders.* London: Centre for Economic Performance, London School of Economics; http://cep.lse.ac.uk/pubs/download/special/depressionreport.pdf.

Layard, R., Clark, D. M., Knapp, M., and Mayraz, G. (2007) *Cost-Benefit Analysis of Psychological Therapy.* London: Centre for Economic Performance, London School of Economics; http://cep.lse.ac.uk/pubs/download/dp0829.pdf.

Lazarus, R. S. (1999) *Stress and Emotion: A New Synthesis.* New York: Springer.

Lazarus, R. S., and Folkman, S. (1984) *Stress, Appraisal and Coping.* New York: Springer.

Legget, J., Hurn, C., and Goodman, W. (1997) Teaching psychological strategies for managing auditory hallucinations: a case report, *British Journal of Learning Disabilities* 25: 158–61.

Leventhal, H., and Cameron, L. (1987) Behavioural therapies and the problem of compliance, *Patient Education and Counselling* 10: 117–38.

Leventhal, H., Benyamini, Y., Brownlee, S., Diefenbach, M., Leventhal, E. A., Patrick-Miller, L., et al. (1997) Illness representations: theoretical foundations, in K. J. Petrie and J. A. Weinman (eds), *Perceptions of Health and Illness.* Amsterdam: Harwood Academic, pp. 19–45.

Leventhal, H., Leventhal, E. A., and Breland, J. Y. (2011) Cognitive science speaks to the 'common-sense' of chronic illness management, *Annals of Behavioural Medicine* 41: 152–63.

Leventhal, H., Mayer, D., and Nerenz, D. R. (1980) The common sense representation of illness danger, in S. Rachman (ed.), *Contributions to Medical Psychology* 2. New York: Pergamon Press, pp. 17–30.

Levine, J., Gordon, N., and Fields, H. (1978) The mechanism of placebo analgesia, *The Lancet* 2, 654–7.

Levine, L., and Munsch, J. (2011) *Child Development: An Active Learning Approach.* Thousand Oaks, CA: Sage.

Ley, P. (1988) *Communication with Patients: Improving Communication, Satisfaction and Compliance.* London: Chapman & Hall.

Li, L., and Moore, D. (1998) Acceptance of disability and its correlates, *Journal of Social Psychology* 138: 13–25.

Lill-Elghanian, D., Schwartz, K., King, L., and Fraker, P. (2002) Glucocorticoid-induced apoptosis in early B-cells from human bone marrow, *Experimental Biology and Medicine* 227(9): 763–70.

Lin, H., and Bauer-Wu, S. (2003) Psycho-spiritual well-being in patients with advanced cancer: an integrative review of the literature, *Journal of Advanced Nursing* 44(1): 69–80.

Lindsay, W., Baty, F., Michie, A., and Richardson, I. (1989) A comparison of anxiety treatments with adults who have moderate and severe mental retardation, *Research in Developmental Disabilities* 10: 129–40.

Lindsay, W., Howells, L., and Pitcaithly, P. (1993) Cognitive therapy for depression with individuals with intellectual disabilities, *British Journal of Medical Psychology* 66: 135–41.

Lindsay, W., Michie, A., Baty, F., and McKenzie, K. (1988) Dog phobia in people with mental handicaps: anxiety management training and exposure treatments, *Mental Handicap Research* 1(1): 39–48.

Lindsay, W., Neilson, C., and Lawrenson, H. (1997) Cognitive-behaviour therapy for anxiety in people with learning disabilities, in B. Stenfert Kroese, D. Dagnan and K. Loumidis (eds), *Cognitive-Behaviour Therapy for People with Learning Disabilities*. London: Routledge.

Lindsay, W., Overend, H., Allan, R., and Williams, C. (1998) Using specific approaches for individual problems in the management of anger and aggression, *British Journal of Learning Disabilities* 26: 44–50.

Lockeridge, S., and Simpson, J. (2013) The experience of caring for a partner with young onset dementia: how younger carers cope, *Dementia: The International Journal of Social Research and Practice* 12(5): 635–51.

Lohne, V., and Severinsson, E. (2005) The power of hope: patients' experiences of hope a year after acute spinal cord injury, *Journal of Clinical Nursing* 15: 315–23.

Lorber, J. (1975) Good patients and problem patients: conformity and deviance in a general hospital, *Journal of Health and Social Behaviour* 16: 213–25.

Luborsky, L., Singer, B., and Luborsky, L., (1975) Comparative studies of psychotherapies, *Archives of General Psychiatry* 23: 995–1008.

Lupton, D. (1997) Consumerism, reflexivity and the medical encounter, *Social Science and Medicine* 45: 373–81.

Lynch, D., Laws, K. R., and McKenna, P. J. (2010) Cognitive behavioural therapy for major psychiatric disorder: does it really work? A meta-analytical review of well-controlled trials, *Psychological Medicine* 40: 9–24.

Ma, A., and Turner, A. (2012) A life without pain: congenital insensitivity to pain due to compound heterozygous SCN9A mutation, *Journal of Paediatrics and Child Health* 48: 285–6.

McCabe, R. (2013) Finding the right words to talk about depression, *Irish Times*, 22 January, p. 5.

McCabe, R., Leudar, I., and Healey, P. G. T. (2005) What do you think I think? Theory of mind and schizophrenia, *Proceedings of the 27th Annual Conference of the Cognitive Science Society*, 21–3.

MacDonagh, J. (2012) Humboldt's parrot and the re-voicing of a dead language: a metaphor for family histories of depression, *History and Philosophy of Psychology* 14(1).

Machin, L. (2009) *Working with Loss and Grief: A New Model for Practitioners*. London: Sage.

Mckay, K., and Narasimhan, S. (2012) Bridging the gap between doctors and nurses, *Journal of Nursing Education and Practice* 2(4): 52–5.

McKay, R. T., and Dennett, D. C. (2009) The evolution of misbelief, *Behavioural and Brain Sciences* 32: 493–561.

McKenna, M., Zevon, M., Corn, B., and Rounds, J. (1999) Psychosocial factors and the development of breast cancer: a meta-analysis, *Health Psychology* 18(5): 520–31.

McNeil, T. F., Cantor-Graae, E., and Weinberger, D. R. (2000) Relationship of obstetric complications and differences in size of brain structures in monozygotic twin pairs discordant for schizophrenia, *American Journal of Psychiatry* 157(2): 203–12.

McRae, R., and Costa, P. (1987) Validation of the five-factor model of personality across instruments and observers, *Journal of Personality and Social Psychology* 52: 81–90.

Manthorpe, J., Alaszewski, A., Motherby, E., Gates, B., and Ayer, S. (2004) Learning disability nursing: a multi-method study of education and practice, *Learning in Health and Social Care* 3(2): 92–101.

Martin, C. H. (2013) Obedience: defying the crowd in midwifery practice, *Journal of Reproductive and Infant Psychology* 31(2): 105–8; doi: 10.1080/02646838.2013.798166.

Martin, G. N., Carlson, N. R., and Buskist, W. (2010) *Psychology*. 4th edn, Harlow: Pearson.

Martin, J. A., and Penn, D. L. (2002) Attributional style in schizophrenia: an investigation in outpatients with and without persecutory delusions, *Schizophrenia Bulletin* 28: 131–41.

Maslach, C. (2007) Burnout in health professionals, in S. Ayers et al. (eds), *The Cambridge Handbook of Psychology, Health and Medicine*. 2nd edn, Cambridge: Cambridge University Press, pp. 427–30.

Maslow, A. (1954) *Motivation and Personality*. 3rd edn, New York: Longman.

Master, S., Eisenberger, N., Taylor, S., Naliboff, B., Shirinyan, D., and Liberman, M. (2009) A picture's worth: partner photographs reduce experimentally induced pain, *Psychological Science* 20: 1316–18.

Mayer, D., Price, D., and Rafii, A. (1977) Antagonism of acupuncture analgesia in man by the narcotic antagonist naloxone, *Brain Research* 121(2): 368–72.

Meissner, K. (2011) The placebo effect and the autonomic nervous system: evidence for an intimate relationship, *Philosophical Transactions of the Royal Society B: Biological Sciences* 366: 1808–17.

Melnyk, B. M., and Fineout-Overholt, E. (2010) *Evidence-Based Practice in Nursing and Healthcare: A Guide to Best Practice.* 2nd edn, Philadelphia: Lippincott Williams & Wilkins.

Messari, S., and Hallam, R. (2003) Cognitive behavioural therapy for psychosis: a qualitative analysis of client's experiences, *British Journal of Clinical Psychology* 42: 171–88.

Meyer, D., Leventhal, H., and Gutmann, M. (1985) Common-sense models of illness: the example of hypertension, *Health Psychology* 4: 115–35.

Michie, S., van Stralen, M., and West, R. (2011) The behaviour change wheel: a new method for characterising and designing behaviour change interventions, *Implementation Science* 6(42); doi: 10.1186/1748-5908-6-42.

Mid Staffordshire NHS Foundation Trust (2013) *Report of the Mid Staffordshire NHS Foundation Trust Public Inquiry.* London: The Stationery Office.

Miesen, B. (1993) Alzheimer's disease, the phenomenon of parent fixation and Bowlby's attachment theory, *International Journal of Geriatric Psychiatry* 8: 147–53.

Milgram, S. (1974) *Obedience to Authority.* New York: Harper & Row.

Miller, W. R., and Rollnick, S. (2013) *Motivational Interviewing: Helping People Change.* 3rd edn, New York: Guilford Press.

Moore, E., Adams, R., Elsworth, J., and Lewis, J. (1997) An anger management group for people with a learning disability, *British Journal of Learning Disabilities* 25: 53–7.

Moos, R. H., and Schaefer, J. A. (1984) The crisis of physical illness: an overview and conceptual approach, in R. H. Moos (ed.), *Coping with Physical Illness,* Vol. 2: *New Perspectives.* New York: Plenum, pp. 3–25.

Morrison, A. P. (2001) The interpretation of intrusions in psychosis: an integrative cognitive approach to hallucinations and delusions, *Behavioural and Cognitive Psychotherapy* 29: 257–76.

Morrow, G. R., Roscoe J. A., Kirshner, J. J., et al. (1998) Anticipatory nausea and vomiting in the era of 5-HT3 antiemetics, *Support Care Cancer* 6(3): 244–7.

Morss, J. (1995) *Growing Critical: Alternatives to Developmental Psychology.* London: Routledge.

Mõttus, R., McNeill, G., Jia, X., Craig, L., Starr, J., and Deary, I. (2013) The associations between personality, diet and body mass index in older people, *Health Psychology* 32(4): 353–60.

Murray, M. (2009) Telling stories and making sense of cancer, *International Journal of Narrative Practice* 1: 23–36.

Murray, R. M., Jones P. B., O'Callaghan, E., and Takei, N. (1992) Genes, viruses and neurodevelopmental schizophrenia, *Journal of Psychiatric Research* 26: 225–35.

Music, G. (2011) *Nurturing Natures: Attachment and Children's Emotional, Sociocultural and Brain Development*. Hove: Psychology Press.

Myers, D. G. (1998) *Psychology*. 5th edn, New York: Worth.

Nagy, S. (1999) Strategies used by burns nurses to cope with the infliction of pain on patients, *Journal of Advanced Nursing* 29: 1427–33.

Nakamura, T., Tomida, M., Yamamoto, T., Ando, H., Takamata, T., Kondo, E., Kurasawa, I., and Asanuma, N. (2013) The endogenous opioids related with antinociceptive effects induced by electrical stimulation into the amygdala, *Open Dentistry Journal* 7: 27–35.

Nakaya, N., Hansen, P., Schapiro, I., Eplov, L., Saito-Nakaya, K., Uchitomi, Y., and Johansen, C. (2006) Personality traits and cancer survival: a Danish cohort study, *British Journal of Cancer* 95(2): 146–152.

National End of Life Care Programme (2009) *Core Competencies for End of Life Care*. London: NELCP.

National Treatment Agency for Substance Misuse (2006) *Models of Care for Treatment of Adult Drugs Misusers: Update 2006*. London: Department of Health.

NCPC (National Council for Palliative Care) (2011) *Commissioning End of Life Care: Initial Actions for New Commissioners*, www.ncpc.org.uk/sites/default/files/AandE.pdf.

Negro-Vilar, A. (1993) Stress and other environmental factors affecting fertility in men and women: overview, *Environmental Health Perspectives* 101: 59–64.

Neimeyer, G. J., and Metzler, A. E. (1994) Personal identity and autobiographical recall, in U. Neisser and R. Fivush (eds), *The Remembering Self*. Cambridge: Cambridge University Press.

NELCIN (National End of Life Care Intelligence Network) (2013) End of life care profiles, www.endoflifecare-intelligence.org.uk/end_of_life_care_profiles/.

Neugebauer, V., Li, W., Bird, G., and Han, J. (2004) The amygdala and persistent pain, *The Neuroscientist* 10(3): 221–34.

NHS Confederation (2012) Investing in emotional and psychological wellbeing for patients with long-term conditions, http://nhsconfed.org/resources/2012/04/investing-in-emotional-and-psychological-wellbeing-for-patients-with-long-term-conditions.

NHS Scotland (2011) *Living and Dying Well: Building on Progress*, www.scotland.gov.uk/Resource/Doc/340076/0112559.pdf.

NICE (2003) Guidance on the use of electroconvulsive therapy, www.nice.org.uk/guidance/TA59.

NICE (2004a) Anxiety: management of anxiety (panic disorder with or without agoraphobia, and generalised anxiety disorder) in adults in primary, secondary and community care, www.nice.org.uk/guidance/cg22.

NICE (National Institute for Clinical Excellence) (2004b) *Improving Supportive and Palliative Care for Adults with Cancer.* London: NICE.

NICE (2005) Post-traumatic stress disorder (PTSD): the management of PTSD in adults and children in primary and secondary care, www.nice.org.uk/guidance/cg26.

NICE (2007) Chronic fatigue syndrome/myalgic encephalomyelitis (or encephalopathy): diagnosis and management of CFS/ME in adults and children, www.nice.org.uk/guidance/cg53.

NICE (National Institute for Health and Clinical Excellence) (2009a) Schizophrenia: core interventions in the treatment and management of schizophrenia in adults in primary and secondary care, www.nice.org.uk/guidance/cg82.

NICE (2009b) Depression in adults: the treatment and management of depression in adults, www.nice.org.uk/guidance/cg90.

NICE (National Institute of Health and Clinical Excellence) (2010) Alcohol-use disorders: preventing harmful drinking, https://www.nice.org.uk/guidance/ph24.

NICE (National Institute for Health and Care Excellence) (2014) Neuropathic pain – pharmacological management: the pharmacological management of neuropathic pain in adults in non-specialist settings, https://www.nice.org.uk/guidance/cg173/ifp/chapter/neuropathic-pain.

NICE/SCIE (2006) *Dementia: Supporting People with Dementia and their Carers in Health and Social Care,* www.scie.org.uk/publications/misc/dementia/dementia-guideline.pdf.

NMC (Nursing and Midwifery Council) (2010) Essential skills clusters (2010) and guidance for their use, Annexe 3 in *Standards for Pre-Registration Nursing Education.* London: Nursing and Midwifery Council.

NMC (Nursing and Midwifery Council) (2015) *The Code: Professional Standards of Practice and Behaviour for Nurses and Midwives.* London: Nursing and Midwifery Council.

Noel, M., Chambers, C., McGrath, P., Klein, R., and Stewart, S. (2012) The influence of children's pain memories on subsequent pain experience, *Pain* 153(8): 1563–72.

Nolen-Hoeksema, S. (2002). Gender differences in depression. In: Gotlib I. H. & Hammen, C. L. (eds.), Handbook of depression. New York, Guilford Press.

Nolen-Hoeksema, S., Wisco, B. E., and Lyubomirsky, S. (2008) Rethinking rumination, *Perspectives on Psychological Science* 3: 400–24.

Norman, I., and Ryrie, I. (2013) *The Art and Science of Mental Health Nursing Principles and Practice,* 3rd edn, Maidenhead: Open University Press.

Novaco, R. W. (1975) *Anger Control: The Development and Evaluation of an Experimental Treatment.* Lexington, MA: D. C. Heath.

Noyes, R., Clarkson, C., Crowe, R. R., Yates, W. R., and McChesney, C. M. (1987) A family study of generalized anxiety disorder, *American Journal of Psychiatry* 144(8): 1019–24.

Nutt, D. J. (2001) The pharmacology of human anxiety, in E. J. L. Griez, C. Faravelli, D. Nutt and J. Zohar (eds), *Anxiety Disorders: An Introduction to Clinical Management and Research*. Chichester: John Wiley.

O'Connor, P., and Brown, G. W. (1984) Supportive relationships: fact or fancy? *Journal of Social and Personal Relationships* 1: 159–75.

Ogden, J. (2007) *Health Psychology: A Textbook*. 4th edn, Maidenhead: Open University Press.

Öhlén, J., Andershed, B., Berg, C., et al. (2007) Relatives in end-of-life care, part 2: a theory for enabling safety, *Journal of Clinical Nursing* 16: 382–90.

Oliver, M. (1990) *The Politics of Disablement*. Basingstoke: Macmillan.

ONS (Office for National Statistics) (2013) *National Bereavement Survey (VOICES), 2012*, www.ons.gov.uk/ons/dcp171778_317495.pdf.

Orentreich, N., Brind, J., Vogelman, J., Andres, R., and Baldwin, H. (1992) Long-term longitudinal measurements of plasma dehydroepiandrosterone sulphate in normal men, *Journal of Clinical Endocrinological Metabolism* 75(4): 1002–4.

O'Sullivan, G., Hocking, C., and Spence, D. (2014) Dementia: the need for attitudinal change, *Dementia: The International Journal of Social Research and Practice* 13(4): 483–97.

Padesky, C. (1993) Socratic questioning: changing minds or guiding discovery? Keynote address delivered at the European Congress of Behavioural and Cognitive Therapies, London, 24 September, http://padesky.com/newpad/wp-content/uploads/2012/11/socquest.pdf.

Pain, C. M., Chadwick P., and Abba, N. (2008) Clients' experience of case formulation in cognitive behaviour therapy for psychosis, *British Journal of Clinical Psychology* 47: 127–38.

Papadatou, D. (2001) The grieving healthcare provider, *Bereavement Care* 20(2): 26–9.

Papadatou, D. (2006) Caregivers in death, dying and bereavement situations, *Death Studies* 30(7): 649–63.

Papadatou, D., Papazoglou, I., Petraki, D., et al. (1998) Mutual support among nurses who provide care to dying children, *Illness, Crisis and Loss* 7: 37–48.

Parkes, C. M. (1972) *Bereavement: Studies of Grief in Late Life*. New York: Basic Books.

Parkes, C. M. (1986) *Bereavement: Studies of Grief in Adult Life*. London: Tavistock.

Parkes, C. M., and Prigerson, H. G. (2010) *Bereavement: Studies of Grief in Adult Life*. 4th edn, London: Penguin.

Parr, H., and Butler, R. (1999) New geographies of illness, impairment and disability: mind and body spaces, in R. Butler and H. Parr (eds), *Geographies of Illness, Impairment and Disability*. London: Routledge.

Parsons, T. (1951) *The Social System*. London: Routledge & Kegan Paul.

Patton, R., and O'Hara, P. (2013) Alcohol: signs of improvement: the 2nd national emergency department survey of alcohol identification and intervention activity, *Emergency Medical Journal* 30: 492–5.

Pavlov, I. P. (1927) *Conditioned Reflexes*. New York: Oxford University Press.

Pennebaker, J. W. (1997) *Opening Up: The Healing Power of Expressing Emotions*. Rev. edn, New York: Guilford Press.

Perreault, A., Fothergill-Bourbonnais, F., and Fiset, V. (2004) The experience of family members caring for a dying loved one, *International Journal of Palliative Nursing* 10: 133–43.

Perrin, K., Daley, E., Naoom, S., Packing-Ebuen, J., Rayko, H., McFarlane, M., and McDermott, R. (2006) Women's reactions to HPV diagnosis: insights from in-depth interviews, *Women's Health* 43(2): 93–110.

Perry, M. J. (1996) The relationship between social class and mental disorder, *Journal of Primary Prevention* 14(1): 17–30.

Petersen, T., and McBride, A. (2008) *Working with Substance Misusers: A Guide to Theory and Practice*. London: Routledge.

Peterson, C., and Seligman, M. E. (1984) Causal explanations as a risk factor for depression: theory and evidence, *Psychological Review* 91: 347–74.

Petrie, K. J., Cameron, L. D., Ellis, C. J., Buick, D., and Weinman, J. (2002) Changing illness perceptions following myocardial infarction: an early intervention, randomized control trial, *Psychosomatic Medicine* 64: 580–6.

Petrie, K. J., Weinman, J. A., Sharpe, N., and Buckley, J. (1996) Role of patients' view of their illness in predicting return to work and functioning after myocardial infarction: longitudinal study, *British Medical Journal* 312: 1191–4.

Peyron, R., García-Larrea, L., Grégoire, M., Costes, N., Convers, P., Lavenne, F., Mauguière, F., Michel, D., and Laurent, B. (1999) Haemodynamic brain responses to acute pain in humans: sensory and attentional networks, *Brain* 122(9): 1765–80.

Phelps, E., and LeDoux, J. (2005) Contributions of the amygdala to emotion processing: from animal models to human behaviour, *Neuron* 48(2): 175–87.

Piaget, J. (1950) *The Psychology of Intelligence*. London: Routledge.

Piaget, J. (1952) *The Origins of Intelligence in Children*. New York: W. W. Norton.

Piaget, J., and Inhelder, B. (1956) *The Child's Conception of Space*. London: Routledge.

Piguet, O., Hornberger, M., Mioshi, E., and Hodges, J. R. (2011) Behavioural-variant frontotemporal dementia: diagnosis, clinical staging, and management, *Lancet Neurology* 10: 162–72.

Popper, K. (1959) *The Logic of Scientific Discovery*. New York: Basic Books.

Priest, H. (2012) *An Introduction to Psychological Care in Nursing and the Health Professions*. Abingdon: Routledge.

Prince, M., Albanese, E, Guerchet, M., and Prina, M. (2014) *World Alzheimer Report 2014: Dementia and Risk Reduction: An Analysis of Protective and Modifiable Factors*. London, Alzheimer's Disease International.

Prince, M., Knapp, M., Guerchet, M., et al. (2014) *Dementia UK: Second edition – Overview*. London: Alzheimer's Society.

Prochaska, J. O., and DiClemente, C. C. (1984) *The Transtheoretical Approach: Crossing Traditional Boundaries of Therapy*. Homewood, IL: Dow Jones/Irwin.

Prochaska, J. O., and DiClemente, C. C. (1992) Stages of change in the modification of problem behaviors, *Progress in Behaviour Modification* 28: 184–218.

Prout, H. T., and Nowak-Drabik, K. M. (2003) Psychotherapy with persons who have mental retardation: an evaluation of effectiveness, *American Journal on Mental Retardation* 108: 82–93.

Racine, M., Tousignant, Y., Laflamme, Y., Kloda, L., Dion, D., Dupuis, G., and Choinère, M. (2012a) A systematic literature review of 10 years of research on sex–gender differences and experimental pain perception, part 1: Are there really differences between women and men? *Pain* 153: 602–18.

Racine, M., Tousignant, Y., Laflamme, Y., Kloda, L., Dion, D., Dupuis, G., and Choinère, M. (2012b) A systematic literature review of 10 years of research on sex–gender differences and experimental pain perception, part 2: Do biopsychosocial factors alter pain sensitivity differently in men and women? *Pain* 153: 619–35.

Raistrick, D., Heather, N., and Godfrey, C. (2006) *Review of the Effectiveness of Treatment for Alcohol Problems*. London: National Treatment Agency for Substance Misuse.

Raistrick, D., Russell, D., Tober, G., and Tindale, A. (2007) A survey of substance use by health care professionals and their attitudes to substance misuse patients (NHS staff survey), *Journal of Substance Use* 13(1): 57–69.

Rank, S. G., and Jacobson, C. K. (1977) Hospital nurses' compliance with medication overdose orders: a failure to replicate, *Journal of Health and Social Behavior* 18: 188–93.

Rasool, G. H. (2008) *Alcohol and Drug Misuse*. London: Routledge.

RCN (Royal College of Nursing) (2004) *Transcultural Health Care Practice with Children and their Families*, www.rcn.org.uk/resources/transcultural/childhealth/sectionone.php.

RCN (Royal College of Nursing) (2013) *Mid Staffordshire NHS Foundation Trust Public Inquiry Report: Response of the Royal College of Nursing*, https://www.rcn.org.uk/_data/assets/pdf_file/0011/530948/004477.pdf

RCP (Royal College of Psychiatrists) (2004) *Psychotherapy and Learning Disability*, Council Report CR116. London: Royal College of Psychiatrists.

RCP (Royal College of Psychiatrists) (2011) *Report of the National Audit of Dementia Care in General Hospitals 2011*, ed. J. Young, C. Hood, R. Woolley, A. Gandesha and R. Souza. London: Royal College of Psychiatrists.

RCP (Royal College of Psychiatrists) (2012) Mental health and growing up factsheet: psychosis: information for parents, carers and anyone who works with young people, www.rcpsych.ac.uk/healthadvice/parentsandyouthinfo/parentscarers/psychosis.aspx.

Read, J., Agar, K., Argyle, N., and Aderhold, V. (2003) Sexual and physical abuse during childhood and adulthood as predictors of hallucinations, delusions and thought disorder, *Psychology and Psychotherapy: Theory, Research and Practice* 76: 1–22.

Read, J., van Os, J., Morrison, A., and Ross, C. A. (2005) Childhood trauma, psychosis and schizophrenia: a literature review with theoretical and clinical implications, *Acta Psychiatrica Scandinavica* 112: 330–50.

Reber, E., Reber, A. S., and Allen, R. (2004). *The Penguin Dictionary of Psychology*. 3rd edn, London: Penguin.

Reitz, C., Brayne, C., and Mayeux, R. (2011) Epidemiology of Alzheimer disease, *Nature Reviews: Neurology* 7: 137–52.

Relf, M., Machin, L., and Archer, N. (2008) *Guidance for Bereavement Needs Assessment in Palliative Care*. London: Help the Hospices.

Rhudy, J., and Meagher, M. (2000) Fear and anxiety: divergent effects on human pain thresholds, *Pain* 84(1): 65–75.

Riley J. (2008) A strategy for end-of-life care in the UK, *British Medical Journal* 337: 185–6.

Riley, J., Robinson, M., Wise, E., Myers, C., and Fillingim, R. (1998) Sex differences in the perception of noxious experimental stimuli: a meta-analysis, *Pain* 74: 181–7.

Ritvanen, T., Louhevaara, V., Helin, P., Halonen, T., and Hanninen, O. (2007) Effect of aerobic fitness on the physiological stress responses at work, *International Journal of Occupational Medicine and Environmental Health* 20(1): 1–8.

Rogers, C. R. (1951) *Client-Centered Therapy: Its Current Practices, Implications and Theory*. Boston: Houghton Mifflin.

Rogers, C. R. (1961) *On Becoming a Person*. London: Constable.

Rogers, C. R. (1965) A humanistic conception of man, in R. E. Farson (ed.), *Science and Human Affairs*. Palo Alto, CA: Science and Behavior Books.

Rohde, P., Lewinsohn, P. M., Klein, D. N., Seeley, J. R., and Gau, J. M. (2013) Key characteristics of major depressive disorder in childhood, adolescence, emerging adulthood, and adulthood, *Clinical Psychological Science* 1(1): 41–53.

Rose, J., West, C., and Clifford, D. (2000) Group interventions for anger in people with intellectual disabilities, *Research in Developmental Disabilities* 12: 211–24.

Rosenman, R., Brand, R., Scholz, R., and Friedman, M. (1976) Multivariate prediction of coronary heart disease during 8.5 year follow up in the Western Collaborative Group Study, *American Journal of Cardiology* 37: 903–10.

Rosenstock, I. M. (1974) The health belief model and preventive health behavior, *Health Education and Behavior* 2(4): 354–86.

Rouch, I., Dorey, J.-M., Boublay, N., et al. (2014) Personality, Alzheimer's disease and behavioural and cognitive symptoms of dementia: the PACO prospective cohort study protocol, *BMC Geriatrics* 14: 110.

Rozema, H., Völlink, T., and Lechner, L. (2009) The role of illness representations in coping and health of patients treated for breast cancer, *Psycho-Oncology* 18: 849–57.

Ruau, D., Liu, L., Clark, J., Angst, M., and Butte, A. (2012) Sex differences in reported pain across 11,000 patients captured in electronic medical records, *Journal of Pain* 13(3): 228–34.

Ruffin, R., Ironson, G., Fletcher, M., Balbin, E., and Schneiderman, N. (2012) Health locus of control and healthy survival with AIDS, *International Journal of Behavioural Medicine* 19(4): 512–17.

Ruggeri, M., Leese, M., Thornicroft, G., Bisoffi, G., and Tansella, M. (2000) Definition and prevalence of severe and persistent mental illness, *British Journal of Psychiatry* 177: 149–55.

Russell, M. A. H. (1971) Cigarette smoking: natural history of a dependence disorder, *British Journal of Medical Psychology* 44: 1–16.

Rutter, M., and Rutter, M. (1993) *Developing Minds: Challenge and Continuity across the Life Span*. London: Penguin.

Sabat, S. R. (2001) *The Experience of Alzheimer's Disease*. Oxford: Blackwell.

Sacco, M., Valenti, G., Corvi, M., Wu, F., and Ray, D. (2002) DHEA, a selective glucocorticoid receptor antagonist: its role in immune system regulation and metabolism, *Journal of Endocrinological Investigation* 25: 81–2.

Saewert, K. (2011) Socialization to professional nursing, in J. L. Creasia and E. E. Friberg (eds), *Conceptual Foundations: The Bridge to Professional Nursing Practice*. St Louis, MO: Mosby, pp. 42–63.

Sapolsky, R. (2004) *Why Zebras Don't Get Ulcers*. 3rd edn, New York: Henry Holt.

Schaefer, J. A., and Moos, R. H. (1992) Life crises and personal growth, in B. N. Carpenter (ed.), *Personal Coping: Theory, Research, and Application*. Westport, CT: Praeger, pp. 149–70.

Scheier, M. F., Matthews, K. A., Owens, J. F., Magouern, G. J., Lefebvre, R. C., Abbott, R. A. et al. (1989) Dispositional optimism and recovery from coronary artery bypass surgery: the beneficial effects on physical and psychological well-being, *Journal of Personality and Social Psychology* 57: 1024–40.

Schon, D. (1990) *Educating the Reflective Practitioner: Toward a New Design for Teaching and Learning in the Professions*. San Francisco: Jossey Bass.

Schore A (2003) Minds in the making: attachment, the self-organising brain, and developmentally oriented psychoanalytic psychotherapy, in J. Corrigall and H. Wilkinson (eds), *Revolutionary Connections: Psychotherapy and Neuroscience*. London: Karnac, ch. 1.

Sedikides, C. (1993) Assessment, enhancement, and verification determinants of the self-evaluation process, *Journal of Personality and Social Psychology* 65: 317–38.

Seligman, M. E. P. (1975) *Helplessness: On Depression, Development, and Death*. San Francisco: W. H. Freeman.

Seligman, M. E. P. (2002) Positive psychology, positive prevention, and positive therapy, in C. R. Snyder and S. J. Lopez (eds), *Handbook of Positive Psychology*. Oxford: Oxford University Press, pp. 3–9.

Shontz, F. C. (1975) *The Psychological Aspects of Physical Illness and Disability*. New York: Macmillan.

Siegel, D. (1999) *The Developing Mind: Towards a Neurobiology of Interpersonal Experience*. New York: Guilford Press.

Siegel, L. J., and Conte, P. (2001) Hospitalization and medical care of children, in C. E. Walker and M. C. Roberts (eds), *Handbook of Clinical Child Psychology*. 3rd edn, New York: Wiley, pp. 895–909.

Silverman, P. R. (2005) Mourning: a changing view, in P. Firth, G. Luff and D. Oliviere (eds), *Loss, Change and Bereavement in Palliative Care*. Maidenhead: Open University Press, pp. 18–37.

Sinason, V. (1992) *Mental Handicap and the Human Condition*. London: Free Association Books.

Skinner, B. F. (1969) *Contingencies of Reinforcement*. New York: Appleton Century Crofts.

Slade, M. (2009) *Personal Recovery and Mental Illness: A Guide for Mental Health Professionals*. Cambridge: Cambridge University Press.

Sloan, T., and Telch, M. J. (2002) The effects of safety-seeking behavior and guided threat reappraisal on fear reduction during exposure: an experimental investigation, *Behaviour Research and Therapy* 40(3): 235–51.

Smith, A. J., Hodgson, R. J., and Shepherd, J. P. (2000) *Reducing Binge Alcohol Consumption in Young Men*. London: Alcohol Education Research Council; http://alcoholresearchuk.org/downloads/final Reports/AERC_FinalReport_0003.pdf.

Smith, B., and Sparkes, A. C. (2005) Men, sport, spinal cord injury, and narratives of hope, *Social Science and Medicine* 61: 1095–105.

Smyth, J. M., Stone, A. A., Hurewitz, A., and Kaell, A. (1999) Effects of writing about stressful experiences on symptom reduction in patients with asthma or rheumatoid arthritis, *Journal of the American Medical Association* 281: 304–9.

Sniehotta, F., Presseau, J., and Araújo-Soares, V. (2014) Time to retire the theory of planned behaviour, *Health Psychology Review* 8(1): 1–7.

Spencer, P.T. (1983) Psychology and utopia: an interview with Don Bannister, *New Ideas in Psychology* 2: 191–5.

Spencer, P. T. (1990a) Exercise as psychotherapy, *Counselling Psychology Quarterly* 3(3): 291–3.

Spencer, P. T. (1990b) The benefits of exercise, *Counselling News for Managers* 7(2): 1–8.

Spencer, P. T. (1998) CFS: A suitable case for treatment, *The Psychologist* 11(5): 223–6.

Spencer, P. T., and Bannister, D. (1983) The personal construction of utopia, *New Ideas in Psychology* 1(2): 201–3.

Spencer, P. T., and Tordoff, S. (1983) Age, self-concept and the adult student, *Adult Education* 56(3): 256–8.

Spiegel, D., Bloom, J., Kraemer, H., and Gottheil, E. (1989) Effect of psychosocial treatment on survival of patients with metastatic breast cancer, *The Lancet* 14(2): 888–91.

Spinelli, M. G., and Broudy, C. (2013) Depression in the context of pregnancy, in J. J. Mann, P. J. McGrath and S. P. Roose (eds), *Clinical Handbook for the Management of Mood Disorders*. Cambridge: Cambridge University Press.

Spitzer, M. (1995) A neurocomputational approach to delusions, *Comprehensive Psychiatry* 36: 83–105.

Sprangers, M. A., Tempelaar, R., van den Heuval, W. J., and de Haes, H. C. (2002) Explaining quality of life with crisis theory, *Psycho-Oncology* 11: 419–26.

Stein, M., Keller, S., and Schleifer, S. (1985) Stress and immunomodulation: the role of depression and neuro-endocrine function, *Journal of Immunology* 135: 827–33.

Stenfert Kroese, B. (1997) Cognitive-behaviour therapy for people with learning disabilities: conceptual and contextual issues, in B. Stenfert Kroese, D. Dagnan and K. Loumidis (eds), *Cognitive-Behaviour Therapy for People with Learning Disabilities*. London: Routledge.

Stern, D. (1985) *The Interpersonal World of the Infant*. New York: Basic Books.

Stewart, M. J. (1993) *Integrating Social Support in Nursing*. Thousand Oaks, CA: Sage.

Strada, E. A. (2013) *The Helping Professional's Guide to End-of-Life Care: Practical Tools for Emotional, Social and Spiritual Support for the Dying*. Oakland, CA: New Harbinger.

Straub, R. O. (2007) *Health Psychology: A Biopsychosocial Approach*. New York, Worth.

Street, R. L., and Haidet, P. (2010) How well do doctors know their patients? Factors affecting physicians' understanding of patients' health beliefs, *Journal of General Internal Medicine* 26(1): 22–7.

Stroebe, M., and Schut, H. (1999) The dual process model of coping with bereavement: rationale and description, *Death Studies* 23: 197–224.

Stroebe, M., and Schut, H. (2010) The dual process model of coping with bereavement: a decade on, *Omega* 61(4): 273–89.

Strupp, H. H. (1978) Psychotherapy research and practice: an overview, in S. Garfield and A. Bergin (eds), *Handbook of Psychotherapy and Behaviour Change*. New York: Wiley.

Stuart-Hamilton, I. (1994) The Psychology of Ageing: An Introduction. 2nd edn, London: Jessica Kingsley.

Sun, F., Ong, R., and Burnette, D. (2012) The influence of ethnicity and culture on dementia caregiving: a review of empirical studies on Chinese Americans, *American Journal of Alzheimer's Disease and Other Dementias* 27(1): 13–22.

Surr, C. (2006) Preservation of self in people with dementia living in residential care: a socio-biographical approach, *Social Science and Medicine* 62(7): 1720–30.

Sutherland, S. (2010) *Breakdown: A Personal Crisis and a Medical Dilemma*. London: Pinter & Martin.

Svanberg, E., Spector, A., and Stott, J. (2011) The impact of young onset dementia on the family: a literature review, *International Psychogeriatrics* 23(3): 356–71.

Tajfel, H., and Turner, J. C. (1979) An integrative theory of intergroup conflict, in W. G. Austin and S. Worchel (eds), *The Social Psychology of Intergroup Relations*. Monterey, CA: Brooks/Cole, pp. 33–47.

Tajfel, H., Billig, M., Bundy, R., and Flament, C. (1971) Social categorization and intergroup behaviour, *European Journal of Social Psychology* 1: 149–78.

Tan, A., Zimmermann, C., and Rodin, G. (2005) Interpersonal processes in palliative care: an attachment perspective on the patient–clinician relationship, *Palliative Medicine* 19: 143–50.

Tanegashima, A., Yamamoto, H., Yada, I., and Fukunega, T. (1999) Estimation of stress in child neglect from thymic involution, *Forensic Science International* 101(1): 55–63.

Taylor, D. M., and Doria, J. R. (1981) Self-serving and group-serving bias in attribution, *Journal of Social Psychology* 113(2): 201–11.

Taylor, S. E. (1979) Hospital patient behaviour: reactance, helplessness, or control? *Journal of Social Issues* 35: 156–84.

Taylor, S. E. (1983) Adjustment to threatening events: a theory of cognitive adaption, *American Psychologist* 38: 1161–73.

Taylor, S. E., and Brown, J. D. (1988) Illusion and well-being: a social psychological perspective on mental health, *Psychological Bulletin* 103: 193–210.

Taylor, S. E., Lichtman, R. R., and Wood, J. V. (1984) Attributions, beliefs about control, and adjustment to breast cancer, *Journal of Personality and Social Psychology* 46: 489–502.

Terunuma, H., Deng, X., Dewan, Z., Fujimoto, S., and Yamamoto, N. (2008) Potential role of NK cells in the induction of immune responses: implications for NK cell-based immunotherapy for cancers and viral infections, *International Reviews of Immunology* 27: 93–110.

Thoits, P. A. (1991) On merging identity theory and stress research, *Social Psychology Quarterly* 54: 101–12.

Thompson, G., et al. (2012) *Olympic Britain: Social and Economic Change since the 1908 and 1948 London Games*. London: House of Commons Library; www.parliament.uk/documents/commons/lib/research/olympic-britain/olympicbritain.pdf.

Thompson, T., Keogh, E., French, C., and Davis, R. (2008) Anxiety sensitivity and pain: generalisability across noxious stimuli, *Pain* 134(1): 187–96.

Tienari, P., Wynne, L. C., Sorri, A., Lahti, I., Laksy, K., Moring, J., Naarala, M., Nieminen, P., and Wahlberg, K. (2004) Genotype-environment interaction in schizophrenia-spectrum disorder: long-term follow-up study of Finnish adoptees, *British Journal of Psychiatry* 184: 216–22.

Tomiyama, T., Uchida, K., Matsushita, M., Ikeura, T., Fukui, T., Takaoka, M., Nishio, A., and Okazaki, K. (2011) Comparison of steroid pulse therapy and conventional oral steroid therapy as initial treatment for autoimmune pancreatitis, *Journal of Gastroenterology* 46(5): 696–704.

Toner, J. (2012) Cognitive behavioural therapy, in S. Weatherhead and G. Flaherty-Jones (eds), *The Pocket Guide to Therapy: A How To of Core Models*. London: Sage.

Torn, A. (2011) Chronotopes of madness and recovery: a challenge to narrative linearity, *Narrative Inquiry* 21: 130–50.

Torrey, E. F. (1986) *Witch Doctors and Psychiatrists*. New York: Harper & Row.

Trevarthen, C. (2003) Neuroscience and intrinsic psychodynamics: current knowledge and potential for therapy, in J. Corrigall and H. Wilkinson (eds), *Revolutionary Connections: Psychotherapy and Neuroscience*. London: Karnac, ch.2.

Trilling, J. (2000) Psychoneuroimmunology: validation of the biopsychosocial model, *Family Practice* 17: 90–3.

Twycross, A. (2008) Does the perceived importance of a pain management task affect the quality of children's nurses' post-operative pain management practices? *Journal of Clinical Nursing* 17: 3205–16.

Ulrich. R. (1984) View through a window may influence recovery from surgery, *Science* 334: 420–2.

Umeh, K., and Jones, L. (2010) Mutually dependent health beliefs associated with breast self-examination in British female university students, *Journal of American College Health* 59(2): 126–31.

Underdown, A. (2007) *Young Children's Health and Well-Being*. Maidenhead: Open University Press.

Vachon, M. (1995) Staff stress in hospice/palliative care: a review, *Palliative Medicine* 9: 91–122.

Van Wormer, K., and Thyer, B. A (2010) *Evidence-Based Practice in the Field of Substance Abuse: A Book of Readings*. London: Sage.

Vanistendael, S. (2007) Resilience and spirituality, in B. Monroe and D. Oliviere (eds), *Resilience in Palliative Care: Achievement in Adversity*. Oxford: Oxford University Press, pp. 115–35.

Vernooij-Dassen, M. (2007) Meaningful activities for people with dementia, *Aging and Mental Health* 11(4): 359–60.

Vits, S., Cesko, C., Enck, P., Hillen, U., Schadendorf, D., and Schedlowski, M. (2011) Behavioural conditioning as the mediator of placebo responses in the immune system, *Philosophical Transactions of the Royal Society B: Biological Sciences* 366: 1799–807.

Volicer, B. J., and Bohannon, M. W. (1975) A hospital rating scale, *Nursing Research* 24: 352–9.

Waddell, M. (1998) *Inside Lives*. London: Tavistock.

Waitman, A., and Conboy-Hill, S. (1992) *Psychotherapy and Mental Handicap*. London: Sage.

Walder, B., Schafer, M., Henzi, I., and Tramer, R. (2001) Efficacy and safety of patient-controlled analgesia for acute postoperative pain: a quantitative systematic review, *Acta Anaesthesiologica Scandinavica* 45(7): 795–804.

Walker, J., Payne, S., Jarrett, N., and Ley, T. (2012) *Psychology for Nurses and the Caring Professions*. 4th edn, Buckingham: Open University Press.

Wallace, P., Cutler, S., and Haines, A. (1988) Randomised controlled trial of general practitioner intervention with excessive alcohol consumption, *British Medical Journal* 297: 663–8.

Wallston, K. A., Wallston, B. S., and DeVellis, R. (1978) Development of the multidimensional health locus of control (MHLC) scales, *Health Education Monographs* 6(2): 160–70.

Walter, T. (1997) Letting go and keeping hold: a reply to Stroebe, *Mortality* 2(3): 263–6.

Wang, R., Chadalavada, K., Wilshire, J., Kowalik, U., Hovinga, K., Geber, A., Fligelman, B., Leversha, M., Brennan, C., and Tabar, V. (2010) Glioblastoma stem-like cells give rise to tumour endothelium, *Nature* 468: 829–33.

Weinberger, D. R., Torrey, E. F., Neophytides, A. N., and Wyatt, R. J. (1979) Lateral cerebral ventricular enlargement in chronic schizophrenia, *Archives of General Psychiatry* 36: 735–9.

Wells, A. (1997) *Cognitive Therapy for Anxiety Disorders*. Chichester: Wiley.

Wells, A. (2000) *Meta-Cognitions and Emotional Disorders*. Chichester: Wiley.

Welsh Government (2013) *Together for Health – Delivering End of Life Care: A Delivery Plan up to 2016 for NHS Wales and its Partners: The Highest Standard of Care for Everyone at the End of Life*, http://wales.gov.uk/docs/dhss/publications/130416careen.pdf.

WHO (World Health Organization) (1992) *The ICD-10 Classification of Mental and Behavioural Disorders: Diagnostic Criteria for Research.* Geneva: WHO.

WHO/ADI (World Health Organization/Alzheimer's Disease International) (2012) *Dementia: A Public Health Priority.* London: WHO.

Wilkinson, S. (1991) Factors which influence how nurses communicate with cancer patients, *Journal of Advanced Nursing* 16: 677–88.

Williams, G. (2004) The genesis of chronic illness, in M. Bury and J. Gabe (eds), *The Sociology of Health and Illness: A Reader.* London: Routledge, pp. 247–55.

Williams, S. (2015) *Recovering from Psychosis: Empirical Evidence and Lived Experience.* Abingdon: Routledge.

Willner, P., Jones, J., Tams, R., and Green, G. (2002) A randomised controlled trial of the efficiency of a cognitive-behavioural anger management group for clients with learning disabilities, *Journal of Applied Research in Intellectual Disabilities* 15: 224–35.

Winnicott, D. W. (1971) *Playing and Reality.* London: Tavistock.

Wolpe, J. (1958) *Psychotherapy by Reciprocal Inhibition.* Stanford, CA: Stanford University Press.

Wood, G. (1983) *The Myth of Neurosis.* London: Macmillan.

Woodgate, R., and Kristjanson, L. (1996) A young child's pain: how parents and nurses 'take care', *International Journal of Nursing Studies* 33: 271–84.

Worden, J. W. (2010) *Grief Counselling and Grief Therapy: A Handbook for the Mental Health Practitioner.* 4th edn, London: Routledge.

Wortman, C. B., and Brehm, J. W. (1975) Responses to uncontrollable outcomes: an integration of reactance theory and the learned helplessness model, in L. Berkowitz (ed.), *Advances in Experimental Social Psychology* 8. New York: Academic Press, pp. 277–336.

Wrenn, R. L., Levinson, D., and Papadatou, D. (1999) Working with dying patients: caregivers need support too! *Texas Nursing* 73(10): 6–8.

Yoo, W., Kwon, M., and Pfeiffer, L. (2013) Influence of communication on colorectal cancer screening: revisiting the health belief model, *Journal of Communication in Healthcare* 6(1): 35–43.

Zimmermann, G., Favrod, J., Trieu, V. H., and Pomini, V. (2005) The effect of cognitive behavioral treatment on the positive symptoms of schizophrenia spectrum disorders: a meta-analysis, *Schizophrenia Research* 77(1): 1–9.

Zinberg, N. E. (1986) *Drug, Set, and Setting: The Basis for Controlled Intoxicant Use.* New Haven, CT: Yale University Press, pp. x–xi.

Index

WITHDRAWN